Health and Wellness IN PEOPLE LIVING WITH Serious Mental Illness

D1423954

Health and Wellness IN PEOPLE LIVING WITH Serious Mental Illness

Edited by

Patrick W. Corrigan, Psy.D.

Sonya L. Ballentine, B.A.

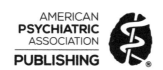

AMERICAN
PSYCHIATRIC
ASSOCIATION
PUBLISHING

Copyright © 2021 American Psychiatric Association Publishing

ALL RIGHTS RESERVED

First Edition

Manufactured in the United States of America on acid-free paper
25 24 23 22 21   5 4 3 2 1

American Psychiatric Association Publishing
800 Maine Avenue SW, Suite 900
Washington, DC 20024-2812
www.appi.org

Library of Congress Cataloging-in-Publication Data
Names: Corrigan, Patrick W., editor. | Ballentine, Sonya L., editor. | American Psychiatric Association, issuing body.
Title: Health and wellness in people living with serious mental illness / edited by Patrick W. Corrigan, Sonya L. Ballentine.
Description: First edition. | Washington, DC : American Psychiatric Association Publishing, [2021] | Includes bibliographical references and index.
Identifiers: LCCN 2020057420 (print) | LCCN 2020057421 (ebook) | ISBN 9781615373796 (paperback ; alk. paper) | ISBN 9781615373802 (ebook)
Subjects: MESH: Mentally Ill Persons | Community-Based Participatory Research | Mental Disorders—complications | Health Status | Health Status Disparities
Classification: LCC RC454 (print) | LCC RC454 (ebook) | NLM WM 29.5 | DDC 616.89—dc23
LC record available at https://lccn.loc.gov/2020057420
LC ebook record available at https://lccn.loc.gov/2020057421

British Library Cataloguing in Publication Data
A CIP record is available from the British Library.

To our mothers,
Eileen Corrigan (P.W.C.) and Pat Ballentine (S.L.B.)

Contents

Contributors xi

Preface xv

Patrick W. Corrigan, Psy.D.
Sonya L. Ballentine, B.A.

1 Breadth and Depth of
Mortality and Morbidity 1

Patrick W. Corrigan, Psy.D.
Carla Kundert, M.S.
Sara Catanese, M.A.

2 Research Considerations and
Community-Based
Participatory Research 23

Lindsay Sheehan, Ph.D.
Katherine Nieweglowski, M.S.
Yu Sun, M.P.H.

3 Effects of Concurrent Substance Use 47

Ayorkor Gaba, Psy.D.
Siu Ping Chin Feman, M.D.
Kelsey M. Clary, B.A.
David Smelson, Psy.D.

4 Health Service Disparities 65

Janis Sayer, Ph.D.
Susan A. Pickett, Ph.D.

5 Consequences of and Life Choices
Related to Living With a
Serious Mental Illness 83

Andrea B. Bink, Ph.D.
Patrick W. Corrigan, Psy.D.

6 Impact of Medication Effects on
Physical Health 103

Marc De Hert, M.D., Ph.D.
Johan Detraux, M.Psy.
Davy Vancampfort, Ph.D.

7 Role of Medical Homes in
Primary Care 131

Evelyn T. Chang, M.D., M.S.H.S.
Alexander S. Young, M.D., M.S.H.S.

8 Shared Decision Making 145

Karina J. Powell, Ph.D.
Patrick W. Corrigan, Psy.D.

9 Healthy Living Skills 163

Erin L. Kelly, Ph.D.
John S. Brekke, Ph.D.

10 Health Navigators to
Address Wellness 221

Lindsay Sheehan, Ph.D.
Carla Kundert, M.S.
Jonathon E. Larson, Ed.D.

11 Smoking 239

Janis Sayer, Ph.D.
Marisa D. Serchuk, M.S.

12 Improving Diet, Activity, and Weight 267

Katherine D. Hoerster, Ph.D., M.P.H.
Alexander S. Young, M.D., M.S.H.S.

13 The COVID-19 Pandemic 285

Patrick W. Corrigan, Psy.D.
Sang Qin, M.S.

14 Final Thoughts: Moving Forward 297

Patrick W. Corrigan, Psy.D.
Sonya L. Ballentine, B.A.

Index 303

Contributors

Sonya L. Ballentine, B.A.
Project Manager, Department of Psychology, Illinois Institute of Technology, Chicago, Illinois

Andrea B. Bink, Ph.D.
Department of Psychology, Illinois Institute of Technology, Chicago, Illinois

John S. Brekke, Ph.D.
Professor of Social Work, Suzanne Dworak-Peck School of Social Work, University of Southern California, Los Angeles, California

Sara Catanese, M.A.
Student, Department of Psychology, Illinois Institute of Technology, Chicago, Illinois

Evelyn T. Chang, M.D., M.S.H.S.
Physician-Investigator, Department of Medicine, VA Greater Los Angeles Healthcare System; Assistant Professor, Department of General Internal Medicine, University of California at Los Angeles, David Geffen School of Medicine, Los Angeles

Kelsey M. Clary, B.A.
M.P.H. Candidate, Department of Health Promotion and Policy, School of Public Health and Health Sciences, University of Massachusetts, Amherst, Massachusetts

Patrick W. Corrigan, Psy.D.
Distinguished Professor, Department of Psychology, Illinois Institute of Technology, Chicago, Illinois

Johan Detraux, M.Psy.
KU Leuven, Department of Neurosciences, Public Health Psychiatry, Leuven, Belgium; University Psychiatric Center, KU Leuven, Kortenberg, Belgium

Siu Ping Chin Feman, M.D.
Medical Director of Substance Use Disorder Services, Edith Nourse Rogers Memorial Veterans Hospital, Bedford, Massachusetts

Ayorkor Gaba, Psy.D.
Professor of Psychiatry, Department of Psychiatry, University of Massachusetts Medical School, Worcester Massachusetts

Marc De Hert, M.D., Ph.D.
KU Leuven, Department of Neurosciences, Center for Clinical Psychiatry, Leuven, Belgium; University Psychiatric Center, KU Leuven, Kortenberg, Belgium; Antwerp Health Law and Ethics Chair, AHLEC University Antwerpen, Antwerp, Belgium

Katherine D. Hoerster, Ph.D., M.P.H.
Investigator and Psychologist, VA Puget Sound Healthcare System, Seattle Division; Assistant Professor, University of Washington Department of Psychiatry and Behavioral Sciences, Seattle, Washington

Erin L. Kelly, Ph.D.
Assistant Professor, Department of Family and Community Medicine, Thomas Jefferson University, Philadelphia, Pennsylvania; Visiting Scholar, Center for Social Medicine and Humanities, University of California, Los Angeles, California

Carla Kundert, M.S.
Clinical Research Associate, Department of Psychology, Illinois Institute of Technology, Chicago, Illinois

Jonathon E. Larson, Ed.D.
Associate Professor, Department of Psychology, Lewis College of Science and Letters, Illinois Institute of Technology, Chicago, Illinois

Katherine Nieweglowski, M.S.
Clinical Research Associate, Department of Psychology, Lewis College of Science and Letters, Illinois Institute of Technology, Chicago, Illinois

Susan A. Pickett, Ph.D.
Deputy Director, Center for Research and Evaluation, Advocates for Human Potential, Inc., Chicago, Illinois

Karina J. Powell, Ph.D.
Rehabilitation Neuropsychology Postdoctoral Fellow, Department of Psychology and Neuropsychology, Rehabilitation Institute of Michigan, Detroit Medical Center, Detroit, Michigan

Sang Qin, M.S.
Department of Psychology, Illinois Institute of Technology, Chiacgo, Illinois

Janis Sayer, Ph.D.
Clinical Research Professional, Department of Psychology, Illinois Institute of Technology, Chicago, Illinois

Marisa D. Serchuk, M.S.
Doctoral Student, Department of Psychology, Illinois Institute of Technology, Chicago, Illinois

Lindsay Sheehan, Ph.D.
Research Assistant Professor, Department of Psychology, Lewis College of Science and Letters, Illinois Institute of Technology, Chicago, Illinois

David Smelson, Psy.D.
Professor of Psychiatry, Department of Psychiatry, University of Massachusetts Medical School, Worcester Massachusetts

Yu Sun, M.P.H.
Research Assistant, Department of Psychology, Lewis College of Science and Letters, Illinois Institute of Technology, Chicago, Illinois

Davy Vancampfort, Ph.D.
University Psychiatric Center KU Leuven, Kortenberg, Belgium; KU Leuven Department of Rehabilitation Sciences, Leuven, Belgium

Alexander S. Young, M.D., M.S.H.S.
Professor and Interim Chair, Department of Psychiatry, David Geffen School of Medicine, University of California, Los Angeles; Associate Director, Health Services, VISN22 MIRECC, Department of Veterans Affairs, Los Angeles, California

Disclosure of Competing Interests

Dr. Corrigan and Ms. Ballentine have indicated that they have no financial interests or other affiliations that represent or could appear to represent a competing interest with their contributions to this book.

Preface

People with serious mental illness (SMI) get sick and die 10–20 years younger than other members of their same-age cohort. Much of this problem is due to the social determinants of health that define disparities which undermine health, wellness, and the system meant to realize these goals. Determinants include the stigma of mental illness, which sways health care providers from offering the best standard of care, and the resulting failure of the health care system to provide services needed by this group. The impact of stigma specific to mental illness is exacerbated by poverty. Some people with SMI, by virtue of their disabilities, lack a health safety net because governments lack commitment to those from this economic class. Poverty is worsened by ethnicity and discrimination. Communities of color often find the breadth and depth of clinics and services that fully support health and wellness absent. In addition, communities of color cannot avail themselves of the kind of culturally sensitive strategies required to meet the needs and expectations of these communities. With poverty and discrimination come the insidious effects of homelessness and crime. Many people with SMI and of color lack stable housing and are often exposed to health challenges that result from living on the streets. Others are victims of crime, often violent and sometimes family based, that interferes with health care. Still others are convicted of crime and involved in the criminal justice system—police, courts, jail, prison, probation, and parole—and are confronted with the challenges involvement with this system brings to rightful health care.

SMI, poverty, and other social determinants lead to an inordinate rate of modifiable health risks. People with mental illness smoke more often than same-age others. They use alcohol and other drugs at higher rates. Substance use increases their morbidity and mortality. People with SMI often have diet and exercise/activity patterns that undermine wellness and worsen health. Chronic levels of stress exacerbate prolonged illnesses. Some people with SMI fail to use safe-sex strategies. On top of this, medications and other psychiatric treatments may have harmful side effects that worsen health.

Interventions have begun to emerge as ways to overcome barriers like these to health challenges. They include medical practices that diminish the iatrogenic effects of psychiatry, psychoeducation to teach people how to manage health and wellness, instrumental and interpersonal supports that help people to navigate their community, and shared decision making that ensures that individuals have ultimate control over their health and wellness plan.

Research is essential for the development and evaluation of strategies at all levels of the public health agenda. Community-based participatory research (CBPR) is the first principle herein. Research meant to test concepts and interventions specific to a community needs to be steeped in that community. That does not mean people from the community are subjects of the research; rather, they are partners in all facets of its conduct. Investigators and members of the community as partners define hypotheses, methods, analyses, and summaries of the research and development effort. CBPR is especially notable "coming in to" and "going out of" the project. "Coming in," members of the community have fundamental insights about what needs to be examined to make sense of their problems and ways to make an impact. "Going out" is ownership. Researchers on the CBPR team often are on to the next grant and research project when data are analyzed and reports are written up. Community members are likely to use the insights to meaningfully impact their neighborhood over time. This kind of ownership gives credibility. The final project is not something developed in an ivory tower by researchers who differ from the community; it is developed by the community itself.

The community comprises people with shared experience relevant to health and wellness. Typically, CBPR focuses on diversity, especially in terms of ethnicity and religious heritage. Public health investigators also may seek to include additional communities of concern, including women, LGBTQ persons, veterans, and rural residents. It is important here to understand that people with SMI are a community worthy of CBPR. They have shared experience and similar needs vis-à-vis the health care system. Some might ask whether people with SMI can capably participate in CBPR given their social and cognitive disabilities. YES, they can! As will be laid out herein, people with SMI are vital members of the CBPR team, especially when reasonable accommodations are provided by team members.

Meet This Book's Editors: Pat Corrigan and Sonya Ballentine

We (Pat and Sonya) met over a National Institute of Mental Health (NIH)–funded project investigating the effects of peer navigators on the health and wellness goals of African Americans with SMI who were also homeless. Pat was the study's principal investigator and Sonya was a member of its CBPR team.

SONYA: In 2012, I finally believed I was in some control of both my drug addictions and mental illness and ready to go beyond weekly groups and counseling sessions to get back into the world. I saw this flyer about a program that was looking for African Americans with lived experience of mental illness to develop a health program for people who were homeless. I signed up thinking this would be an easy first transition because it would be one and done, and then on to something else. No need for long commitment. I made the second meeting, where I met the team of people with lived experience—many I knew from the neighborhood—and these university scientists. The scientists were a bit of a surprise. Sue was very patient for a researcher, more like a liberal white lady than a number cruncher. Pat was laid back and over-accommodating; I thought he should have been more in control. "Sometimes you just need to cut 'Mary' off." But frankly, I didn't think it would matter. We'd sit around the table a few times talking about health and then the researchers would be elsewhere on something else.

My greatest surprise was that this was serious, something was actually going to get done, not just pretending. We developed a 130-page treatment manual, and then we hired three peer navigators to use the manual to help African Americans with SMI. Honestly, that freaked me out.

PAT: The project with Sonya was the first I led on health and wellness concerns of people with SMI. I had written the proposal months earlier, was funded by NIH, had my team in place, and was ready to go. After all, I was an expert in SMI and thought the research plan would be easy to throw down on paper. But also, to be honest, I wondered whether working with a CBPR team—African Americans with mental illness who had been homeless—would be helpful or actually a hindrance to my wisdom.

It was a lot of work; first, we had to come to know and trust each other. I remember an icebreaker at an early meeting: "Turn to the person on your left and tell them one fun thing about you." I greeted Lee to my left with a smile and fun story about my golden retriever, Cleo. Flat reaction; almost no response. "So what does that have to do with me being here?" What Sonya says about going through the motions resonates for me. Was this something that was really going to lead to a change or just hollow talk? Our proposal included CBPR-led "windshield tours" within the first 3 months of start-up. We split up researchers and people with lived experience into small groups to walk and learn from the community. I ended up with Lee, who proudly walked me around his neighborhood introducing me to people he talked with every day. He introduced me to friends who had cocaine addiction and still called the streets home. He walked me into the north end of Lincoln Park and showed me where people live. One good spot was a large bush where people could not be seen by passing drivers on Lake Shore Drive, nor be rushed by fellow angry travelers. He said that when staying in the park "it's best to put personal belongings up a tree and make sure they are wrapped in garbage bags.

That way they won't get wet." That single afternoon stroll advanced my knowledge about project challenges exponentially.

SONYA: I remember the windshield tour too. I was the lead of a small group that included Dana [the research project director] and Curlee. I began to understand how this research partnership stuff was really supposed to go. I was in my comfort zone. I was the professor teaching Dana what it meant to be where I come from. I got to introduce them to people I know on the street and hand out gift cards for their participation.

Things have changed immensely since then. Pat first offered me a part-time job on a PCORI [Patient-Centered Outcomes Research Institute] grant and then a position as project manager of an NIMHD [National Institute on Minority Health and Health Disparities] grant on peer navigators for the diet and exercise needs of African Americans with SMI. Moving to part-time, and then full-time, work was frightening, a huge challenge given my past few years, but also a great success for me. I had been on the streets for more than 5 years, overwhelmed with my illnesses, and never thought I could do this. But now I am a university employee and actually run a CBPR team made up of investigators and people with lived experience. I've been there. I know what it means when figuring out the needs of people with mental illness. We are now 4 years into a manualized diet and exercise program, with a goal of recruiting 270 people with SMI into the program.

Just last week, I was doing my monthly calls, getting process information about research participant activity during the preceding 4 weeks. I was talking to "Ken" on the phone, asking him the standard questions. "Ken, in the past month, has your drug use changed at all?" He responded like most respondents: "No." "Ken! You're on 45th and Halsted and I can hear you making a heroin deal. Don't give me that." I don't think Pat would have gotten that kind of info.

I should not understate the joy I get in this job. I'm making a difference in the community, people who are disadvantaged in terms of health and health services. And it's my community. Not some abstract textbook notion of "disadvantaged population." These are the streets I grew up on, that I still walk through. These are people I know, their smiles and frowns and stories. These are people I sit next to at church on Sunday or stand in line with at the local store. I am privileged and honored to be working for their well-being.

PAT: I struggle here to put my real thoughts into words on a page. I have learned and continue to learn from Sonya each day. Health challenges and disparities are so much more than numbers in a book. They are meaningful relationships that lead to enduring change. Sonya is my muse.

Who This Book Is For

This book is written for professionals and students of psychiatry—providers who are often the first line in addressing the physical health and wellness needs of people with SMI. Psychiatrists working in community settings have come to endorse integrated care as an essential goal for comprehensive services. Partnerships with primary care providers are a first step in meeting integrated service goals. Allied health professionals—nurses, nurse practitioners, physician assistants, psychologists, social workers, and community health workers—are a second group of readers that would benefit from the content herein. The book was crafted, as well, for policy makers and others working in the public health sector, to provide insights on how to realize state-of-the-art programs discussed herein. Finally, this book is written for people with lived experience like Sonya, those who advocate at the grassroots for better health and wellness services.

Outline and Organization

The book has two goals: to describe the challenges of health and wellness for people with mental illness and then to explore ways to address these challenges. Chapter 1 summarizes research on mortality and morbidity in this group as well as information about the status quo on wellness. Chapter 2 sets out research priorities for advancing concepts and interventions in this area. CBPR has a central role in this research agenda.

The next four chapters address causal factors related to health and wellness concerns of people with SMI. Chapter 3 summarizes health challenges experienced by people with co-occurring mental illness and substance use disorder. Chapter 4 notes how ethnic health disparities account for many of the health problems. Chapter 5 summarizes life choices (e.g., smoking, poor diet, little exercise, unsafe sex) and life consequences (e.g., homelessness, involvement in the criminal justice system) that worsen health. Chapter 6 describes the iatrogenic effects of psychiatric medication that harm physical health.

Solutions to these health challenges are reviewed in the next six chapters. Chapter 7 summarizes the promise of integrated services and patient care medical homes. Chapter 8 then, to set the ground for all other interventions, introduces the concept of shared decision making. Patients and care providers partner together so that patients are able to make choices about services that meet their priorities. This approach can involve a different dynamic from the hierarchical relationship—doctor and patient—that has defined the medical system in the past. Chapter 9 describes the wide range of psychoeducation programs meant to teach people better ways to manage their health and obtain wellness goals. Chapter 10 reviews the benefits of health navigators. Specifically, it describes how navigators might assume the hands-on role for walking people with SMI around their health care system. Chapter 11 reviews the extensive research about how people with SMI might manage smoking. Chapter 12 describes exercise and diet as key ingredients in wellness. Chapter 13 further considers the impact of the COVID-19 pandemic. We end the book, in Chapter 14, with future considerations for moving forward.

Acknowledgments

This book was made possible with the support and inspiration of many. We started this journey with Sue Pickett, who has been a steady partner throughout. Many thanks to people with lived experience who have been vital partners on our CBPR teams:

- Peer navigators for African Americans with mental illness who are homeless: Curlee Jenkins, Joyce Johnson, Robert Johnson, Christina Jones, Rodney Lewis, Lee Taylor, Monica Williams.
- Peer navigators for Latinxs with mental illness who are homeless: MavisLinda Lehmann, Patricia Munoz, Judith Ortiz, Marilyn Perez-Aviles, Timoteo Rodriguez, Nelson Santiago, Rudy Suarez.
- Community partners involved in developing a "how to" manual to conduct CBPR in African American communities: LaShelle Agnew, Yusuf Ali, Mark Canser, John Connor, Renee Jones, Edward Laster, Khalilah Muhammad, Scott Noble, Rhonda Smith, Gary Walley.
- Community partners involved in developing a "how to" manual for peer leaders in CBPR teams: Sylvia Cole, Christopher Ervin, Jamie Eskridge, Cheryl Metcalf, Scott Noble, John Owens, Helen Wakefield.
- Peer navigators to address diet and activity needs of African Americans with mental illness: Kenneth Bledsoe, Alicia Carter, Chantee Evans, Lora Flowers, LaToya Glover, DeAndre Hill, Howard Rosing, Paul Williams.

Peer members of CBPR teams are balanced by partners from service organizations, including, from Heartland Alliance Health, Ed Stellon, Erin Hantke, Christopher Ervin, Stephanie Brown, Elizabeth Brown, and Chris Robinson; and, from Trilogy Behavioral Healthcare, John Mayes and Susan Doig. Thanks to Lisa Razzano from Thresholds, Dani Lazar from ACCESS Community Health, and Pastor Chris Harris from Bright Star Church.

Several colleagues from our own research team have been important partners. Jon Larson has been working alongside Pat Corrigan for almost 20 years. Our Chicago Health Disparities research team includes Janis Sayer, Deysi Paniagua, Sang Qin, and Katherine Niewoglowski. Lindsay Sheehan is the anchor on which we rest.

Thanks for financial support from and guidance from the National Institute on Minority Health and Health Disparities and the Patient-Centered Outcomes Research Institute.

Finally, we acknowledge all those unsung people with lived experience who have either implemented or participated in our services.

Patrick W. Corrigan, Psy.D.
Sonya L. Ballentine, B.A.

CHAPTER 1

Breadth and Depth of Mortality and Morbidity

Patrick W. Corrigan, Psy.D.
Carla Kundert, M.S.
Sara Catanese, M.A.

Serious mental illness (SMI) has a deep and broad impact on the physical health of many people. People with SMI frequently get sick and die about 20 years younger than same-age peers. We seek to describe the overall problem in this chapter. First, we begin with a brief "definition" of psychiatric disability. Next, we review research on the extent of mortality in this population. We then seek to make sense of varying morbidities by organ systems. SMI also undermines wellness, the next topic reviewed in the chapter. We end the chapter by summarizing the key issues as a foundation for the remainder of the book.

Who Are People With Psychiatric Diagnoses?

Many people experience a mental illness in their lifetime. In some cases, the illness becomes serious. Approximately one in five adults in the United States have symptoms that meet criteria for mental illness during their lifetime; 24% of those individuals experience SMI (National Institute of Mental Health 2019). Seriousness is defined by diagnosis, persistence, and disability. Several diagnoses in DSM-5 are typically viewed as serious—schizophrenia spectrum and other psychotic disorders, mood disorders (bipolar and depressive), and trauma- and stressor-related disorders—though diagnosis per se does not equal severity (American Psychiatric Association 2013). Schizophrenia, which is often viewed as the prototypical disorder, actually has a more benign course than that originally described by Emil Kraepelin in the early twentieth century and later incorporated into versions of DSM. A rough rule of thirds seems to emerge from long-time follow-up research on schizophrenia: about one-third of persons with the disorder seem to recover altogether, one-third are able to meet life goals with relatively low treatment demands (e.g., regular visits to a psychiatrist and corresponding medication), and one-third—those we typically think of—are seriously disabled by the recurring illness (Harding et al. 1987; Huber et al. 1975; Ogawa et al. 1987). Hence, it is the recurring and challenging nature of mental illness that makes it disabling. For example, anxiety disorders, considered less pernicious than schizophrenia, can be persistently disabling and thus serious. Let us consider these two concepts more thoroughly.

Serious Mental Illness

SMI is persistent; its effects tend to be chronic. For some people, the course of symptoms and dysfunctions may be unchanging. For others, especially those with mood disorders, symptoms may wax and wane. It is not clear from the criteria how long the illness must harm someone for it to be considered persistent. Persistence is best understood from the perspective of people with lived experience, and where they find themselves in their development. Young adults, for example, may find a course of mental illness lasting just a year to be persistent. Conversely, elders in their 60s might not consider a couple of months of schizophrenia recurring every 5 years or so to be chronic. Like most ideas in this book, chronicity and persistence are defined by the person.

Key to "seriousness" is disability: people are not able to achieve significant life goals because of the symptoms and dysfunctions of their mental illness. The standard for "significant life goal" is defined by culture: goals in one ethnic group may differ from those in another. Under Title XVI, the U.S. Social Security Administration defines disability in terms of work: "the inability to engage in any substantial gainful activity" (U.S. Code §§1381–1383f, Subchapter XVI, Chapter 7, Title 42). In addition to work, common life goals impeded by SMI include education, independent living, relationships, and health. Specific to this book, people with SMI are disabled in terms of health when their symptoms and dysfunctions undermine accomplishing these goals.

Co-occurring Disorders

The disabilities of people with the index psychiatric diagnoses summarized above—for example, schizophrenia spectrum and other psychotic disorders, mood disorders, and anxiety disorders—are worse when there are co-occurring disorders, especially those related to substance use disorder. Epidemiological research suggests that the lifetime prevalence of substance use disorders can be as high as 50% in persons with these index conditions (Kenneson et al. 2013). Co-occurring disorders may lead to greater rates of relapse, violence, incarceration, homelessness, and HIV infection; in Chapter 3 of this book, Gaba and colleagues more thoroughly unpack this issue in terms of health.

Illness Leading to Death

Co-occurring Physical Illness

People with psychiatric disabilities show inordinate rates of co-occurring physical illnesses that worsen disabilities or lead to death. As explored in more detail later in this chapter, they have a higher incidence and prevalence of cardiovascular and respiratory illness, gastrointestinal disorders, neurological disorders, cancer, blood-borne illnesses, and orthopedic illnesses, including those due to accident. As a result, people with SMI are hospitalized for physical health problems at much higher rates (Mai et al. 2011). They overutilize emergency rooms both for exacerbated chronic conditions and for relatively benign primary care evaluations (Kêdoté et al. 2008).

The physical functioning of people with SMI resembles that of people in the general population who are 10–20 years older (Chafetz et al. 2006). Individuals with SMI are vulnerable to early institutionalization in nursing homes (Bartels et al. 2004). They enter nursing homes several years earlier than do their non–mentally ill counterparts in the population. Medical problems exacerbate mental health conditions. Finally, people with SMI experience high levels of early death; on average, people with SMI have a 20% shorter life span than others in the general population (Newman and Bland 1991).

Mortality

Mortality rates due to physical illness among people with mental illness are catastrophic across the globe. A meta-analysis of studies from around the world showed that medical diseases account for almost 70% of deaths among people with mental illness (Walker et al. 2015). Large-scale epidemiological studies have documented this more fully within individual countries. A 17-year nationally representative epidemiology study in the United

States revealed that the life span of people with SMI is shortened, on average, by 8.2 years compared with the general population; 95.4% of deaths could be attributed to physical illnesses (Druss et al. 2011). In the United Kingdom, the ratio between observed and expected death rates for people with SMI ranges from 2.2 to 3.2, with bipolar and mood disorders being the lowest and psychotic disorders being the highest (John et al. 2018). Those living with SMI in the United Kingdom were 2.2–3.2 times more likely to die compared with the general population. In Australia, the life expectancy gap between people with and without mental illness is estimated to be 14–16 years; physical diseases contributed to 80% of this excess mortality (Lawrence et al. 2013). Although relatively few national epidemiological studies on comorbidities of mental and physical disorders have been conducted in developing countries, a similar pattern has been observed. Researchers investigating the Chinese population in rural communities showed that depression and anxiety significantly increased mortality rates for persons with chronic obstructive pulmonary disease (COPD), with a 3.8- to 4.5-fold elevated risk of premature death (Lou et al. 2014).

Morbidities

People with SMI exhibit morbidities in each of the 12 organ systems. We summarize the research on this in Table 1–1. In this section, we review epidemiological data on differing morbidities, describing incidence or prevalence across specific diagnoses. We also examine how physical illnesses might occur as an iatrogenic effect of treatment.

Integumentary, Muscular, and Skeletal Systems

These body systems constitute the foundations of human anatomy and include skin, hair, nails, bones, cartilage, teeth, ligaments, and muscles. Conditions involving these body systems can severely interrupt functioning as well as appearance of individuals who experience them. Links between comorbid conditions of the integumentary and skeletal systems and SMI, as well as possible etiology and impacts, are delineated below. (Of note, we were unable to find a connection between SMI and musculature.)

Integumentary System

An investigation by Mookhoek et al. (2010) noted increased risk of skin infection for individuals with SMI and comorbid diabetes (risk of diabetes in

TABLE 1–1.   Common morbidities experienced by people with mental illness, by organ system

Organ system	Examples
Integumentary, muscular, and skeletal systems	Integument
	Increased risk of skin infection in the presence of comorbid diabetes and obesity relative to those without diabetes and obesity (Mookhoek et al. 2010)
	Link between clozapine use and benign skin neoplasms (Mookhoek et al. 2010)
	Skeleton
	Risk of decreased bone mineral density associated with antipsychotic use (Leucht et al. 2007) and diagnosis of depression (Cizza et al. 1996)
	Greater likelihood (three times greater) of experiencing edentulousness and higher prevalence of tooth decay among people with psychiatric disability compared with people without psychiatric disability (Kisely et al. 2011)
Cardiovascular, nervous, and respiratory systems	Cardiovascular system
	Greater likelihood of experiencing cardiovascular disease and of dying compared with people without psychiatric disability (Leucht et al. 2007)
	Greater likelihood (two times greater) of having an elevated coronary heart disease score compared to people without psychiatric disability due to increased rates of smoking, cholesterol, diabetes mellitus, and hypertension (Osborn et al. 2006)
	Greater likelihood (4.9 times greater) of sudden cardiac death among people with schizophrenia (Ruschena et al. 2003)
	Association between depression and heart disease (Leucht et al. 2007)
	Link between anxiety disorders, including panic disorder, and heart disease such as stroke, arrhythmia, cardiomyopathy, high blood pressure, and mitral valve prolapse (Kahn et al. 1990)
	Nervous system
	Link between epilepsy and schizophrenia (Qin et al. 2005)
	Increased risk of obstructive sleep apnea due to weight gain as a side effect of antipsychotic medications (Winkelman 2001)

TABLE 1–1.   Common morbidities experienced by people with mental illness, by organ system *(continued)*

Organ system	Examples
Cardiovascular, nervous, and respiratory systems *(continued)*	Nervous system *(continued)* More frequent reports of migraines among people with serious mental illness, with greater likelihood of poorer health outcomes among individuals with both migraines and a mental health diagnosis compared with those reporting just one of those conditions (Jette et al. 2008) Higher rates of Alzheimer's disease among older adults with schizophrenia compared with estimates in the general population (Prohovnik et al. 1993) Link between preceding diagnosis of depression or anxiety and Parkinson's disease (Ishihara and Brayne 2006) Higher prevalence of hypoalgesia, or decreased sensitivity to pain, experienced in people with schizophrenia (reported in 37%–91% of schizophrenia patients) (Singh et al. 2006) Respiratory system Increased risk of chronic obstructive pulmonary disease and asthma among people with schizophrenia compared with the general population (Partti et al. 2015) Potential genetic link between asthma and bipolar disorder (Wu et al. 2019) Increased risk of pneumonia among people with bipolar disorder with antipsychotic use compared with people with bipolar disorder not receiving antipsychotics (Yang et al. 2013)
Digestive, reproductive, and urinary systems	Digestive system Increased prevalence of irritable bowel syndrome in schizophrenia and major depression compared with rates in the general population (Garakani et al. 2003) Increased prevalence of celiac disease in individuals with schizophrenia and their relatives (Eaton et al. 2006) Reproductive system Increased prevalence of sexual dysfunction in individuals with schizophrenia compared with the general population (Meyer and Nasrallah 2009) Association between medication-induced prolactin elevation and sexual dysfunction in schizophrenia (Knegtering et al. 2008)

TABLE 1–1.   Common morbidities experienced by people with mental illness, by organ system *(continued)*

Organ system	Examples
Digestive, reproductive, and urinary systems *(continued)*	Reproductive system *(continued)* Higher prevalence of amenorrhea in women using antipsychotic medication compared with those not using antipsychotic medication (Bargiota et al. 2013) Urinary system Increased lifetime prevalence of chronic kidney disease (linked with cardiovascular disease and death) in individuals with bipolar disorder partially mediated by chronic lithium and/or anticonvulsant use (Kessing et al. 2015)
Endocrine, immune, and lymphatic systems	Endocrine system Increased lifetime risk for affective disorder in individuals with hypothyroid disorder (Thomsen et al. 2005) Immune system Higher prevalence of autoimmune disease in individuals presenting with onset of schizophrenia compared with matched control subjects (Eaton et al. 2006)

people with SMI is explored more later in this chapter) and in patients experiencing obesity. Pharmacological treatment of SMI could prove an added risk factor for developing integumentary conditions among individuals with SMI. In a study of 108 participants enrolled in psychiatric outpatient services in Hong Kong, the 51 participants prescribed lithium, typically for bipolar disorder, were significantly more likely than the 57 prescribed other psychotropic medications to develop skin conditions ($P=0.025$); there was no significant difference between the two groups in terms of rate of cutaneous conditions before commencing medication. Cutaneous conditions reported included psoriasis, acne, maculopapular eruption, folliculitis, and seborrheic dermatitis (Chan et al. 2000). A possible link between use of clozapine and benign skin neoplasms has been reported, though the nature of this relationship is, as of yet, undetermined (Mookhoek et al. 2010).

Skeletal System

Long-term psychopharmacological treatment of SMI, specifically through the use of typical antipsychotics, may have an impact on bone mineral density (BMD) and thus increase risk for skeletal system damage such as osteoporosis, fractures, and sprains (Leucht et al. 2007). The relationship is often attributed in research to increased levels of prolactin caused by antipsychotic use and its effect on the dopamine$_2$ receptors in the hypothalamic-pituitary axis. This can lead to hypogonadism in both men and women, resulting in decreased levels of testosterone and estrogen, respectively. Estrogen deficiency has been linked to decreased BMD and osteoporosis in women and men, and testosterone deficiency to profound osteopenia in men, though the latter has been less studied than estrogen deficiency in women. There is also evidence of a link between depression and osteoporosis, but the nature of this link is not clearly elucidated yet in the literature; the positive association between depression and osteoporosis is believed to involve hypercortisolism that leads to decreased bone formation, hypogonadism, and increased levels of interleukin-6 (Cizza et al. 1996).

Risk of falls and subsequent fractures is also increased among individuals with mental illness because of several factors. In addition to the potential for decreased BMD associated with certain types of psychiatric medications, as described above, several classes of medications are related to incidences of falls and fractures: antidepressants, sedatives, and hypnotics are specifically linked to fall risk among adults (Leipzig et al. 1999). In a case-control study by Liu et al. (1998), researchers investigated the link between use of differing classes of antidepressants and risk of hip fracture among elderly men and women in the hospital. The odds ratio (OR) of hip fracture among those taking tertiary tricyclic antidepressants was 1.5; among those taking selective serotonin reuptake inhibitors, the OR was 2.4 (Liu et al. 1998).

An area often treated as distinct entirely from physical or mental health is dental health. Aside from the obvious impacts dental disease can have on one's daily functioning (e.g., eating, appearance, speech), evidence repeatedly indicates that dental disease increases individuals' risk of systemic illnesses such as diabetes mellitus and cardiovascular disease, and makes it more likely that those comorbidities will result in death (Nazir 2017). This is especially important when considering the health and wellness of individuals with SMI. A meta-analysis looking at dental disease among people with SMI indicated that those with SMI were more than three times as likely as people without SMI to experience edentulousness (toothlessness), and the prevalence of dental caries (tooth decay) was significantly higher among people with SMI compared with people without SMI. These differences in dental health may be linked to less frequent access to and use of preventive dental care such as cleanings and treatments (Kisely et al. 2011).

There is an increased risk of unintentional injury among those with SMI (Wan et al. 2006). Wan and colleagues (2006) examined medical records of individuals admitted to a trauma center in San Francisco for unintentional injury; the rate of admission due to injury for those with SMI was twice as high as the rate for those without SMI, and the rate of repeated injuries (injury recidivism) for individuals with SMI was 4.5 times the rate for individuals without SMI. These findings indicate not only that mental illness may be an independent risk factor for hospitalization due to unintentional injury such as falls and accidents at home, but also that the risk of injury could complicate and/or exacerbate other comorbid conditions.

Cardiovascular, Nervous, and Respiratory Systems

Cardiovascular System

People with SMI are more likely to experience cardiovascular disease and are more likely to die due to heart disease than people without SMI. Several factors may contribute to this increased risk, including increased exposure to cardiac risk factors (e.g., smoking, obesity, diabetes mellitus), antipsychotic side effects, systemic barriers, stigma, and social barriers (Leucht et al. 2007). In a cross-sectional study by Osborn et al. (2006), people with SMI were two times more likely to have coronary heart disease compared with participants without SMI. Risk factors in the SMI group in this study included increased smoking rates, cholesterol risk factors, diabetes mellitus diagnosis, and hypertension risk (Osborn et al. 2006). Furthermore, varying treatments for SMI, including antipsychotic medications, can lead to significant weight gain. Increased adiposity, like that which can be caused or exacerbated by antipsychotic treatment, is often linked to increased risk of type 2 diabetes and cardiovascular disease. Insulin insensitivity that can result from increased adiposity is also associated with cardiovascular risk factors such as hypertension, increased likelihood of blood clots, and increases in blood low-density lipoprotein levels. There is also a demonstrated link between schizophrenia and sudden cardiac death; risk of sudden cardiac death in people with schizophrenia is 4.9 times the risk in the general population (Ruschena et al. 2003). Other risk factors contributing toward sudden cardiac death among people with schizophrenia include increased use of substances such as alcohol and cocaine.

Depression alone can be an independent risk factor for heart disease; for those with depression and comorbid heart disease, increased risk of morbidity and mortality has been found. Studies indicate that increased platelet reactivity among individuals with depression may be linked to changes in serotonin binding mechanisms at the platelet level (Schins et al. 2003) as well as changes in endothelial cells, which make up the lining of blood vessels. Anxiety and panic disorders have also been noted to increase risk of heart diseases such as stroke, arrhythmia, cardiomyopathy, hypertension, and mitral valve prolapse (Kahn et al. 1990). Additionally, there is a potential link between heart rate variability, mental illness, and heart disease; normal levels of heart rate variability are an indicator of balanced sympathetic and parasympathetic input from the nervous system to the cardiovascular system. Decreased heart rate variability, which is a risk factor for heart disease, has been observed in people with depression, anger/hostility, panic, and anxiety (Kemp and Quintana 2013).

Nervous System

The relationship between mental illness and neurological disorders is complicated. Many mental health conditions have neurological symptoms, psychiatric medications may have neurological side effects such as dyskinesia, and neurological disorders can have symptoms that mimic mental health symptoms (e.g., affective disruptions experienced by people with multiple sclerosis). The subtleties of the complex relationship between neurological diagnoses and SMI are beyond the scope of this text. However, we discuss below some of the connections and comorbidities among mental illness and acute neurological disorders, neurodegenerative conditions, and an important neurological symptom experienced by many individuals with SMI.

A number of studies indicate a relationship, though not clearly delineated, between epilepsy (temporal lobe epilepsy specifically) and schizophrenia or psychosis. A study including about 2.1 million people confirmed this relationship and identified a link between family history of epilepsy and increased risk of schizophrenia; the etiology of this connection is not well understood, but it may be indicative of genetic association between the two (Qin et al. 2005).

Use of psychiatric medications can often lead to weight gain, an often-mentioned risk factor for several comorbidities and systemic health conditions. Obesity is a primary risk factor in the development of sleep apnea, characterized by repeated obstruction of the upper airway during sleep. People with schizophrenia are at particular risk because of the significant causal relationship between antipsychotic use and weight gain; individuals with schizophrenia were more likely than individuals with other mental health diagnoses to present with obstructive sleep apnea (Winkelman 2001).

A robust study utilizing the data from the 2002 Canadian Community Health Survey—Mental Health and Well-Being identified a significant positive association between a mental health diagnosis and chronic migraines. Particularly important to note, the study also measured health outcomes, including quality of life, 2-week disability, restriction of activity, and mental health care utilization. Individuals who reported both migraines and a mental health diagnosis were more likely to have poorer health outcomes, compared with those who reported just one of those conditions, indicating that the combination of both illnesses has a significant impact on broader health and functioning (Jette et al. 2008).

There are also links between SMI and neurodegenerative diseases, though the connections are not clearly understood. For example, a study by Prohovnik et al. (1993) identified a high number of Alzheimer's disease diagnoses among patients living with schizophrenia, especially in significantly older adults (≥90 years old), among whom prevalence rates reach about 50%. The authors speculated that this increased prevalence may have been due to the cognitive side effects of long-term antipsychotic use, though further research is necessary to explore the relationship (Prohovnik et al. 1993). Additionally, a 2006 study by Ishihara and Brayne identified a link between prevalence of mental illness—specifically depression and anxiety—and subsequent diagnosis of Parkinson's disease. Again, the cause of this relationship has not yet been identified, but researchers supposed that it might be related to depletion of neurotransmitters involved in both mental illness and Parkinson's disease (Ishihara and Brayne 2006).

Finally, an important feature of note is altered pain perception among individuals with schizophrenia. There is an extensive amount of literature that indicates decreased sensations of pain (hypoalgesia) among individuals with schizophrenia. A review of the literature indicated that from 37% to 91% of people with schizophrenia experience reduced levels of pain (Singh et al. 2006). The cause of the hypoalgesia is not well understood. Hypoalgesia may contribute to morbidity and mortality in other areas of health and wellness. If, for example, people with schizophrenia are not aware of or responsive to pain or discomfort, or do not report pain or discomfort to health care providers, proper diagnosis and treatment of comorbid health conditions may be impeded.

Respiratory System

The respiratory system is responsible for the exchange of oxygen and carbon dioxide between the air and the human body. The primary organs of the respiratory system are the lungs. Swelling or inflammation of the airways in the lungs can lead to various respiratory diseases, such as asthma, COPD, or pneumonia.

According to the few existing studies, SMI may be associated with an increased risk of COPD and asthma. The most important cause of COPD is smoking, which is highly prevalent in individuals with SMI. In a recent study, individuals with schizophrenia and other nonaffective psychoses had significantly lower lung function values when compared with the general population, and the association remained significant for schizophrenia after adjustment for smoking and other potential confounders. Schizophrenia was associated with increased odds of pneumonia, COPD, and chronic bronchitis (Partti et al. 2015).

Studies on the genetic linkages between respiratory diseases and SMI are limited. In a Swedish population-based cohort study, children with hospitalizations for asthma during adolescence (11–15 years) had increased rates for bipolar disorder and schizophrenia spectrum disorders. Researchers also found an association between both maternal and paternal asthma and bipolar disorder, suggesting that there is potentially a shared genetic vulnerability between the two (Wu et al. 2019).

Similar to the effect of antipsychotics in the development of diabetes, antipsychotics have also been shown to increase risk for pneumonia. Current use of atypical antipsychotics in individuals with schizophrenia—clozapine in particular—is associated with a dose-dependent increased risk for pneumonia. The possible mechanisms for drug-induced pneumonia remain speculative. Histamine H_1 receptor antagonism by clozapine and olanzapine (inducing sedation) and muscarinic M_1 receptor antagonism (resulting in dryness of the mouth, esophageal dilatation, and hypomotility) may be involved, as well as an additive sedating effect by carbamazepine or valproic acid (Yang et al. 2013).

Depression is associated with a 43% increased risk of asthma (Gao et al. 2015). Wamboldt and colleagues (2000) found evidence supporting a genetic linkage between asthma and depression. They assessed the prevalence of atopic disease and depressive symptomatology in Finnish twin pairs and found a within-person correlation between atopic and depressive symptoms; using a best-fit model, they estimated that 64% of this association was due to shared familial vulnerability, mainly genetic factors (Wamboldt et al. 2000).

Digestive, Reproductive, and Urinary Systems

Digestive System

Although diseases of the digestive system in people with SMI are relatively understudied, irritable bowel syndrome (IBS) and celiac disease have received significant attention in individuals with SMI. The prevalence of IBS in schizophrenia was reported to be 19% (Garakani et al. 2003). Individuals with major depression have a higher prevalence, at 29%, although no significant associations were found between bipolar disorder and IBS. Additionally, Eaton et al. (2006) found that individuals with schizophrenia and their relatives tend to have higher-than-expected prevalence of celiac disease (0.05

vs. 0.01 in comparison groups). Research into celiac disease and schizophrenia has found support for shared genetic susceptibility. Highly significant differences in allele frequencies were observed in the intron of *MYO9B* between individuals with schizophrenia and healthy control subjects, providing preliminary evidence for a correlation between celiac disease and schizophrenia (Jungerius et al. 2008).

Reproductive System

Prevalence of sexual dysfunction varies but has been historically reported to affect 50%–75% of individuals with schizophrenia, a rate significantly higher than that reported in the general population (Meyer and Nasrallah 2009). Effects of psychotropic medications vary considerably, but these medications are thought to most directly induce this effect via their impact on the dopaminergic, serotonergic, cholinergic, adrenergic, and/or histaminergic systems. Of particular concern are elevated prolactin levels, or hyperprolactinemia, which may be largely a downstream effect of dopamine antagonism. Prolactin-elevating antipsychotic drugs are associated with abnormalities in libido, erectile function, and menstruation. Knegtering et al. (2008) reported that medication-induced hyperprolactinemia accounted for 40% of all sexual dysfunction present in a sample of individuals with schizophrenia.

Psychotropic medication has also been associated with reproductive hormone abnormalities in women, and this has implications for fertility in individuals with SMI. According to a review by Bargiota et al. (2013), the prevalence of menstrual abnormalities ranges from 15% to 97% in women using antipsychotic agents. Given that hyperprolactinemia may mediate the production of abnormally low levels of estrogen or no estrogen, manifesting in abnormal menstruation, and given the clinical significance of low estrogen in cardiovascular disease and osteoporosis, research regarding best prescribing practices for long-term antipsychotic regimens is critical (Leucht et al. 2007).

Urinary System

Bipolar disorder has been associated with an increased lifetime prevalence of chronic kidney disease (CKD), though this relationship appears to be partially mediated by long-term use of lithium and/or anticonvulsants (Kessing et al. 2015). An analysis comparing a random sample of patients from the Clinical Practice Research Datalink Registry with patients with SMI who had first psychiatric contact between 1994 and 2012 revealed an increased likelihood of CKD (defined as glomerular filtration rate of <60 mL/min/

1.732 m^2 for ≥3 months or confirmed renal replacement therapy) among those with SMI (Kessing et al. 2015). Those with SMI with no history of lithium use were 1.5 times more likely to develop CKD than the general population, and those with a history of lithium use were 6.5 times more likely, indicating the extent to which lithium use may mediate the strong correlation between CKD and SMI. Because CKD is independently and strongly associated with cardiovascular disease and mortality, relevant systemic disorders (i.e., hypothyroid-related kidney dysfunction) versus environmental factors (i.e., medication use) need to be captured with more specificity. The prevalence of other diseases of the urinary system, such as urological disease, systemic lupus erythematosus, and polycystic kidney disease, was not significantly different between SMI and No SMI groups.

Endocrine and Immune Systems

Endocrine System

In a British registry study following individuals with schizophrenia between 1981 and 1994, standard mortality ratio for diabetes-related death and all endocrine disease–related death was 9.96 and 11.66, respectively. Abnormalities in circulating thyroid hormones are related to glucose homeostasis and, by extension, the development of diabetes. Using population-level data obtained by linking three Danish registers—the Danish National Hospital Register, the Danish Psychiatric Central Research Register, and the Danish Register of Causes of Death—Thomsen et al. (2005) found that individuals hospitalized for hypothyroidism were significantly more likely to have a future psychiatric hospitalization for an affective disorder than were individuals hospitalized for either osteoarthritis or nontoxic goiter.

Immune System

In a population-based, retrospective case-control study conducted by linking the Danish National Patient Registry with the Danish Psychiatric Registry, Eaton et al. (2006) reported an association between the prevalence of autoimmune disease in individuals presenting with onset of schizophrenia (first contact with psychiatric care) compared with matched control subjects. History of thyrotoxicosis, intestinal malabsorption, acquired hemolytic anemia, interstitial cystitis, and Sjögren's syndrome was significantly more prevalent in individuals presenting with onset of schizophrenia compared with matched controls. Prevalence of these autoimmune disorders in patients' parents compared with parents of matched controls was significantly higher, lending some credence to the suggestion that heritability of predisposition to autoimmune diseases may exert a predisposition to physical disease that may confer significantly greater risk for the development of schizophrenia throughout the life span.

Considerations for Psychiatric Providers

To begin conceptualizing the risks of complex comorbidities and psychiatric providers' role in reducing morbidity and mortality, consider the case of Charlotte.

> Charlotte is an African American woman living in the rural United States who, 10 years ago, was diagnosed with schizoaffective disorder, which has been treated with antipsychotics for many years, contributing to her obesity. She has also developed type 2 diabetes mellitus. Charlotte lives in an apartment with her partner, works at the local library, and sees a provider at the clinic every 3 months for monitoring of her mental health. Unfortunately, she experiences an injury to her foot in an accident at home; however, because of neuropathy secondary to her diabetes, she is unable to feel the extent of this injury and does not seek proper treatment quickly. She does not complete regular foot checks as recommended by her doctor because of her challenges with planning and executive functioning related to her SMI, and she is geographically quite far from her primary care doctor. By the time Charlotte mentions the wound on her foot to her psychiatrist several months later, she is already at risk for complications such as local infection, irreversible tissue damage, septicemia, amputation, and death.

In treating someone like Charlotte, psychiatric providers should remain mindful of the potential health complications related to her mental illness. Communication and collaboration with patients and their physical health care providers are key to closely monitoring health risks and complications. In addition, understanding the links between mental health diagnosis and physical health conditions, delineated in this chapter, is crucial. Not only may her risk for additional health conditions increase because of genetic linkage to mental illness, psychiatric medication, and lifestyle factors, the functional limitations due to her mental illness may pose an additional challenge in managing physical health conditions. Because not all primary care and specialty health care providers are well versed in providing accessible, welcoming care to patients with SMI, psychiatric providers may consider collaborating to ensure the patients' specific health care needs are met and appropriate accommodations are considered. In Charlotte's case, these accommodations may include making a referral to occupational therapy to increase adherence to and efficacy of foot checks and wound care; inviting significant others who will provide support to Charlotte to attend follow-up appointments and to help her perform self-care; providing care instructions and appointment reminders in alternative formats that are more adaptive to her needs; speaking with Charlotte about peer navigator/community health worker or care management services; recommending that Charlotte obtain wound care supplies through the mail to reduce the likelihood that she will run out; and the like.

Another consideration in the morbidity and mortality of people with SMI is the impact a patient's mental health diagnosis may have on the quality of treatment he or she receives from other providers. Health service disparities among people with SMI exist in both primary and specialized medicine for various reasons, explored in greater detail in Chapter 4 of this book. While some of the barriers to high-quality treatment may be related to systemic issues and diminished engagement and adherence in care, there are also considerations to be made about the providers and potential bias in treating people with SMI. Indeed, some primary care providers find patients with mental illness to be disruptive or challenging to engage, feel uncomfortable providing services, and may be less likely to recommend more advanced or intensive treatments (Lawrence and Kisely 2010). As such, psychiatric providers should remain ever mindful of the lifelong impact of diagnosis on each patient, especially within the health care system.

These, and other, considerations and potential solutions are unpacked in later chapters of this book, particularly in Chapters 7–13. However, in short, by establishing an alliance with Charlotte as a trusted psychiatric provider who acknowledges how her physical and mental health are connected, one may be able to help her manage, arrest, improve, or even prevent her comorbid physical health conditions and reduce mortality. Although fragmentation of physical and mental health care can make it particularly challenging to address comorbid physical health conditions, psychiatrists are well positioned to have crucial conversations with patients and other providers to ensure high-quality care to the patient as a whole person.

The Impact on Wellness

Absence of illness does not make for quality of life per se. The Centers for Disease Control and Prevention (CDC) and the National Institutes of Health in the United States, as well as the World Health Organization on the international stage, have added wellness and well-being as essential domains to a total definition of health. Steinberg (2007), from the CDC, described wellness as an active process of decisions and choices in pursuit of a healthy and fulfilling life. It is a dynamic process leading to physical, mental, and social well-being, and not merely the absence of disease or infirmity.

A position paper from the Boston University Center of Psychiatric Rehabilitation (2019) outlined eight dimensions of wellness specific to the person with SMI:

1. Emotional—coping with life and developing satisfying relationships
2. Environmental—finding stimulating settings that promote well-being
3. Financial—achieving satisfaction with income and entitlements
4. Intellectual—finding enjoyable ways to expand one's knowledge and understanding
5. Occupational—finding satisfaction with one's employment
6. Physical—engaging in activities that promote healthy foods, exercise, and sleep
7. Social—having a sense of connectedness and a satisfactory support system
8. Spiritual—meeting one's sense of purpose and finding meaning in life

As is evident from this list, wellness is more than what happens in the organ systems. It also implies the overall impact on a person's sense of well-being (however that person defines well-being). All the chapters in this book consider wellness and well-being where appropriate.

Key Points

- Morbidity and mortality are clear concerns for the life and well-being of people with serious mental illness (SMI). Almost every organ system in the body seems to be impacted by mental illnesses.

- SMI is defined by impact on functioning (disability), developmental considerations, and persistence/chronicity of symptoms.

- The life expectancy gap for individuals with SMI compared with those without SMI ranges from 8.2 to 16 years.

- Both having a SMI and taking psychiatric medications can increase risk for integumentary and skeletal systems, including skin sensitivities, decreased bone density, edentulousness, and unintentional injury.

- People with SMI have high rates of cardiovascular disease related to increased exposure to risk factors as well as physiological changes to the cardiac structures.

- Psychiatric medications may contribute to some comorbid neurological conditions, though there is also indication of genetic and physiological links between mental health and neurological diseases.

- Rates of chronic obstructive pulmonary disease and other respiratory diseases among those with SMI are significantly higher than in the general population and contribute to the premature mortality of people with SMI.

- Research indicates a relation between digestive conditions (such as irritable bowel disease and celiac disease) and mental health diagnosis.

- Sexual and reproductive dysfunction and chronic kidney disease affect a disproportionate amount of people with SMI, with the increased prevalence often attributed to use of psychotropic medications.

- Endocrine disease, including diabetes, contributes to around 1 in 10 deaths of people with schizophrenia.

- Symptoms of comorbid mental illness and physical conditions often exacerbate one another, perhaps because of genetic linkage, exposure to risk factors, psychiatric medications, and related functional limitations.

- Providers who diagnose and prescribe medications for the psychiatric care of people with SMI should remain mindful of health risks and disparities to help their patients manage comorbidities, reduce risk and harm, and access health care providers who are competent and considerate in working with individuals with mental illness.

References

American Psychiatric Association: Diagnostic and Statistical Manual of Mental Disorders, 5th Edition. Arlington, VA, American Psychiatric Association, 2013

Bargiota SI, Bonotis KS, Messinis IE, et al: The effects of antipsychotics on prolactin levels and women's menstruation. Schizophr Res Treatment 2013:502697, 2013

Bartels SJ, Forester B, Mueser KT, et al: Enhanced skills training and health care management for older persons with severe mental illness. Community Ment Health J 40(1):75–90, 2004

Boston University Center of Psychiatric Rehabilitation: Eight dimensions of wellness. 2019. Available at: https://cpr.bu.edu/resources-and-information/eight-dimensions-of-wellness. Accessed October 20, 2020.

Chafetz L, White MC, Collins-Bride G, et al: Predictors of physical functioning among adults with severe mental illness. Psychiatr Serv 57(2):225–231, 2006

Chan HH, Wing Y, Su R, et al: A control study of the cutaneous side effects of chronic lithium therapy. J Affect Disord 57(1–3):107–113, 2000

Cizza G, Nieman LK, Doppman JL, et al: Factitious Cushing syndrome. J Clin Endocrinol Metab 81(10):3573–3577, 1996

Druss BG, Zhao L, Von Esenwein S, et al: Understanding excess mortality in persons with mental illness: 17-year follow up of a nationally representative US survey. Med Care 49(6):599–604, 2011

Eaton WW, Byrne M, Ewald H, et al: Association of schizophrenia and autoimmune diseases: linkage of Danish national registers. Am J Psychiatry 163(3):521–528, 2006

Gao YH, Zhao HS, Zhang FR, et al: The relationship between depression and asthma: a meta-analysis of prospective studies. PLoS One 10(7):e0132424, 2015

Garakani A, Win T, Virk S, et al: Comorbidity of irritable bowel syndrome in psychiatric patients: a review. Am J Ther 10(1):61–67, 2003

Harding CM, Brooks GW, Ashikaga T, et al: The Vermont longitudinal study of persons with severe mental illness, I: methodology, study sample, and overall status 32 years later. Am J Psychiatry 144(6):718–726, 1987

Huber G, Gross G, Schüttler R: A long-term follow-up study of schizophrenia: psychiatric course of illness and prognosis. Acta Psychiatr Scand 52(1):49–57, 1975

Ishihara L, Brayne C: A systematic review of depression and mental illness preceding Parkinson's disease. Acta Neurol Scand 113(4):211–220, 2006

Jette N, Patten S, Williams J, et al: Comorbidity of migraine and psychiatric disorders—a national population-based study. Headache 48(4):501–516, 2008

John A, McGregor J, Jones I, et al: Premature mortality among people with severe mental illness—new evidence from linked primary care data. Schizophr Res 199:154–162, 2018

Jungerius BJ, Bakker SC, Monsuur AJ, et al: Is MYO9B the missing link between schizophrenia and celiac disease? Am J Med Genet Part B Neuropsychiatr Genet 147(3):351–355, 2008

Kahn JP, Gorman JM, King DL, et al: Cardiac left ventricular hypertrophy and chamber dilatation in panic disorder patients: implications for idiopathic dilated cardiomyopathy. Psychiatry Res 32(1):55–61, 1990

Kêdoté MN, Brousselle A, Champagne F: Use of health care services by patients with co-occurring severe mental illness and substance use disorders. Ment Health Subst Use 1(3):216–227, 2008

Kemp AH, Quintana DS: The relationship between mental and physical health: insights from the study of heart rate variability. Int J Psychophysiol 89(3):288–296, 2013

Kenneson A, Funderburk JS, Maisto SA: Substance use disorders increase the odds of subsequent mood disorders. Drug Alcohol Depend 133(2):338–343, 2013

Kessing LV, Gerds TA, Feldt-Rasmussen B, et al: Use of lithium and anticonvulsants and the rate of chronic kidney disease: a nationwide population-based study. JAMA Psychiatry 72(12):1182–1191, 2015

Kisely S, Quek LH, Pais J, et al: Advanced dental disease in people with severe mental illness: systematic review and meta-analysis. Br J Psychiatry 199(3):187–193, 2011

Knegtering H, van den Bosch R, Castelein S, et al: Are sexual side effects of prolactin-raising antipsychotics reducible to serum prolactin? Psychoneuroendocrinology 33(6):711–717, 2008

Lawrence D, Kisely S: Inequalities in healthcare provision for people with severe mental illness. J Psychopharmacol 24(4 suppl):61–68, 2010

Lawrence D, Hancock KJ, Kisely S: The gap in life expectancy from preventable physical illness in psychiatric patients in Western Australia: retrospective analysis of population based registers. BMJ 346:f2539, 2013

Leipzig RM, Cumming RG, Tinetti ME: Drugs and falls in older people: a systematic review and meta-analysis, I: psychotropic drugs. J Am Geriatr Soc 47(1):30–39, 1999

Leucht S, Burkard T, Henderson J, et al: Physical Illness and Schizophrenia: A Review of the Evidence. New York, Cambridge University Press, 2007

Liu B, Anderson G, Mittmann N, et al: Use of selective serotonin-reuptake inhibitors or tricyclic antidepressants and risk of hip fractures in elderly people. Lancet 351(9112):1303–1307, 1998

Lou P, Chen P, Zhang P, et al: Effects of smoking, depression, and anxiety on mortality in COPD patients: a prospective study. Respir Care 59(1):54–61, 2014

Mai Q, Holman D, Sanfilippo F, et al: Mental illness related disparities in potentially preventable hospitalisations: a population-base cohort study from 1990 to 2006. J Epidemiol Community Health 65(suppl 1):A267, 2011

Meyer J, Nasrallah H: Medical Illness and Schizophrenia, 2nd Edition. Washington, DC, American Psychiatric Publishing, 2009

Mookhoek EJ, Van De Kerkhof PC, Hovens JE, et al: Skin disorders in chronic psychiatric illness. J Eur Acad Dermatol Venereol 24(10):1151–1156, 2010

National Institute of Mental Health: Statistics on mental illness. 2019. Available at: www.nimh.nih.gov/health/statistics/mental-illness.shtml. Accessed October 28, 2020.

Nazir M: Prevalence of periodontal disease: its association with systemic diseases and prevention. Int J Health Sci (Qassim) 11(2):72–80, 2017

Newman SC, Bland RC: Mortality in a cohort of patients with schizophrenia: a record linkage study. Can J Psychiatry 36(4):239–245, 1991

Ogawa K, Miya M, Watarai A, et al: A long-term follow-up study of schizophrenia in Japan—with special reference to the course of social adjustment. Br J Psychiatry 151:758–765, 1987

Osborn DPJ, Nazareth I, King MB: Risk for coronary heart disease in people with severe mental illness: cross-sectional comparative study in primary care. Br J Psychiatry 188(3):271–277, 2006

Partti K, Vasankari T, Kanervisto M, et al: Lung function and respiratory diseases in people with psychosis: population-based study. Br J Psychiatry 207(1):37–45, 2015

Prohovnik I, Dwork AJ, Kaufman MA, et al: Alzheimer-type neuropathology in elderly schizophrenia patients. Schizophr Bull 19(4):805–816, 1993

Qin P, Xu H, Laursen TM, et al: Risk for schizophrenia and schizophrenia-like psychosis among patients with epilepsy: population based cohort study. BMJ 331(7507):23, 2005

Ruschena D, Mullen PE, Palmer S, et al: Choking deaths: the role of antipsychotic medication. Br J Psychiatry 183:446–450, 2003

Schins A, Honig A, Crijns H, et al: Increased coronary events in depressed cardiovascular patients: 5-HT 2A receptor as missing link? Psychosom Med 65(5):729–737, 2003

Singh MK, Giles LL, Nasrallah HA: Pain insensitivity in schizophrenia: trait or state marker? J Psychiatr Pract 12(2):90–102, 2006

Steinberg K: Wellness in every stage of life: a new paradigm for public health programs. Prev Chronic Dis 4(1):A02, 2007

Thomsen AF, Kvist TK, Andersen PK, et al: Increased risk of developing affective disorder in patients with hypothyroidism: a register-based study. Thyroid 15(7):700–707, 2005

Walker ER, McGee RE, Druss BG: Mortality in mental disorders and global disease burden implications: a systematic review and meta-analysis. JAMA Psychiatry 72(4):334–341, 2015

Wamboldt MZ, Hewitt JK, Schmitz S, et al: Familial association between allergic disorders and depression in adult Finnish twins. Am J Med Genet 96(2):146–153, 2000

Wan JJ, Morabito DJ, Khaw L, et al: Mental illness as an independent risk factor for unintentional injury and injury recidivism. J Trauma 61(6):1299–1304, 2006

Winkelman JW: Schizophrenia, obesity, and obstructive sleep apnea. J Clin Psychiatry 62(1):8–11, 2001

Wu Q, Dalman C, Karlsson H, et al: Childhood and parental asthma, future risk of bipolar disorder and schizophrenia spectrum disorders: a population-based cohort study. Schizophr Bull 45(2):360–368, 2019

Yang SY, Liao YT, Liu HC, et al: Antipsychotic drugs, mood stabilizers, and risk of pneumonia in bipolar disorder: a nationwide case-control study. J Clin Psychiatry 74(1):e79–e86, 2013

CHAPTER 2

Research Considerations and Community-Based Participatory Research

Lindsay Sheehan, Ph.D.
Katherine Nieweglowski, M.S.
Yu Sun, M.P.H.

Health care for people with psychiatric disabilities includes a history of coercive treatment in segregated settings such as state hospitals, nursing homes, and jails (Fakhoury and Priebe 2007) as well as community practices such as overmedication and outpatient commitment (Link et al. 2008). Stigma and paternalistic attitudes toward people with psychiatric disabilities have led people with psychiatric disabilities to become alienated from communities and to be lacking in social power that could influence public health agendas (Bhui et al. 2006; Kidd and Davidson 2007; Pelletier et al. 2009). Experiences of disenfranchisement and disempowerment lead to apathy, resignation, and the "why try" effect (Corrigan and Rao 2012; Corrigan et al. 2009). Individuals with psychiatric disabilities may think, "Why even try to stay healthy? Nobody cares about people like me."

Despite these challenges, people with psychiatric disabilities, catalyzed by their dissatisfaction with mental health services, have developed a consumer movement of people with psychiatric disabilities focusing on recovery, empowerment, and transformation of the mental health system (Myrick and del Vecchio 2016). This movement has included former or current service users (i.e., peers) not only as health care providers but also as advocates serving on consumer advisory boards and as leaders of grassroots advocacy organizations. Peer-provided services have become increasingly common and accepted, as evidenced by the recent development of national peer service certification (Mental Health America 2020). Likewise, research funding has called for greater involvement of patients in research, such as through the Patient-Centered Outcomes Research Institute (Case et al. 2014), and inclusion of patient reviewers on research grant proposals. In this chapter, we focus on the application of one method of including people with psychiatric disabilities in research on health and wellness: community-based participatory research (CBPR).

What Is Community-Based Participatory Research?

CBPR emerged in response to increasing calls for more power-sharing in research (Green and Mercer 2001; Institute of Medicine 2003) and was developed to incorporate community participation and local practices into research efforts (Minkler and Wallerstein 2008; Wallerstein and Duran 2006). Defined by the W.K. Kellogg Foundation's Community Health Scholars Program (2001) as a "collaborative approach to research that equitably involves all partners in the research process and recognizes the unique strengths that each brings" (p. 2), CBPR is a powerful tool to challenge health disparities, such as those that exist for people with psychiatric disabilities (Israel et al. 2010). Mental and physical health disabilities are recognized as a complex system that shapes individuals' behaviors and influences their health and well-being. Interventions must be developed based on the understanding of the context of people's lives and how they encounter these circumstances in daily life (Institute of Medicine 2003; Lasker et al. 2001). CBPR provides a means for researchers to improve their understanding of how the system works through knowledge sharing and co-learning. CBPR moves the marginalized population, along with its lived experience, to the center of the research process (Hall 1992; Israel et al. 2010). Green and Mercer (2001) described this change as "a restriking of the power balance between the observers and the observed" (p. 1,926). More than being research subjects, local people become active partners and play an essential role in formulating research questions, developing and evaluating programs, and advocating policies that benefit them (Green and Mercer 2001). By doing so, CBPR is likely to create "partnership synergy," where the outcome is greater than the sum of the individual resources and skills (Lasker et al. 2001; Minkler 2005).

Other terms, such as *community partnered participatory research* (CPPR), *participatory action research* (PAR), and *community-engaged research* (CER), have all been used to describe research approaches similar to CBPR. These research strategies share an emphasis on empowering marginalized groups and recognizing the value of engaging participants, with the collective goal of generating social changes. For example, CPPR highlights the central role of the academic-community partnership (Baum et al. 2006; Cornwall and Jewkes 1995), while PAR purports to empower disenfranchised citizens to conduct projects with limited involvement from the academic side (Chevalier and Buckles 2013). Similarly, CER aims to engage the community in research, with level of involvement varying from activities such as interviewing community members or consulting community leaders, to the full engagement and equitable partnership with community, much as in CBPR (Kubicek et al. 2013).

The collaborative approach used in CBPR is essential to the improvement of psychiatric services in several ways. First, CBPR informs services by identifying treatment outcomes that are important to service users. Patients who are members of a CBPR team evaluating a new medication may decide, for example, that social or quality-of-life outcomes are more important than a reduction in hallucinations. New research findings on patient-centered outcomes can allow clinicians to compare possible treatments on these outcomes, leading to greater patient satisfaction. In addition, patients bring their lived experience to research projects, spawning new ideas for services or service delivery mechanisms that are more relevant to patients and thus more likely to be utilized. In traditional patient-doctor interactions, there is often a power dynamic that discourages honest patient feedback. Rather than expressing dissatisfaction directly, patients may simply stop seeking psychiatric treatment or choose another provider. Thus, psychiatrists who are directly involved in CBPR have an opportunity to interact with patients in a more equitable environment, while learning from patient experiences. Research that uses CBPR principles can better incorporate voices of patients, providing a vital level of understanding to psychiatrists and other health care professionals.

Principles of Community-Based Participatory Research

Minkler and Wallerstein (2008) have outlined the key principles of CBPR, as summarized below.

CBPR Recognizes Community as a Unit of Identity

The concept of community is central (Israel et al. 1998) and can be defined alternately in terms of geographical location, common history, collective identity, shared interests, values and norms, common symbols, or combinations of these dimensions (Schulz et al. 1998). Whereas psychology and psychiatry usually consider the individual as the primary unit of action, CBPR acknowledges that individuals live in communities that shape their strengths and challenges, and thus treats community as a single unit of identity, or "a larger socially constructed identity," for research purposes (Collins et al. 2018).

CBPR Holds an Ecological Perspective in Considering Research Questions

The ecological perspective embraces biomedical, economic, social, *and* cultural factors as determinants of health (Israel et al. 1998) and recognizes how these factors contribute to the existence of health disparities. For example, when low-income neighborhoods (often populated by people of color) are food and activity deserts, residents' inability to access fresh food and outdoor exercise may lead to reduced health. Considering research questions from an ecological perspective allows the research team to explain residents' health challenges and develop corresponding solutions.

CBPR Acknowledges Community's Strengths and Embraces Its Resources

The acknowledgment of each community member's knowledge, skills, and experiences as assets is foundational to CBPR (Collins et al. 2018). CBPR emphasizes the role of nonacademic participants in creating knowledge and takes advantage of these assets through active partnership to formulate the research process and generate meaningful results for the community (Chevalier and Buckles 2013; Israel et al. 1998). Community members with lived experience of health care conditions bring their knowledge of how that condition affects their lives, the barriers to getting care, and their connections with other community members who are potential research participants and activists for change. Similarly, health care providers who become involved in CBPR projects bring their unique knowledge of how their patients utilize the health care system and how changes can be implemented within that system.

CBPR Facilitates Collaborative and Equitable Partnership in All Research Phases

CBPR requires an academic-community partnership throughout the research process, from problem definition, data collection, and interpretation of results, to application and dissemination. Researchers and participants from the community share the control over each step to ensure that development and implementation of the research are based on mutual agreement and are a result of shared decision making (Minkler and Wallerstein 2008).

CBPR Is an Iterative Process That Fosters Co-learning and Capacity Building

In the process of CBPR, academic researchers shift their role from outside experts to learners. They share knowledge, skills, and resources with the community partners and meanwhile learn from the community's perspective on health issues. Community members may sometimes consider themselves inadequate research partners, so certain types of training are delivered before and during the research process to foster confidence. This is a co-learning process that emerges throughout the project (Baum et al. 2006; Minkler 2005). Both parties repeatedly reflect on what they know and what they have learned, to create new knowledge. For example, the researcher learns from community members that dental care is difficult to access, while community members learn what randomized controlled trials are. The new knowledge, in turn, nurtures each party and enhances the capacity to practice research, not only for the current study but also for future endeavors (Green and Mercer 2001).

CBPR Is Contextually Bound

In CBPR, research topics should come from the community and reflect its main interests (D'Alonzo 2010; Minkler 2005). Research design should consider local perspectives in order to develop culturally applicable methods and measurements. The interpretation of data must consider the specific context of the community in order to be culturally logical and appropriate. Dissemination of the findings should address the local audience and emphasize actions that the community might take (Collins et al. 2018; Israel et al. 1998).

These principles serve as core CBPR strengths that have great value for psychiatrists. CBPR not only enhances the comprehensive understanding of a given issue for psychiatrists but also increases the practical viability and the possibility for successful psychiatric interventions (Cornwall and Jewkes 1995; Israel et al. 1998). Since CBPR tailors research designs to community context, psychiatric interventions developed through CBPR efforts are more likely to be implemented with fewer barriers in the community, to be accepted by the community members, and to produce effective and meaningful health outcomes.

Summary of the Community-Based Participatory Research Health Literature

The overall purpose of CBPR is to actively employ community members and other local stakeholders during the research process. Nevertheless, it is important to understand various ways in which this involvement is utilized in the health literature. To illustrate this, we identified studies that observed or addressed physical *and* mental health needs of various communities. Search terms included "community-based participatory research (CBPR)," "participatory action research (PAR)," "community-based research," "mental illness," "mental health," "physical illness," "physical health," and "health disparities." Of the 44 total articles that we found, 32 were excluded because they did not describe research on both physical and mental health outcomes. Here we summarize the 12 articles that specifically investigated CBPR to address both physical and mental health (see Table 2–1).

Eight of the 12 studies investigated health outcomes in racial minority populations: Chinese (Dong et al. 2010), Latinos (Corrigan et al. 2017b, 2017c; Michael et al. 2008), and African Americans/Black minorities (Corrigan et al. 2015, 2017a; Muzik et al. 2016; Salihu et al. 2016). One study broadly investigated female immigrants and refugees (Krieger et al. 2002). Schulz and colleagues (1998) did not specifically target a racial minority. However, their sample population (women and children on the east side of Detroit) was described as primarily African American such that representative interviewers were employed accordingly by the CBPR team. These studies demonstrate that CBPR is heavily utilized among minority populations that are usually not provided with voices and would otherwise lack representation in research. Two study groups (Krieger et al. 2002; Poleshuck et al. 2018) conducted CBPR health research to investigate outcomes for survivors of domestic violence. The final study did so with adult male college students, many of whom identified as gay or bisexual, who "cruised" for sexual interactions (Reece and Dodge 2004).

TABLE 2–1. Review of community-based participatory research (CBPR) literature addressing mental and physical health outcomes

Study	Target population and health outcomes	Study methodology and findings	CBPR team involvement
Poleshuck et al. 2018	Intimate partner violence (IPV) survivors in New York State; chronic pain and depression	Qualitative focus group data ($N=31$) indicated that existing IPV services ignore many health concerns of survivors; there is too much focus on medical model. IPV advocates lack mental health training. Results were intended to be used to inform a new intervention by a community advisory board that included IPV survivors.	CBPR team comprised IPV survivors; they identified needs of IPV victims and survivors in the community and developed corresponding focus group questions, collected data, and analyzed results.
Corrigan et al. 2017b	Latinos with serious mental illness (SMI) in Chicago; physical and mental health care needs, barriers, and solutions	Participants were randomly assigned to either treatment as usual (control) or a peer navigation (PN) intervention. Quantitative survey data ($N=110$) indicated that PN intervention participants showed better health care engagement and greater improvement in recovery, more empowerment, and better quality of life.	CBPR team from qualitative portion of the study defined inclusion criteria and helped to recruit participants for PN intervention by passing out flyer to mental health clinics and community centers.
Corrigan et al. 2017c	Latinos with SMI in Chicago; physical and mental health care needs, barriers, and solutions	Qualitative focus group data ($N=122$) indicated health care needs and barriers. Needs included mental health services, substance use services, and preventive screenings. Barriers included financial constraints, language barriers, and immigration status. One identified solution included the implementation of PNs.	CBPR team worked to reach a consensus on major health care problems for Latino Chicagoans with SMI, develop a corresponding interview guide, make decisions on focus group logistics, and analyze findings.

TABLE 2–1. Review of community-based participatory research (CBPR) literature addressing mental and physical health outcomes (*continued*)

Study	Target population and health outcomes	Study methodology and findings	CBPR team involvement
Corrigan et al. 2017a	Homeless African Americans with SMI in Chicago; physical and mental health care needs, barriers, and solutions	Participants were randomly assigned to either treatment as usual (control) or PN intervention. Based on quantitative survey data (*N*=67), the PN intervention group showed small-to-moderate effect sizes in general health status, psychological experience of physical health, recovery, and quality of life.	CBPR team from qualitative portion of the study helped to recruit participants for PN intervention by passing out flyer to mental health clinics and homeless shelters. Team members were also involved in developing the PN intervention, including contrasting PN guidelines from the research literature with results from the qualitative study.
Salihu et al. 2016	Low-income African American women living in Tampa, Florida; physical health–related quality of life, physical fitness, nutrition, and depression	Qualitative focus group and interview data (no sample size reported) indicated needs such as lack of physical activity, sleep, poor nutritional status, and stress. Fortified dietary intervention (FDI) (*N*=49) was then designed from these results and led to higher physical health–related quality of life, smaller waist circumference, and lower depression.	Community member team helped to design an FDI to address effects of health disparities on physical and mental health. Design included conducting needs assessments, focus groups, and interviews.

TABLE 2–1. Review of community-based participatory research (CBPR) literature addressing mental and physical health outcomes (*continued*)

Study	Target population and health outcomes	Study methodology and findings	CBPR team involvement
Corrigan et al. 2015	Homeless African Americans with SMI in Chicago; physical and mental health care needs, barriers, and solutions	Qualitative focus group and interview data ($N=42$) showed that failure to attend to onset of acute illness may lead to chronic illness and disabling conditions. Additional issues stemming from psychiatric disorder and homelessness serve as barriers. One explored solution included the implementation of PNs.	CBPR team worked to reach consensus on major health care problems for homeless African American Chicagoans with SMI, develop a corresponding interview guide, make decisions on focus group logistics, and analyze findings.
Muzik et al. 2016	Teenage mothers of Black and minority ethnic origin in western Wayne County in metropolitan Detroit; use of pre- and postnatal health care services and support for physical and mental health	Qualitative focus group data ($N=19$) and semistructured interviews ($N=21$) indicated inadequate knowledge and accessibility to perinatal health services; need for family-focused services, especially for mental health.	Steering committee composed of two teenage mothers, one parent of a teenage mother, and local organizations met monthly to discuss recruitment strategies and inform the development of focus group questions.

TABLE 2–1. Review of community-based participatory research (CBPR) literature addressing mental and physical health outcomes (*continued*)

Study	Target population and health outcomes	Study methodology and findings	CBPR team involvement
Dong et al. 2010	Chinese older adults in Chicago's Chinatown; focus group questions focused on healthy aging, which involved both physical and mental health topics	Qualitative focus group data (*N*=78) indicated that Chinese older adults believe aging leads to irreversible deterioration in physical health and the realization of this is unwelcome; experiences of loneliness and boredom lead to psychological distress.	Community advisory board was established between Rush University Medical Center and Chinese American Service League to involve Chinese community members in identifying needs assessment topics, examining research instruments for cultural appropriateness, and reviewing findings.

TABLE 2–1. Review of community-based participatory research (CBPR) literature addressing mental and physical health outcomes (*continued*)

Study	Target population and health outcomes	Study methodology and findings	CBPR team involvement
Michael et al. 2008	Latino and African American communities in Multnomah County, Oregon; self-rated physical health and depressive symptoms	Qualitative interviews (*N*=14) and quantitative surveys (*N*=113) identified and measured health outcomes and social capital of participants. Following the community health worker intervention, data showed that social support and self-rated physical health increased, while depressive symptoms decreased.	A CBPR organization called Poder es Salud/Power for Health recruited study participants, constructed research surveys, developed in-depth interviews, selected community interviewers, and employed community health workers to survey and educate individuals from the target population about ways to identify and address health disparities.
Reece and Dodge 2004	Adult male college students who "cruise" for sexual interactions on campus; HIV transmission/ infection risks and mental health/social well-being	This paper focused on the CBPR process rather than the study results. A follow-up article was written to describe study methodology and findings. A mixed methods design including semi-structured interviews and quantitative survey data (*N*=30) found that cruising for sex presents challenges to physical health (i.e., sexually transmitted infections), mental health (i.e., sexual compulsivity, body image issues), and social well-being.	CBPR team members helped develop research and interview questions, make decisions on study design, plan and carry out recruitment strategies, collect and analyze data, and disseminate findings.

TABLE 2–1. Review of community-based participatory research (CBPR) literature addressing mental and physical health outcomes *(continued)*

Study	Target population and health outcomes	Study methodology and findings	CBPR team involvement
Krieger et al. 2002	Female immigrant and refugee domestic violence (DV) survivors in Seattle; physical health, mental health, and trauma	Qualitative interview and focus group data (sample size not reported) indicated that there is a lack of social support that leads to poor physical and mental health outcomes, especially due to immigration status and language barriers. The findings led to the development of a Refugee Women's Alliance group to increase social support.	A CBPR organization, Seattle Partners for Healthy Communities, formed a qualitative research team that included bilingual and bicultural community members from DV agencies; the team clarified research questions, recruited participants, and collected and analyzed data.
Schulz et al. 1998	Women and children on the east side of Detroit; infant physical health, maternal chronic health problems (e.g., diabetes, hypertension), and psychological outcomes (e.g., lack of emotional support, worry) resulting from environmental stressors	This article focused on describing the CBPR process rather than on reporting research findings. The authors published a follow-up article about how the results informed the development of a village health worker (VHW) intervention. Qualitative focus groups and interviews ($N=50$) and existing survey data ($N=700$) indicated that VHW interventions should consider the different complexities between providing services in urban versus rural areas.	A CBPR organization, East Side Village Health Worker Partnership, designed and conducted a survey to obtain data from the target population; this included defining survey items, choosing the sample, recruiting and training interviewers, and dissemination.

Altogether, racial/ethnic minorities, domestic violence survivors, and campus cruisers are vulnerable to negative physical and mental health outcomes. It is important to note that only 4 of the 12 articles specifically identified their target populations as "people with mental illness" (Corrigan et al. 2015, 2017a, 2017b, 2017c). The remaining 8 articles simply identified mental health outcomes as important variables. For example, trauma, chronic pain, and depression were some of the specific mental health measures associated with the domestic violence survivor studies (Krieger et al. 2002; Poleshuck et al. 2018). The campus cruiser study detailed social well-being, sexual compulsivity, and body image issues as important psychological variables for its population (Reece and Dodge 2004). Other mental health outcomes measured in the literature included lack of emotional support, loneliness, quality of life, recovery, and empowerment. Physical health outcomes were often measured generally through self-report. However, specific data included information regarding fitness, nutrition, waist circumference, and sexual health risks.

All 12 studies in this review utilized qualitative focus groups and/or interviews as their preliminary study methodology, and four of them constructed additional quantitative surveys to measure physical and mental health outcomes of participants (Corrigan et al. 2015, 2017c; Michael et al. 2008; Reece and Dodge 2004). Schulz and colleagues (1998), however, utilized a large-scale survey from a previous study ($N=700$) to conduct their analyses and construct their focus group and interview questions. Five studies applied their data to inform a future community health worker intervention through randomized controlled trials (RCTs) (Corrigan et al. 2015, 2017b; Michael et al. 2008; Poleshuck et al. 2018; Schulz et al. 1998), and one study created a fortified dietary intervention (Salihu et al. 2016). Results from the RCT interventions demonstrated overall positive effects on health outcomes within the selected target populations. Those studies that did not use their results for behavioral interventions instead set out to identify important health care needs and barriers within their designated communities as an important exploratory process to inform future research. For example, Muzik and colleagues (2016) sought to understand, on the basis of their qualitative data, the level of knowledge and needs for perinatal and mental health services among Black and minority ethnic teenage mothers in Detroit. Three other studies had similar agendas for health among Chinese older adults (Dong et al. 2010), campus cruisers (Reece and Dodge 2004), and female immigrant and refugee domestic violence survivors (Krieger et al. 2002). Although Krieger and colleagues (2002) did not set out to test a behavioral intervention, they did use the results to form an alliance group for domestic violence survivors. We can see from these study characteristics that CBPR is utilized to improve the lives of groups that may be disadvantaged and consequently experience health care disparities.

Critical Assessment of Community-Based Participatory Research Studies

Our examination of the 12 studies also allows us to summarize the involvement of CBPR team members and the perceived benefits and limitations of CBPR in these research projects.

CBPR Team Member Involvement

Project leads were primarily university researchers or medical doctors. Noticeably absent was involvement from psychiatrists in the CBPR process. This may have occurred because mental health was often a study outcome rather than an inclusion criterion. CBPR leaders and organizers frequently partnered with social service agencies, community networks, and local health care networks. Although the outcomes of the studies are important, it is also critical to understand how CBPR team members are involved throughout the research process to produce these results. The most common task identified among the studies was developing research questions, which included, for example, focus group and interview questions as well as quantitative survey items. The next most common task involved both collecting and analyzing data. Data collection included conducting focus groups, carrying out interviews, and distributing surveys, while analysis of data varied, from using statistical procedures to assessing the appropriateness of the research questions. In some cases, *analysis* also referred to developing and informing the corresponding health care interventions (i.e., intervention design, training providers).

Identifying the needs of the target population appeared as the third most common CBPR task. This was typically achieved through formal CBPR meetings with the entire team, with special emphasis on input from community members. Without such involvement, CBPR team members may not be as prepared to develop or assess research questions and data. CBPR teams are also by definition composed of members from the target population, so it is key for them to help the academic representatives (who may not be from the designated communities) to understand what should be addressed. Related to this is recruitment and identification of participants. Members from the community likely have the connections and resources to help select participants who fit the eligibility criteria of the study and are best able to inform the research questions. Dissemination of results is a crucial task that was only explicitly mentioned in two studies (Reece and Dodge 2004; Schulz et al. 1998); however, such efforts demonstrate that CBPR involvement does not have to end after data have been collected and analyzed. CBPR team members, especially those from the community, should continue to use their connections to distribute results directly into the community and lead the way for future research (Minkler 2005).

Benefits

Authors of the studies we reviewed reported that including members from the community as researchers has significant advantages. Obtaining local perspectives, defining relevant questions, and ensuring cultural sensitivity (i.e., respect, ethics, safety) are all positives that emerge at the very early stages of study development. CBPR has additional benefits for the community members who are involved because it facilitates engagement and empowers them to make strides toward their own health and wellness (as well as within their communities). For example, Corrigan et al. (2017a) noted that CBPR allows persons with serious mental illness to engage and be included in all phases of the research process. CBPR also helps to maintain a balance between research and action, which is something that may not be achieved without active involvement of community stakeholders, because they are uniquely able to use their connections and resources to facilitate direct change. CBPR team members from the Krieger et al. (2002) study conducted research to inform the development of an alliance group for refugee women. Such a benefit goes back to the importance of disseminating results directly back into the community.

Limitations

Many of the authors reported that CBPR is a time-consuming process that may prevent members from staying committed throughout the entire project (Krieger et al. 2002; Reece and Dodge 2004; Schulz et al. 1998). Such attrition may present an obstacle for disseminating results because academic researchers may lose their direct connections to the community before data have been completely analyzed. Another limitation is that it may be difficult to balance research interests and opinions of all CBPR team members, and this may be especially damaging if academic researchers do not maintain trust with local community members (Reece and Dodge 2004). Lack of trust may further lead to discontinued involvement or lower levels of commitment (Krieger et al. 2002). Other concerns include the ambiguity or breadth of CBPR principles and the potential for researcher bias. For example, academic researchers in these studies have concerns that CBPR may sometimes lack scientific rigor. Including community members from a specific locale may lead to nongeneralizability of results to similar groups throughout the general population (Corrigan et al. 2015, 2017a).

Implementation of Community-Based Participatory Research: A Case Study

We describe here a CBPR project that addressed health issues of homeless African Americans with serious mental illness in the Edgewater neighborhood of Chicago (hereinafter referred to as "the community") to illustrate how CBPR is conducted in practice. Our intention is to show a real-world example rather than a standardized procedure. Researchers should customize each CBPR project to the local context through a mutual process with all parties (Minkler and Wallerstein 2008). Figure 2–1 depicts the stages of the CBPR process for this example.

The research idea stemmed from primary concerns expressed by the community through the consumer advisory board at a local community organization serving a large population of urban homeless people. To address the health concerns of homeless African Americans, researchers from the university worked with the director at the community organization to come up with a proposal for submission to a nationwide CBPR initiative. Once the project was funded, a CBPR team was assembled by the university principal investigator and community organization. The team consisted of two academic researchers, a research staff, a peer research leader (an African American with lived experience of homelessness and mental illness who was hired by the university), a health care provider from the community organization, and eight community members who were African Americans with experiences of homelessness and mental illness. During the first 1.5 years of the 3-year project, the CBPR team met every week, and thereafter every month. Community members were paid hourly for attending each meeting and for recruitment efforts on the project (Corrigan et al. 2015).

After defining research questions, the team decided to conduct a needs assessment. To begin, they took a tour through the neighborhood, where community members introduced the environment to the other team members to facilitate better understanding of the target population (Corrigan et al. 2017a). One possible solution that emerged was to utilize peer health

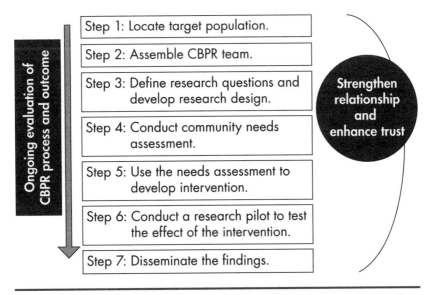

FIGURE 2–1. Case study: steps of the peer navigator community-based participatory research (CBPR) project.

navigators to facilitate access to and engagement in health care. Peer navigators, who would be African Americans with lived experience of mental illness and homelessness, could help patients get to medical appointments and manage their chronic illnesses. With this idea in mind, focus group and key informant interviews were used to collect information and gain insights into available resources and the community's readiness for the project. Team members collaborated with one another in identifying key stakeholders, recruiting participants for focus groups, and developing interview questions. One academic investigator and one community member co-led the focus groups and interviews.

Focus groups and key informant interviews with 42 individuals (33 homeless African Americans and 9 health care providers) resulted in three broad categories: health care problems, health care solutions, and the potential of peer navigators. The category of health care problems highlighted many chronic medical conditions, such as diabetes, heart disease, and arthritis, as well as deficiencies in ancillary care for eyes, teeth, and feet. Other prominent problems that emerged included wait times for health care, underfunded systems, and barriers in traveling to appointments. Health care solutions focused on increasing the number of clinics, drop-in programs, and housing options and the availability of integrated mental and physical health care. Another theme for solutions centered around the need for people with lived experience to self-manage their chronic conditions in their everyday lives. Results yielded a list of values in hiring peer navigators as well as skills and resources they would need to be successful.

Using the findings from the needs assessment, the CBPR team developed a peer navigator program as the intervention to address the mental and physical health concerns. The team members collectively developed the curriculum to train peer navigators, who were paraprofessionals with lived experience similar to that of the target population. Peer navigators work with a caseload of homeless individuals to help them navigate the complex health care system, including activities such as helping them make doctor appointments, enroll in health insurance, obtain prescriptions, and communicate with medical professionals (Corrigan et al. 2015, 2017a). The manualized curriculum included didactics, role-playing and worksheets around reflective listening, goal setting, motivational interviewing, advocacy, time management, and emphasis on using a strengths-based model. The curriculum also covered harm reduction, cultural competence, problem solving, crisis management, and trauma-informed care. The "Managing My Role" chapter provided information about relationship boundaries, management of burnout, and self-disclosure of lived experience. Three African Americans who were in recovery from serious mental illness and formerly homeless were hired by the community agency to fulfill the peer navigator role. Two community members and project research staff conducted a 2-week training with the newly hired peer navigators.

The CBPR team also designed and conducted a pilot to examine the efficacy of the program. Team members specified the inclusion and exclusion criteria and developed measurements based on the suggestions from the community members. With help from the community members, the team was able to recruit 97 participants and randomly assigned 67 individuals to the intervention group or the treatment-as-usual group for comparison. With consensus from the team regarding dissemination, the project was presented at a local conference with the presence of the entire CBPR team, and the results were published in academic journals (Corrigan et al. 2015, 2017a). The results were also distributed within the community organization.

This study exemplifies the CBPR approach through highlighting collaboration, equitable involvement, and shared decision making. During the course of the project, each party brought in strengths and resources, including the community members' lived experience and connections, the technical skills and resources from the academic members, and the supportive service and historical perspectives on the community from the health care organization. The project consisted of a co-learning process during which community members gained skills in conducting research and the academic members developed a better understanding of what life is like for a homeless African American experiencing serious mental illness and the challenges they face every day. The perspectives of both parties evolved throughout, especially in relation to contributing health factors. In addition, the project enhanced trust between the community and researchers and, as a result, strengthened the academic-community relationship. After the project, one community member of the CBPR team was hired by the university, and is now managing other CBPR projects. Other team members have also continued to engage in and contribute to CBPR projects.

An ongoing evaluation was conducted to assess the CBPR process and outcome. All team members shared their experience with the CBPR team, such as the challenges they encountered and their opinions on how to improve CBPR implementation. The evaluation provided valuable feedback to guide the CBPR team while the project continued. One limitation of this project was that the community organization was not able to continue the peer navigator program after the grant period ended, because of lack of funding.

Future Considerations for Community-Based Participatory Research

Given the stark health inequities for people with psychiatric disabilities and intersectional disadvantages such as socioeconomic or racial status, health research should continue to include community members, especially those with lived experience in the research and program development process. However, some might hesitate to involve people with psychiatric disabilities out of the misconception that they are too disabled to contribute substantially to research. Similarly, people with psychiatric disabilities risk being involved as token members of the team. Surmounting these obstacles requires commitment of the investigator and the entire research team. Team members with lived experience may enter projects with clear disadvantages in terms of social power, education, and research experience, which may cause them to become frustrated and disengaged. Our research group brought together a CBPR team to explore these disadvantages and learn how researchers might address them. The result of that project, the Inspiring Change CBPR curriculum, suggests ways to engage disenfranchised individuals in the CBPR process (Sheehan et al. 2015). One key to engagement for people with disabilities is reasonable accommodations. Just as employers are called upon by the Americans with Disabilities Act to make accommodations for employees in the workplace, CBPR teams can accommodate members by providing individualized instruction and feedback, allowing for additional breaks, and formatting the meeting to alleviate situations that might trigger psychiatric symptoms.

Involvement of People With Psychiatric Disabilities in Leadership Roles

Another way to challenge tokenistic involvement in CBPR is to involve lived-experience representatives as co-leaders on research projects. However, these lived experience leaders will have challenges of their own that should be recognized and supported by institutions and funders. First, lived experience leaders will transition from roles of service recipients, with an inherent power imbalance relative to the health care provider and researcher. The lived experience leader must navigate this power imbalance and transition into the role of partner rather than recipient. The leader is required to be able to identify and develop his or her strengths going into the project and become confident in the important roles (e.g., mentor and coach) that he or she will fulfill when working with the other community members on the research team. This also requires the lived experience leader to tactfully communicate with the academic lead and assert opinions that ensure community voices are reflected in the project. The lived experience leader will set the tone for the group and model socially appropriate ways of challenging authority embedded in traditional research structures.

Second, people with psychiatric disabilities might be at a disadvantage in terms of formal education and experience with the basics of conducting research. Lived-experience research leaders have important knowledge to bring to projects but can misunderstand or misinterpret jargon used by service providers and researchers. The lived experience leader must be able to directly acknowledge any lack of understanding to the other leaders and seek clarification and explanation. If information conveyed by the academic researcher is not expressed in words that a layperson (i.e., research participant or CBPR team member) would understand, then the spirit of CBPR is not preserved and the research risks losing a culturally competent approach. If the researcher, for example, tells the CBPR team that the project needs IRB approval, the lived experience leader can jump in and say, "Hold on, now what is this IRB thing that you're talking about...can you explain more?"

Third, lived experience leaders may struggle to understand and navigate workplace culture and norms. Because of limited experience working in health care settings or large gaps in work history due to psychiatric disabilities, lived experience leaders can benefit from extra support in navigating effectively in professional work environments and may need help in advocating for organizational resources and supports. Experiences of racial discrimination and stressors related to working in unfamiliar or white-dominated environments could compromise the confidence and effectiveness of lived-experience research leaders.

Finally, lived experience research leaders, despite being in recovery, may still experience periodic psychiatric symptoms or require reasonable accommodations to be effective leaders. This could require, for example, extra support from other leaders in planning or structuring research tasks or debriefing after team sessions. Our research group developed a curriculum that includes training in leadership concepts, CBPR, and long-term mentorship activities intended to address challenges faced by lived-experience leaders (Sheehan et al. 2017). Psychiatrists and other health care providers can be attuned to the obstacles facing people with lived experience and be prepared to advocate for more active roles by lived-experience researchers.

Key Points

Given the benefits of and moral imperatives for community-based participatory research (CBPR), researchers and clinicians should

- Consider greater inclusion of people with lived experience in research and program evaluation efforts meant to reduce health inequities for people with psychiatric disabilities.

- Tailor CBPR efforts to the specific culture of the local community.

- Intentionally design research and services in true collaboration with patients.

- Be willing to learn from people with lived experience.

- Be willing to commit time and resources to CBPR projects.

- Anticipate and proactively manage CBPR challenges.

References

Baum F, MacDougall C, Smith D: Participatory action research. J Epidemiol Community Health 60(10):854–857, 2006

Bhui K, Shanahan L, Harding G: Homelessness and mental illness: a literature review and a qualitative study of perceptions of the adequacy of care. Int J Soc Psychiatry 52(2):152–165, 2006

Case AD, Byrd R, Claggett E, et al: Stakeholders' perspectives on community-based participatory research to enhance mental health services. Am J Community Psychol 54(3–4):397–408, 2014

Chevalier JM, Buckles DJ: Participatory Action Research: Theory and Methods for Engaged Inquiry. London, Routledge, 2013

Collins SE, Clifasefi SL, Stanton J, et al: Community-based participatory research (CBPR): towards equitable involvement of community in psychology research. Am Psychol 73(7):884–898, 2018

Cornwall A, Jewkes R: What is participatory research? Soc Sci Med 41(12):1667–1676, 1995

Corrigan PW, Rao D: On the self-stigma of mental illness: stages, disclosure, and strategies for change. Can J Psychiatry 57(8):464–469, 2012

Corrigan PW, Larson JE, Ruesch N: Self-stigma and the "why try" effect: impact on life goals and evidence-based practices. World Psychiatry 8(2):75–81, 2009

Corrigan PW, Pickett SA, Kraus DJ, et al: Community-based participatory research examining the health care needs of African Americans who are homeless with mental illness. J Health Care Poor Underserved 26(1):119–133, 2015

Corrigan PW, Kraus DJ, Pickett SA, et al: Using peer navigators to address the integrated health care needs of homeless African Americans with serious mental illness. Psychiatr Serv 68(3):264–270, 2017a

Corrigan PW, Sheehan L, Morris S, et al: The impact of a peer navigator program in addressing the health needs of Latinos with serious mental illness. Psychiatr Serv 69(4):456–461, 2017b

Corrigan PW, Torres A, Lara JL, et al: The healthcare needs of Latinos with serious mental illness and the potential of peer navigators. Adm Policy Ment Health 44(4):547–557, 2017c

D'Alonzo KT: Getting started in CBPR—lessons in building community partnerships for new researchers. Nurs Inq 17(4):282–288, 2010

Dong X, Chang E-S, Wong E, et al: Assessing the health needs of Chinese older adults: findings from a community-based participatory research study in Chicago's Chinatown. J Aging Res 2010:124246, 2010

Fakhoury W, Priebe S: Deinstitutionalization and reinstitutionalization: major changes in the provision of mental healthcare. Psychiatry 6(8):313–316, 2007

Green LW, Mercer SL: Can public health researchers and agencies reconcile the push from funding bodies and the pull from communities? Am J Public Health 91(12):1926–1929, 2001

Hall BL: From margins to center? The development and purpose of participatory research. Am Sociol 23(4):15–28, 1992

Institute of Medicine: Who Will Keep the Public Healthy? Educating Public Health Professionals for the 21st Century. Washington, DC, National Academy Press, 2003

Israel BA, Schulz AJ, Parker EA, et al: Review of community-based research: assessing partnership approaches to improve public health. Annu Rev Public Health 19(1):173–202, 1998

Israel BA, Coombe CM, Cheezum RR, et al: Community-based participatory research: a capacity-building approach for policy advocacy aimed at eliminating health disparities. Am J Public Health 100(11):2094–2102, 2010

Kidd SA, Davidson L: "You have to adapt because you have no other choice": the stories of strength and resilience of 208 homeless youth in New York City and Toronto. J Community Psychol 35(2):219–238, 2007

Krieger J, Allen C, Cheadle A, et al: Using community-based participatory research to address social determinants of health: lessons learned from Seattle Partners for Healthy Communities. Health Educ Behav 29(3):361–382, 2002

Kubicek K, Beyer WH, McNeeley M, et al: Community-engaged research to identify house parent perspectives on support and risk within the house and ball scene. J Sex Res 50(2):178–189, 2013

Lasker RD, Weiss ES, Miller R: Partnership synergy: a practical framework for studying and strengthening the collaborative advantage. Milbank Q 79(2):179–205, 2001

Link B, Castille DM, Stuber J: Stigma and coercion in the context of outpatient treatment for people with mental illnesses. Soc Sci Med 67(3):409–419, 2008

Mental Health America: National certified peer specialist (NCPS) certification—get certified! 2020. Available at: www.mentalhealthamerica.net/national-certified-peer-specialist-ncps-certification-get-certified. Accessed June 22, 2020.

Michael YL, Farquhar SA, Wiggins N, et al: Findings from a community-based participatory prevention research intervention designed to increase social capital in Latino and African American communities. J Immigr Minor Health 10(3):281–289, 2008

Minkler M: Community-based research partnerships: challenges and opportunities. J Urban Health 82(2 suppl 2):ii3–ii12, 2005

Minkler M, Wallerstein N: Community-Based Participatory Research for Health: From Process to Outcomes, 2nd Edition. San Francisco, CA, Jossey-Bass, 2008

Muzik M, Kirk R, Alfafara E, et al: Teenage mothers of black and minority ethnic origin want access to a range of mental and physical health support: a participatory research approach. Health Expectations 19(2):403–415, 2016

Myrick K, del Vecchio P: Peer support services in the behavioral healthcare workforce: State of the field. Psychiatr Rehabil J 39(3):197–203, 2016

Pelletier J, Davidson L, Roelandt J, et al: Citizenship and recovery for everyone: a global model of public mental health. Int J Ment Health Promot 11(4):45–53, 2009

Poleshuck E, Mazzotta C, Resch K, et al: Development of an innovative treatment paradigm for intimate partner violence victims with depression and pain using community-based participatory research. J Interpers Violence 33(17):2704–2724, 2018

Reece M, Dodge B: A study in sexual health applying the principles of community-based participatory research. Arch Sex Behav 33(3):235–247, 2004

Salihu HM, Adegoke KK, Das R, et al: Community-based fortified dietary intervention improved health outcomes among low-income African-American women. Nutr Res 36(8):771–779, 2016

Schulz AJ, Parker EA, Israel BA, et al: Conducting a participatory community-based survey for a community health intervention on Detroit's east side. J Public Health Manag Pract 4(2):10–24, 1998

Sheehan L, Ballentine S, Agnew L, et al: The Inspiring Change Manual: A Community-Based Participatory Research Manual for Involving African Americans With Serious Mental Illness in Research. Chicago, Illinois Institute of Technology, 2015

Sheehan L, Ballentine S, Cole S, et al: Inspiring Change Leadership Training: A Curriculum for Preparing African American Lived Experience Research Leaders: Instructors Manual. Chicago, Illinois Institute of Technology, 2017

Wallerstein NB, Duran B: Using community-based participatory research to address health disparities. Health Promotion Practice 7(3):312–323, 2006

W.K. Kellogg Foundation Community Health Scholars Program: Stories of Impact (brochure). Ann Arbor, University of Michigan, School of Public Health, Community Scholars Program, National Program Office, 2001

CHAPTER 3

Effects of Concurrent Substance Use

Ayorkor Gaba, Psy.D.
Siu Ping Chin Feman, M.D.
Kelsey M. Clary, B.A.
David Smelson, Psy.D.

Approximately 11 million American adults experience serious mental illness (SMI). Of those, over a quarter also have a substance use disorder (SUD) (Substance Abuse and Mental Health Services Administration 2018). The combination of any mental illness, including SMI, and SUD, referred to as *co-occurring disorders*, contributes to poorer outcomes in a multitude of areas as compared with SUD or SMI alone. Examples of poor outcomes include frequent hospitalization, premature death, higher rate of infectious diseases, unemployment, homelessness, and incarceration (Substance Abuse and Mental Health Services Administration 2018). In addition, individuals with co-occurring disorders tend to have worse treatment outcomes and increased treatment costs (McCauley et al. 2010). Physical illness frequently co-occurs with mental health disorders and SUD. Research has shown disproportionate medical comorbidities and premature death among people with SMI alone or with co-occurring disorders (Roshanaei-Moghaddam and Kanton 2009), and over half of the medical comorbidities in this population are preventable (Chang et al. 2011).

Unfortunately, the physical health of people with co-occurring disorders is less often the focus of treatment, resulting in significant disparities in the wellness of people with co-occurring disorders compared with those without co-occurring disorders (Saxena and Maj 2017). In this chapter we explore *multimorbidity* (the presence of two or more long-term conditions), specifically defined as the co-occurrence of SMI (i.e., schizophrenia, schizoaffective disorder, or bipolar disorder with psychotic features), substance use, and physical conditions. This chapter excludes individuals with co-occurring disorders who do not have SMI. We describe the prevalence, etiology, course, and associated outcomes of comorbid SMI, substance use, and physical conditions. We also review evidence-based approaches to inform psychiatric practice to better address these comorbid conditions.

Prevalence of Co-occurring Serious Mental Illness, Substance Use Disorder, and Physical Illness

Serious Mental Illness and Substance Use

Co-occurring disorders are quite common in the United States. Among American adults age 18 or older, approximately 11.2 million (4.5%) had an SMI and 3.1 million (1.3%) had an SMI and an SUD (co-occurring disorders) in the past year (Substance Abuse and Mental Health Services Administration 2018). Individuals with SMI are at higher risk for developing an SUD. For example, a large nationally representative study found that compared with people without SMI, people with SMI were about 4 times more likely to drink alcohol heavily (four or more drinks per day), 3.5 times more likely to use cannabis regularly (21 times per year), 5.1 times more likely to smoke tobacco daily, and 4.6 times more likely to use other drugs at least 10 times in their lives (Hartz et al. 2014). This study replicated findings from various smaller studies indicating a higher risk for substance use for individuals with SMI (Substance Abuse and Mental Health Services Administration 2018).

The elevated risk for SUD for those with SMI is particularly concerning as we are in the midst of an opioid epidemic. Co-occurring disorders have been linked to increased risk for opioid misuse and overdose (Campbell et al. 2018). Data from 170,300 adults participating in the 2015–2017 National Surveys on Drug Use and Health indicated that between 2015 and 2017, 1.1% or approximately 2,083,400 Americans ages 18–64 had a past-year opioid use disorder, 0.7% had a prescription opioid use disorder, and 0.3% had a heroin use disorder (Jones and McCance-Katz 2019). Of the adults with past-year opioid use disorder, 64.3% had any mental illness in the past year and 26.9% (over 1 in 4) had SMI in the past year. Prevalence of co-occurring SMI was similar for adults with prescription opioid use disorder and those with heroin use disorder (Jones and McCance-Katz 2019). Correlates of opioid use disorder among people with SMI include being male, younger age, marital status (never married), cannabis use before age 18, and ease of obtaining other drugs (Prince 2019).

With the growing number of states loosening restrictions related to cannabis use, there is growing concern about the high prevalence of cannabis use among individuals with SMI. Lifetime prevalence of cannabis use among adults with SMI is approximately 2–3.5 times higher than in the general population (Hartz et al. 2014). The link between cannabis use and psychiatric conditions has been investigated many times but with somewhat mixed results (Blanco et al. 2016). Research suggests a link between cannabis use and an increased risk for schizophrenia. For example, heavy cannabis use among those with schizophrenia has been linked to significantly worsened psychiatric symptoms, including more severe psychotic episodes (Brunette et al. 2018).

Another significant area of concern is tobacco use; roughly 60% of those with SMI smoke tobacco. People with SMI who smoke tobacco have 25 years of reduced life expectancy compared with the general population (Ilyas et al. 2017). Because of the critical impact of tobacco use on this population, co-occurring SMI and tobacco use will be explored separately in Chapter 11 of this book.

Serious Mental Illness, Substance Use, and Medical Comorbidities

Physical illness frequently co-occurs with SMI and substance use. Approximately 50%–80% of individuals with SMI have one or more comorbid medical conditions (Roshanaei-Moghaddam and Kanton 2009). A recent study examining medical comorbidities among patients with SMI in a large integrated health system found that having SMI was associated with higher odds of medical comorbidities, including chronic pain, hepatitis C, HIV, chronic kidney disease, chronic obstructive pulmonary disease, diabetes, and heart disease (Bahorik et al. 2017). Two types of medical conditions have received substantial attention in the psychiatric literature: metabolic syndrome and blood-borne viruses, specifically HIV and hepatitis B and C.

First, the concept of metabolic syndrome—a cluster of conditions that occur together and that include abdominal obesity (also known as central obesity), high blood pressure, low high-density lipoprotein cholesterol, elevated triglycerides, and hyperglycemia, predisposing to the development of cardiovascular disease and diabetes—is of significant concern (Penninx and Lange 2018). A meta-analysis showed that the prevalence of metabolic syndrome is 58% higher in psychiatric patients than in the general population (Vancampfort et al. 2015). SUD is considered a prominent risk factor for metabolic syndrome. In the largest meta-analysis to date examining rates of metabolic syndrome in people with alcohol use disorder, researchers found that higher metabolic syndrome frequency was moderated by a higher percentage of psychiatric comorbidity. These findings suggest that psychiatric comorbidity may have a critical role in metabolic syndrome in people with alcohol use disorder (Vancampfort et al. 2015).

Second, decades of research have suggested that SMI is a risk factor for contracting blood-borne viruses, including HIV, hepatitis B, and hepatitis C (Wainberg and Dixon 2017). Studies have found that hepatitis C is more prevalent among people with SMI than in the general population (Hughes et al. 2016). Furthermore, up to 50% of patients with hepatitis C have a history of mental illness and nearly 90% have a history of SUD. Risk factors for hepatitis C include sharing of needles and use of injection drugs and crack cocaine. Research estimates that the prevalence of HIV among individuals with SMI is much higher than in the general population, ranging up to 24% (De Hert et al. 2011). Frequently, these individuals are also diagnosed with an SUD (Parry et al. 2007). Because of the high prevalence of physical illness, including metabolic syndrome and infection with blood-borne viruses, and associated mortality in the SMI population, psychiatrists play a critical role in screening for medical conditions, and referring to and participating in the coordination of care for this high-risk group.

Case Vignette 1

Client background: The client is a 47-year-old Vietnamese male refugee with a history of alcohol and opioid use disorders, depression, severe trauma, hepatitis C infection, cirrhosis complicated by variceal bleeding and hepatic encephalopathy, and osteoarthritis limiting ambulation. The client receives psychiatric care through his local federally qualified health center (FQHC).

Brief description of interventions: The client is living alone in a rented room, with little income and no local family or friends. Additionally, the client is primarily using emergency medical care, with intermittent engagement with his outpatient psychiatrist and therapist, and does not have an identified primary care provider (PCP).

The psychiatrist begins by introducing the client to the medical team at the FQHC by doing a warm hand-off. Through engagement with primary care, the client is able to connect with a PCP, and later to medication-assisted treatment for opioid use disorder with buprenorphine/naloxone. With ongoing opioid and alcohol use, as well as cirrhosis, it is difficult for a psychiatrist to clarify whether the client's depressed mood and isolation are due to substances, medical illness, psychiatric illness, or a combination of all of these.

Although the client's opioid and alcohol use decreases and the client is more engaged with care, he continues to struggle with keeping appointments and taking medications as prescribed, because the client's encephalopathy results in intermittent confusion, making medication adherence and attending appointments difficult. The client's encephalopathy, inconsistency with medications and appointments, and intermittent opioid use all contribute to his continued symptoms of depression and make addressing them more difficult. The client's prior trauma contributes to his difficulty in trusting providers. Through gradual, persistent visits, he begins to slowly engage in care, allowing visiting nurses and home health aides into his home, which improves his medication adherence and encephalopathy, allowing him to feel more supported, and thus increasing his engagement with medical and psychiatric care and improving his psychiatric and medical conditions while supporting his sobriety.

The psychiatrist is challenged to build an alliance with this client, while also collaborating with other specialties to address the client's unmet needs regarding treatment of medical conditions and addiction. Medical diagnoses, addiction, and mental illness all interact and affect the client's health and quality of life.

Etiology of Co-occurring Serious Mental Illness, Substance Use Disorder, and Physical Illness

Etiology of comorbidity in this area is complex and multidirectional. For example, SMI and/or SUD may place a person at risk for medical conditions, and all three disorders may share common risk factors. To effectively treat not only one but all of these disorders, practitioners need a comprehensive understanding of the underlying contributing factors. There have been several theories about the etiology of substance use and medical conditions in individuals with SMI.

First, according to the diathesis-stress model, genetic predisposition interacts with environmental stressors, and this interaction results in the onset of SMI, substance use, and medical conditions. Some assert that exposure to stressors is linked to a weakening of the immune system and an increase in the inflammatory response, which are risk factors for medical disorders (Black 2006). Psychiatric disorders have been linked to altered immune function (Kiecolt-Glaser and Glaser 2002), as has use of alcohol and drugs (Sarkar et al. 2015). The inflammatory response is critical for dealing with injury or infection; therefore, the combined impact of mental illness and substance use on immune functioning increases vulnerability to medical conditions.

Second, the self-medication hypothesis suggests that individuals with SMI develop an SUD because they use the substance to manage their mental health symptoms (Substance Abuse and Mental Health Services Administration 2018). A medical condition, such as hepatitis C, may then come about as a result of activities related to the SUD (e.g., intravenous drug use, sharing needles).

Third, SMI, SUD, and medical conditions may be influenced by a common pathophysiology (e.g., shared genetic mechanisms). One example of this is chronic pain, a medical condition associated with severe emotional distress that dysregulates the brain's stress and reward circuitry. In turn, this dysregulation increases the risk for misusing opioids to mitigate the chronic pain and associated emotional distress and may lead to the development of an opioid use disorder.

Fourth, common treatments for diseases may actually worsen the comorbid mental health, substance use, or medical problems. For example, antipsychotic medications can cause weight gain, obesity, and type 2 diabetes (Muench and Hamer 2010), laying the foundation for the development of metabolic syndrome. In addition, treatments for common medical conditions may have psychological side effects that may exacerbate or complicate underlying psychiatric conditions. For example, interferon-alfa, a drug used to treat hepatitis C, can cause depression and psychosis (Lucaciu and Dumitrascu 2015). An individual may then use substances to address these side effects. In addition, many chronic medical conditions are related to "lifestyle choices or inadequate self-care," such as lack of exercise, poor diet, and lack of effective stress relief/management. These lifestyle choices impact mood, emotional regulation, and management of serious mental health symptoms, which may then put individuals at risk for using substances. Unfortunately, many of these "choices" are closely linked to key social determinants of health.

Finally, social determinants of health contribute to the development of comorbidity. As defined by the World Health Organization, social determinants are the conditions in which we "are born, grow, work, live, and age" (www.who.int/social_determinants/sdh_definition/en). Examples of social determinants include poverty, adverse childhood experiences, discrimination, and food insecurity. Social determinants have been described as "the causes of the causes" of ill health (Sederer 2016). Social determinants force individuals into difficult choices based on limited options, and can lead to severe psychiatric distress, substance use, and/or physical illness. For example, circumstances such as housing insecurity put individuals at increased risk for mental health, substance use, and medical problems (de Similien 2017). Alternatively, an individual living in poverty with chronic physical conditions can be at risk for developing and exacerbating mental health problems because of the stress of living in poverty and potential barriers to care. In these difficult circumstances, individuals may increase substance use to try to manage mental and medical health symptoms. Both illness and wellness are highly influenced by social determinants.

Mortality, Costs, and Treatment Implications

The combination of SMI, substance use, and medical conditions is associated with increased risk for mortality, higher health care costs, and poorer treatment engagement and outcomes.

Mortality

As previously mentioned, individuals with SMI, SUD, and medical conditions are at higher risk for premature death. Compared with the general population, individuals with SMI alone, SUD alone, or co-occurring disorders have increased mortality rates. The highest mortality rates have been found in clinical samples and among individuals with co-occurring SMI (psychosis) and SUD (Walker et al. 2015). Physical diseases account for the overwhelming majority of premature mortality in this population (Walker et al. 2015). Among physical conditions, cardiovascular disease is the main preventable contributor to early death in patients with co-occurring SMI and SUD (Charlson et al. 2016). One of the first meta-analyses in this area identified that individuals with SMI have an 85% higher risk for death from cardiovascular disease compared with the regionally matched general population (Correll et al. 2017).

Costs

Co-occurring substance use, SMI, and medical disorders are particularly costly to the health care system. First, individuals with all three conditions are hospitalized at a higher rate than the general population. Second, these patients have longer lengths of stay than the general population. Third, people with SMI and SUD are the heaviest utilizers of emergency department services (Edwards et al. 2013). These increased rates of hospitalization and long lengths of stay have a significant impact on increasing medical expenditures and costs (Edwards et al. 2013).

According to state Medicaid studies, Medicaid beneficiaries with co-occurring SMI, SUD, and medical conditions have higher total Medicaid costs (e.g., inpatient hospital, skilled nursing facility, pharmacy) than beneficiaries without SMI (Substance Abuse and Mental Health Services Administration 2010). A substantial portion of spending for Medicaid enrollees with SUDs is for services to address significant physical and behavioral health issues. Among this population, opioid use disorder in particular accounts for large discrepancies in health care costs. Individuals with opioid use disorder who are on Medicaid are estimated to have annual health care costs that are much higher than those incurred by their counterparts without opioid use disorder (Hsien-Yen et al. 2018). Because of the growing opioid crisis and rising related health care costs, there has been a call for psychiatrists to receive training in the assessment and treatment of patients with opioid use disorder. A recent study specifically encouraged psychiatrists and psychiatric residents to complete the required 8-hour training needed to prescribe buprenorphine (Muvvala et al. 2019). Medication-assisted treatment training and subsequent medication-assisted treatment service delivery by psychiatrists will drive down health care costs associated with opioid use disorder.

Treatment Implications

Studies have found that 60% of the medical comorbidities among persons with SMI are preventable (Chang et al. 2011). However, individuals experiencing SMI, SUD, and physical illness are less likely than the general population to receive preventive medical services such as immunizations and cancer screenings and smoking cessation counseling (Razanno et al. 2015). They also experience poorer access to primary care and lower quality of primary care received relative to those without all three conditions (Richmond 2017). Furthermore, these individuals report more stigmatizing and discriminatory experiences in primary care settings (Sapag et al. 2018), potentially leading to high utilization of emergency medical services with little to no follow-up care to address primary care needs (Levinson Miller et al. 2003).

Of more concern, many individuals with co-occurring SMI and SUD do not seek treatment for these conditions, let alone seek treatment for their medical comorbidities. Studies show that only 7.4% of individuals with SMI and SUD receive treatment for these disorders in their lifetime (Priester et al. 2016). When seeking co-occurring disorders treatment, individuals experience barriers similar to those experienced in the primary care system, including under-identification and undertreatment of medical problems and fragmented care, leading to higher utilization of crisis services and higher dropout rates. Systems of care and individual providers, such as psychiatrists, often do not have adequate training, infrastructure, and processes in place to successfully screen and coordinate care across these areas. Finally, stigmatizing attitudes of psychiatrists toward individuals with diagnosed co-occurring disorders have a particularly potent adverse impact on treatment engagement (Adams 2008). Several studies suggest that psychiatrists possess more stigmatizing attitudes toward individuals with SMI and SUD than toward individuals with other mental and medical illnesses (Adams 2008; Avery et al. 2013). Specialized training for psychiatrists is needed to reduce stigmatizing attitudes that impact treatment seeking and engagement in this high-risk group.

Evidence-Based Practice to Inform Psychiatric Practice

Integrated care services have been proposed as the most viable, efficient, and cost-effective way to deliver health care to treat co-occurring conditions. *Integrated care* is defined as "the care that results from a practice team of primary care and behavioral health clinicians, working together with patients and families, using a systematic and cost-effective approach to provide patient-centered care for a defined population" (Peek and National Integration Academy Council 2013, p. 2). A team usually consists of a PCP, behavioral health care provider, and consulting psychiatrist, but may also include a case manager (CM), peer support specialist (PSS), and/or nurse. Hallmarks of integrated care models include co-located providers (all team members working together within the same physical space) and utilization of techniques such as joint treatment planning, shared records, joint patient sessions, and case conferencing to enhance communication and collaboration. Integrated care models can improve outcomes of substance use, medical, and mental health conditions and improve quality of care for those with both SMI and SUD. For example, research shows that patients who received services in behavioral health–based integrated care programs experienced increased primary care visits, improved attainment of performance measures related to metabolic and cardiovascular risk, and reduced emergency department use (Pirraglia et al. 2012).

Further specific adaptations of the integrated care model result in better outcomes during delivery of care for a population with SMI and co-occurring substance use. One adaptation is assertive outreach and engagement, including visits in the home and community, which are the cornerstones to enhanced engagement in treatment in a population where retention is low (Drake et al. 2001). Another effective adaptation involves modifying interventions to fit this specific population—for example, incorporating social skills training that may facilitate prosocial relationship building, which is necessary for recovery as well as for avoiding situations that may present a risk for relapse. Furthermore, substance use treatment may need to be tailored for cognitive deficits, negative symptoms, and a greater need for support, which may be needed to treat individuals with both SMI and SUDs. Studies incorporating adaptations of integrated treatment of SMI and SUDs have demonstrated multiple positive outcomes in spheres such as psychiatric symptoms, substance use, hospitalization, arrests, and quality of life (Drake et al. 1998).

Psychiatrists play a critical role on integrated care teams. A study surveying 52 psychiatrists working in integrated care programs in diverse practice settings found that being on an integrated care team enhanced their ability to effectively engage and treat more patients (Norfleet et al. 2016). The American Psychiatric Association (APA) is in full support of this approach to care and has fully endorsed the collaborative care model (Vanderlip et al. 2016), which is a type of integrated care model. The collaborative care model uses a team-based, interdisciplinary approach to screen, diagnose, treat, and provide follow-up care to an identified patient population. In the collaborative care model, a primary care practice establishes a disorder-specific registry of patients within the practice. For example, this registry may include adults who have been identified as having a co-occurring disorder who are not improving under routine primary care. A behavioral health care manager within the primary care practice coordinates screenings, evaluations, and follow-up calls for each patient on the registry. In addition, the behavioral health care manager also meets weekly (in person or by telephone) with a consulting psychiatrist to discuss the patients' progress and explore whether other interventions such as changes in medications need to be recommended. The consulting psychiatrist rarely, if ever, sees a patient, but instead reviews charts and registry data, looks at progress, and makes recommendations to the PCP through the behavioral health care manager. This type of model and service delivery has been associated with lowered costs, improved access, improved clinical outcomes, and increased patient satisfaction (Ward et al. 2016). Specifically having a psychiatrist as part of the care team has been found to be an essential element of the model, impacting outcomes (Vanderlip et al. 2016). The APA strongly promotes the collaborative care model and encourages psychiatrists and organizations to utilize its core principles in practice.

One example of an effective integrated, wraparound co-occurring disorders care model is Maintaining Independence and Sobriety through Systems Integration, Outreach, and Networking (MISSION) (Smelson et al. 2019). MISSION integrates coordinated co-occurring disorders treatment, case management, peer support, and other wraparound recovery supports, such as vocational and housing supports. MISSION services are delivered by a care team, including a CM and PSS, and have been found to reduce psychiatric and substance use symptoms, hospitalizations, and incarceration (Smelson et al. 2019). A recent adaptation of MISSION expanded the care team to include a nurse as well as coordination with and connection to a patient-centered medical home (PCMH). A pilot study of this expanded MISSION care team found that from program intake to discharge, individuals experienced fewer mental health and SUD symptoms and had significant reductions in medical problems and utilization of emergency department services for physical problems. More research is currently under way using an expanded MISSION care team.

Case Vignette 2

Client background: The client is a 66-year-old male veteran who is currently experiencing homelessness, with a history of schizophrenia, chronic lymphocytic leukemia, cardiac disease, and diabetes and who is showing early-onset symptoms of dementia. The client has been known to the PCMH for almost 20 years. Although "known," he is very difficult to engage in care because of his dementia symptoms and suspicion of medical personnel. Many years ago, the client developed a trusting relationship with a PCP at the PCMH, but when the PCP left the organization some years later, the client was lost to PCMH follow-up.

Brief description of interventions: The MISSION psychiatrist, case manager (CM), and peer support specialist (PSS) work closely to develop a plan for engaging the client in care that may lead to a safe-housing opportunity and engagement in medical and psychiatric care. The PSS begins with weekly shelter visits and is able to build a trusting relationship with the client. At this point, a new PCP and medical case manager from the PCMH start to accompany the PSS into the shelter to establish medical care with the client and begin building a relationship via assertive outreach. However, the client is not open to psychiatric treatment.

The PSS, CM, and primary care team consult with the MISSION psychiatrist around methods to best engage and support this client, given that paranoia resulting from his schizophrenia as well as memory impairment is an obstacle to engagement. The psychiatrist also provides consultation to the PCP around appropriate medications for treatment of the client's schizophrenia.

Because the client is a veteran, the CM and PSS start to work with the U.S. Department of Veterans Affairs (VA) to obtain indicated documents for housing, although he is not eligible for VA services. Over a 10-month period, the PSS accompanies the client to follow-up with hematology, cardiology, podiatry, and oncology, as well as housing- and benefits-related appointments. The PSS also communicates weekly with clinic staff at the shelter to make sure the client is receiving medical care as needed. As the client accepts antipsychotic medication from his PCP, his suspiciousness decreases and he is able to receive treatment from the MISSION psychiatrist, as well as individual therapy.

Visiting nurse and other referrals are put in place by the PSS in anticipation of housing. Appropriate housing types are discussed in a case conference between the primary care team at the PCMH and the MISSION team. Ten months into the client's enrollment in MISSION, he is hospitalized for a life-threatening infection, followed by several months in a nursing home for rehabilitation. The PCMH team and MISSION team collaborate to ensure preservation of the client's housing, and assist him with managing his finances, while also providing his inpatient teams with support, consultation, and collateral information to ensure that his medical and psychiatric care are not disrupted through multiple transitions. The client is able to obtain safe housing, to continue to recuperate with appropriate supports, and to continue to increase his level of functioning toward independence.

Psychiatrists in Private Practice

Approximately 50% of psychiatrists in the United States work in private practice (Staff Care 2015); therefore, many psychiatrists are not working in organizations and systems that utilize the collaborative care model. This leads many to question if there is a role for the private practitioner in integrated care practice. The answer is a resounding yes! There are two avenues for inclusion of the private practitioner in integrated care practice. The first avenue is for the private practitioner to work part-time as a consulting psychiatrist in the integrated models described above. The second avenue is to bring the principles of integration into the private practice model, taking a holistic approach in assessing SMI, SUD, medical domains, social determinants, and wraparound support needs of patients. This integration is critical, because each of these factors has been found to be related to treatment engagement and outcomes. Within this holistic view, if the patient or provider identifies unmet needs in any areas, such as housing, the psychiatrist will first make referrals for appropriate supports. After the referrals have been made, the psychiatrist will follow up with the patient to assess engagement with the referrals and coordinate care with the provider. To be sure they are addressing these needs, psychiatrists in a private practice setting can track outcomes using registries, as in the collaborative care model, to ensure that patients are recovering, and reevaluate those who are not progressing.

Another principle of integration is communication, in which developing a reliable system to communicate patients' clinical and treatment status to their other providers is key. This includes a practice of identifying and obtaining releases of information for a patient's providers and routinely contacting them. For example, a psychiatrist may see a patient in private practice who is presenting with bipolar disorder, alcohol use disorder, and peptic ulcer disease. The psychiatrist treats the mental illness and substance use using motivational enhancement along with medications to stabilize mood and reduce alcohol cravings, while a psychologist provides cognitive-behavioral therapy to address the co-occurring disorders, and a medical provider treats the peptic ulcer disease. At intake, the psychiatrist will have the patient sign a release of information to allow contact with the other providers. At each subsequent visit, the psychiatrist will confirm care providers for the patient, and the patient will also complete brief measurement tools assessing mood symptoms and substance use. Results from this tool are then integrated into the visit, as well as recorded in the registry and compared with prior registry data, to inform potential adjustments to the treatment plan and coordination of care. After each visit, if needed, rapid communication with the patient's other providers is made, providing a brief synopsis of issues, the psychiatric care plan, and suggestions regarding coordination of care.

At present, these contacts between private practice psychiatrists and other providers are rare, because there is no reimbursement or policy mandate for this communication, and electronic medical records extremely rarely interface to facilitate this exchange. These challenges reflect the reality that health care is only gradually catching up to the need for collaboration among providers, with ongoing reforms of the Patient Protection and Affordable Care Act to include billing codes for psychiatric collaborative care management, and provision of enhanced care coordination services in accountable care organizations (Press et al. 2012). Although the current care environment presents challenges, and these steps do not approximate the level of comprehensive integration outlined in the collaborative care model, they move the private practice psychiatrist one step closer to providing more integrated care that could enhance patient outcomes.

Case Vignette 3

Client background: The client is a 59-year-old man who is disabled from a work-related back injury, complicated by rheumatoid arthritis. The client has a history of depression and is nearly homebound because of panic disorder. He has just begun seeing a psychiatrist and therapist who work together in a private practice, but stopped seeing his PCP 2 years ago after his

PCP discontinued opioid treatment for pain because of the client's illicit benzodiazepine use. The client is now struggling with use of both illicit opioids and illicit benzodiazepines.

Brief description of interventions: The psychiatrist identifies the client's avoidance of anxiety-inducing situations; lack of coping skills for difficult emotions, complicated by intermittent opioid and benzodiazepine withdrawal; and untreated chronic pain as all contributing to the client's depressed mood and panic attacks. Anxiety and low mood improve somewhat after appropriate medications, as well as cognitive-behavioral therapy and exposure therapy, are started.

As the client's alliance with his psychiatrist strengthens, the client accepts referral to an external office-based addictions treatment program, where he receives medication-assisted treatment with buprenorphine/naloxone for his opioid use disorder, and engages in group therapy and monitoring with toxicology screening. The support and structure of this treatment enable the client to gradually cease illicit opioid and benzodiazepine use, improving both his mood and his panic symptoms. Additionally, the reduction in pain through buprenorphine treatment improves his mobility and decreases his depressive symptoms.

After approximately 6 months of OBAT participation, the client accepts referral back to primary care at a different practice. With primary care, his rheumatoid arthritis is treated, and his mobility and pain improve further. The client completes releases allowing for collaboration between his three treatment teams—psychiatric, medical, and addictions.

The client demonstrates improved management of medical problems and reduced mental health and SUD symptoms.

Key Points

- Individuals with comorbid serious mental illness (SMI), substance use, and medical conditions are a high-risk group.

- Most medical comorbidity that these individuals experience is preventable.

- Psychiatrists, including private practice providers, are uniquely positioned to improve access, quality of care, and patient outcomes via the utilization of integrated models of care and principles.

- To enhance the utilization of integrated models of care, national effort is needed in three areas:
  - **Education and training:** Graduate and medical programs should ensure that trainees develop core competencies in working with patients with co-occurring SMI, substance use disorders, and physical illness.

- **Organizational and systems change:** Organizational and cultural shifts driven by strong leadership, integration of consumer feedback, and continuous performance improvement are needed to create and sustain change.

- **Policy:** Efforts toward education and training and organizational and systems change cannot occur without the support of policy. For example, Medicaid policy changes can have a significant impact on standardizing and implementing integrated models of care. Changing Medicaid policy to mandate all aspects of integrated care, including reimbursement mandates to allow for coverage of all components of integrated care (e.g.,care coordination between private practice psychiatrists and other providers), and provision of "whole person–centered" care, may increase access to treatment and reduce costs and mortality.

References

Adams MW: Comorbidity of mental health and substance misuse problems: a review of workers' reported attitudes and perceptions. J Psychiatr Ment Health Nurs 15(2):101–108, 2008

Avery J, Dixon L, Adler D, et al: Psychiatrists' attitudes toward individuals with substance use disorders and serious mental illness. J Dual Diagn 9(4):322–326, 2013

Bahorik AL, Satre DD, Kline-Simon AH, et al: Serious mental illness and medical comorbidities: findings from an integrated health care system. J Psychosom Res 100:35–45, 2017

Black PH: The inflammatory consequences of psychologic stress: relationship to insulin resistance, obesity, atherosclerosis and diabetes mellitus, type II. Med Hypotheses 67(4):879–891, 2006

Blanco C, Hasin DS, Wall MM, et al: Cannabis use and risk of psychiatric disorders: prospective evidence from a US national longitudinal study. JAMA Psychiatry 73(4):388–395, 2016

Brunette MF, Borodovsky JR, Myers M, et al: Important questions about the impact of medical marijuana on people with serious mental illness. Psychiatr Serv 69(11):1181–1183, 2018

Campbell CI, Bahorik AL, VanVeldhuisen P, et al: Use of a prescription opioid registry to examine opioid misuse and overdose in an integrated health system. Prev Med 110:31–37, 2018

Chang CK, Hayes RD, Perera G, et al: Life expectancy at birth for people with serious mental illness and other major disorders from a secondary mental health care case register in London. PLoS One 6(5):e19590, 2011

Charlson FJ, Baxter AJ, Dua T, et al: Excess mortality from mental, neurological, and substance use disorders in the Global Burden of Disease Study 2010, in Mental, Neurological, and Substance Use Disorders: Disease Control Priorities, 3rd Edition, Vol 4. Washington, DC, The International Bank for Reconstruction and Development/The World Bank, 2016. Available at: www.ncbi.nlm.nih.gov/books/NBK361935. Accessed June 22, 2020.

Correll CU, Solmi M, Veronese N, et al: Prevalence, incidence and mortality from cardiovascular disease in patients with pooled and specific severe mental illness: a large-scale meta-analysis of 3,211,768 patients and 113,383,368 controls. World Psychiatry 16(2):163–180, 2017

De Hert M, Cohen D, Bobes J, et al: Physical illness in patients with severe mental disorders, II: barriers to care, monitoring and treatment guidelines, plus recommendations at the system and individual level. World Psychiatry 10(2):138–151, 2011

de Similien RH: Accounting for the social determinants in psychiatric care delivery. Am J Psychiatry Resid J 12(6):11–13, 2017

Drake RE, McHugo GJ, Clark RE, et al: Assertive community treatment for patients with co-occurring severe mental illness and substance use disorder: a clinical trial. Am J Orthopsychiatry 68(2):201–215, 1998

Drake RE, Goldman HH, Leff HS, et al: Implementing evidence-based practices in routine mental health service settings. Psychiatr Serv 52(2):179–182, 2001

Edwards JN, Lyon KV, Montanez J, et al: Financing and Policy Considerations for Medicaid Health Homes for Individuals With Behavioral Health Conditions: A Discussion of Selected States' Approaches. Rockville, MD, Substance Abuse and Mental Health Services Administration–HRSA Center for Integrated Health Solutions, 2013

Hartz SM, Pato CN, Medeiros H, et al: Comorbidity of severe psychotic disorders with measures of substance use. JAMA Psychiatry 71(3):248–254, 2014

Hsien-Yen C, Kharrazi H, Bodycombe D, et al: Healthcare costs and utilization associated with high-risk prescription opioid use: a retrospective cohort study. BMC Med 16(1):69–80, 2018

Hughes E, Bassi S, Gilbody S, et al: Prevalence of HIV, hepatitis B, and hepatitis C in people with severe mental illness: a systematic review and meta-analysis. Lancet Psychiatry 3(1):40–48, 2016

Ilyas A, Chesney E, Patel R: Improving life expectancy in people with serious mental illness: should we place more emphasis on primary prevention? Br J Psychiatry 211(4):194–197, 2017

Jones CM, McCance-Katz EF: Co-occurring substance use and mental disorders among adults with opioid use disorder. Drug Alcohol Depend 197:78–82, 2019

Kiecolt-Glaser JK, Glaser R: Depression and immune function: central pathways to morbidity and mortality. J Psychosom Res 53(4):873–876, 2002

Levinson Miller CL, Druss BG, Dombrowski EA, et al: Barriers to primary medical care among patients at a community mental health center. Psychiatr Serv 54(8):1158–1160, 2003

Lucaciu LA, Dumitrascu DL: Depression and suicide ideation in chronic hepatitis C patients untreated and treated with interferon: prevalence, prevention, and treatment. Ann Gastroenterol 28(4):440–447, 2015

McCauley JL, Killeen T, Gros DF, et al: Posttraumatic stress disorder and co-occurring substance use disorders: advances in assessment and treatment. Clin Psychol (New York) 19(3):1–27, 2010

Muench J, Hamer AM: Adverse effects of antipsychotic medications. Am Fam Physician 81(5):617–622, 2010

Muvvala SB, Edens EL, Petrakis IL: What role should psychiatrists have in responding to the opioid epidemic? JAMA Psychiatry 76(2):107–108, 2019

Norfleet KR, Ratzliff ADH, Chan YF, et al: The role of the integrated care psychiatrist in community settings: a survey of psychiatrists' perspectives. Psychiatr Serv 67(3):346–349, 2016

Parry CD, Blank MB, Pithey AL: Responding to the threat of HIV among persons with mental illness and substance abuse. Curr Opin Psychiatry 20(3):235–241, 2007

Peek CJ; National Integration Academy Council: Lexicon for Behavioral Health and Primary Care Integration: Concepts and Definitions Developed by Expert Consensus (AHRQ Publ No 13-IP001-EF). Rockville, MD, Agency for Healthcare Research and Quality, 2013. Available at: www.innovations.ahrq.gov/quality-tools/lexicon-behavioral-health-and-primary-care-integration-concepts-and-definitions. Accessed June 22, 2020.

Penninx BWJH, Lange SMM: Metabolic syndrome in psychiatric patients: overview, mechanisms, and implications. Dialogues Clin Neurosci 20(1):63–73, 2018

Pirraglia PA, Rowland E, Wu WC, et al: Benefits of a primary care clinic co-located and integrated in a mental health setting for veterans with serious mental illness. Prev Chronic Dis 9:E51, 2012

Press MJ, Michelow MD, MacPhail LH: Care coordination in accountable care organizations: moving beyond structure and incentives. Am J Manag Care 18(12):778–780, 2012

Priester MA, Browne T, Iachini A, et al: Treatment access barriers and disparities among individuals with co-occurring mental health and substance use disorders: an integrative literature review. J Subst Abuse Treat 61:47–59, 2016

Prince JD: Correlates of opioid use disorders among people with severe mental illness in the United States. Subst Use Misuse 54(6):1024–1034, 2019

Razanno LA, Cook JA, Yost C, et al: Factors associated with co-occurring medical conditions among adults with serious mental disorders. Schizophr Res 161(2–3):458–464, 2015

Richmond L: Patients with serious mental illness need better primary care integration, health advocacy. December 26, 2017. Available at: https://psychnews.psychiatryonline.org/doi/full/10.1176/appi.pn.2018.1a21. Accessed June 22, 2020.

Roshanaei-Moghaddam B, Kanton W: Premature mortality from general medical illnesses among persons with bipolar disorder: a review. Psychiatr Serv 60(2):147–156, 2009

Sapag JC, Sena BF, Bustamante IV, et al: Stigma towards mental illness and substance use issues in primary health care: challenges and opportunities for Latin America. Glob Public Health 13(10):1468–1480, 2018

Sarkar D, Jung MK, Wang HJ: Alcohol and the immune system. Alcohol Res 37(2):153–155, 2015

Saxena S, Maj M: Physical health of people with severe mental disorders: leave no one behind. World Psychiatry 16(1):1–2, 2017

Sederer LI: The social determinants of mental health. Psychiatr Serv 67(2):234–235, 2016

Smelson D, Farquhar I, Fisher W, et al: Integrating a co-occurring disorders intervention in drug courts: an open pilot trial. Community Ment Health J 55(2):222–231, 2019

Staff Care: Psychiatry: "the silent shortage." 2015. Available at: www.staffcare.com/uploadedFiles/psychiatry-shortage-mental-health-white-paper.pdf. Accessed June 22, 2020.

Substance Abuse and Mental Health Services Administration: Mental health and substance abuse services in Medicaid, 2003: charts and state tables. (DHHS Publ No SMA 10-4590). Rockville, MD, Center for Mental Health Services, Substance Abuse and Mental Health Services Administration, 2010

Substance Abuse and Mental Health Services Administration: Key Substance Use and Mental Health Indicators in the United States: Results From the 2017 National Survey on Drug Use and Health (HHS Publ No SMA-18-5068, NSDUH Series H-53). Rockville, MD, Center for Behavioral Health Statistics and Quality, Substance Abuse and Mental Health Services Administration, 2018

Vancampfort D, Stubbs B, Mitchell AJ, et al: Risk of metabolic syndrome and its components in people with schizophrenia and related psychotic disorders, bipolar disorder and major depressive disorder: a systematic review and meta-analysis. World Psychiatry 14(3):339–347, 2015

Vanderlip ER, Rundell J, Avery M, et al: Dissemination of integrated care within adult primary care settings: the collaborative care model. Report on dissemination of integrated care. American Psychiatric Association and Academy of Psychosomatic Medicine, 2016. Available at: www.psychiatry.org/File%20Library/Psychiatrists/Practice/Professional-Topics/Integrated-Care/APA-APM-Dissemination-Integrated-Care-Report.pdf. Accessed June 22, 2020.

Wainberg M, Dixon L: Ending HIV, hepatitis B, and hepatitis C: what about people with severe mental illness? Lancet Psychiatry 4(9):651–653, 2017

Walker ER, McGee RE, Druss BG: Mortality in mental disorders and global disease burden implications: a systematic review and meta-analysis. JAMA Psychiatry 72(4):334–341, 2015

Ward MC, Miller BF, Marconi VC, et al: The role of behavioral health in optimizing care for complex patients in the primary care setting. J Gen Intern Med 31(3):265–267, 2016

CHAPTER 4

Health Service Disparities

Janis Sayer, Ph.D.
Susan A. Pickett, Ph.D.

People with serious mental illness (SMI) die decades earlier than same-age peers, partly because of disparities in the access, utilization, and quality of health services. Although health service disparities have been documented for decades, little progress has been made in closing the disparity gap between persons with SMI and the general population. Multiple factors contribute to health service differences, including insufficient organization and financing of health care resources, provider bias and training, symptoms and consequences of mental illness, and socioeconomic barriers. These disparities may be worsened depending on factors such as race/ethnicity, socioeconomic status, neighborhood conditions, homelessness, and criminal justice involvement. We begin this chapter with a discussion of the types of health service disparities experienced by persons with SMI, and the magnitude of the problem. We then focus on factors contributing to health service disparities. The chapter concludes with a case vignette exemplifying the health care disparities experienced by persons with SMI.

Access to Care

Many persons with SMI lack access to health care. Access to health care is defined as "the timely use of personal health services to achieve the best health outcomes" (Institute of Medicine 1993, p. 33). This includes gaining access to the health care system, receipt of services at the time they are needed, and availability of qualified health care providers. Although care varies by personal characteristics, insurer, and setting, available evidence indicates that persons with SMI are burdened by disparities in access to health services.

Health Care Coverage

Health insurance reduces cost-based barriers to care. Persons without insurance are less likely to obtain medical care for health problems and are less likely to receive care to prevent health problems from occurring (Kaiser Family Foundation 2018). They are also less likely to receive recommended services for injuries and health conditions and obtain prescription medications (Kaiser Family Foundation 2018). Although the Patient Protection and Affordable Care Act (ACA) increased access to health insurance coverage for persons with SMI (Sherrill and Gonzales 2017), there are still disparities in insurance coverage between persons with and without SMI, with a higher proportion of persons with mental illness uninsured compared with those without (Kaiser Family Foundation 2017). Medicaid beneficiaries are more likely to have a mental illness than individuals with private insurance. In 2015, Medicaid covered 26% of adults with SMI and 21% of adults with mental illness (Kaiser Family Foundation 2017). Persons with SMI who have Medicaid report better access to care than those without insurance, and they are more likely to have a usual source of care and to be able to obtain needed services (Kaiser Family Foundation 2012).

Obtaining Care

Studies have shown differences in access to medical care for persons with SMI depending on study population and setting. Research suggests that persons with psychotic disorders and bipolar disorder are less likely to have a primary care provider than are persons who do not have a mental illness (Bradford et al. 2008). Persons with a psychotic, bipolar, or major depressive disorder are significantly more likely to report difficulties accessing medical care, including needing medical care but being unable to obtain it, needing a prescription but being unable to obtain it, and delaying medical care because of concerns about cost (Bradford et al. 2008). Disappointingly, recent data from the National Health Interview Survey demonstrate that among persons with "severe mental illness," the ACA has not increased the percentage of persons with a usual source of care or decreased the percentage of persons who delay getting medical care (Sherrill and Gonzales 2017).

Persons with SMI are more likely than the general population to use hospital and emergency department (ED) services to address concerns related to primary care (Bergamo et al. 2016). Persons who are homeless and have both a mental illness and substance use disorder are at a particularly high risk (Lin et al. 2015). In a study of adults with SMI who were chronically homeless, a lack of health insurance during the previous year was the strongest predictor of using an ED as a regular source of medical care (Chwastiak et al. 2012). However, homeless Medicaid beneficiaries with mental health and substance use disorders still have high rates of hospital and ED use (Lin et al. 2015).

The Agency for Healthcare Research and Quality (AHRQ) has developed Prevention Quality Indicators, or PQIs, composed of 16 ambulatory care–sensitive conditions (ACSCs) for which "good outpatient care can potentially prevent the need for hospitalization, or for which early intervention can prevent complications or more severe disease" (Agency for Healthcare Research and Quality 2001, pp. 20–21). These conditions include hypertension, dehydration, adult asthma, and uncontrolled diabetes (Agency for Healthcare Research and Quality 2001). Research examining factors associated with increased rates of hospitalization for ACSCs among persons with mental illness has shown that poverty and system factors (e.g., health care provider shortages) increase rates of potentially preventable hospitalizations. For example, a study conducted in California uncovered increased rates of preventable hospitalizations among persons with mental disorders and substance use disorders that were associated with geographies with higher rates of poverty, higher rates of primary care safety net use, and fewer mental health providers (Schmidt et al. 2018). Variation in odds of potentially preventable hospitalizations for persons with mental illness has been found by mental health diagnosis, age, race, insurance status, and geographic income level. A study using Texas administrative data showed that a diagnosis of almost any mental disorder (with the exception of posttraumatic stress disorder) increased the odds of having a preventable hospitalization diagnosis. Bipolar disorder and schizophrenia were associated with increased odds of most types of preventable hospitalizations. Additional factors that were associated with preventable hospitalizations were being older, being Black, being uninsured or dual-eligible for Medicare and Medicaid, and living in a low-income area (Medford-Davis et al. 2018).

Medical Screening Tests

Medical screening tests are conducted to identify health conditions early. With early detection, lifestyle changes and/or treatments can potentially address medical problems soon enough to treat them most effectively. Research demonstrates that persons with SMI do not get screened for many common conditions as often as they should. Screening and monitoring for metabolic syndrome are important for some persons with SMI. *Metabolic syndrome* refers to the diagnosis of three of five risk factors—abdominal obesity, high triglyceride levels, low high-density lipoprotein cholesterol level, high blood pressure, and high fasting blood sugar—that increase the likelihood for heart disease, diabetes, and stroke. Screening and monitoring are critical because some second-generation antipsychotic medications increase the risk for metabolic syndrome (Chaplain and Taylor 2014), and further, cardiovascular disease is a leading cause of death among persons with SMI (Walker et al. 2015). About 40% of persons with SMI have metabolic syndrome (Newcomer 2007).

The American Psychiatric Association, American Diabetes Association, American Association of Clinical Endocrinologists, and North American Association for the Study of Obesity (American Diabetes Association et al. 2004) recommend baseline metabolic screening and monitoring for persons taking second-generation antipsychotic medications. This includes initial screening of body mass index (BMI), waist circumference, blood pressure, fasting blood glucose, and fasting lipids. According to guidelines, following initiation of medications, BMI should be monitored every 3 months, waist circumference should be monitored annually, and fasting lipids should be monitored at least every 5 years. However, it is estimated that as many as 70% of persons taking antipsychotic medications are not screened for metabolic syndrome (Mangurian et al. 2016). For example, in a study of New York State Medicaid beneficiaries taking second-generation antipsychotic medications, 60% of individuals taking these medications with at least a moderate risk of metabolic abnormalities had not received such monitoring in the past year (Essock et al. 2009).

Studies looking specifically at rates of screening for cardiovascular disease risk factors for persons with SMI have shown varying rates of screening depending on population and setting. A review of screening rates for persons with schizophrenia or bipolar disorder receiving services in the United States showed wide ranges for diabetes (8%–75%) and cholesterol (8%–85%), with a narrower range of rates of screening for high blood pressure (79%–88%) (Baller et al. 2015).

There is evidence that persons with SMI have inadequate rates of screening for some cancers, with most studies examining breast and cervical cancer screening in women (Xiang 2015). Comparisons of respondents to the

Household Component of the Medical Expenditure Panel Survey demonstrated that women with serious psychological distress had significantly lower odds of getting screened for breast cancer and cervical cancer than did women without serious psychological distress. This included lower rates of clinical breast exam (67.56% compared with 81.93%), mammography (59.94% vs. 75.56%), and Pap tests (72.27% vs. 85.37%) among persons with serious psychological distress (Xiang 2015). All in all, women with serious psychological distress were 40% less likely to be current on their mammogram, breast exam, and Pap smear, after adjustment for demographic characteristics, health insurance, health behaviors, comorbidity, and service utilization, than were other women (Xiang 2015).

Persons with SMI are at higher risk for blood-borne viral infections such as HIV, hepatitis B, and hepatitis C. The risk is exacerbated by multiple factors, including those related to low socioeconomic status, substance use disorders, and psychiatric symptoms and factors (Hughes et al. 2016). Despite these risks, persons with SMI have low rates of screening for these diseases. In a study utilizing California Medicaid data, 4.7% of persons with SMI receiving care at community health mental health centers were screened for hepatitis C between October 2010 and September 2011, as compared with 12.7% in the general U.S. population (Trager et al. 2016). Mangurian et al. (2017) found that only 6.7% of this group received testing for HIV.

Persons with SMI have increased odds of dental decay compared with the general population (Kisely et al. 2018). However, persons with schizophrenia and others with psychiatric disorders have been shown to have low rates of oral health screening. Some research finds that only about one-third of patients with schizophrenia have seen a dentist within the last 3 years (De Hert et al. 2011).

Standard of Care and Quality Treatments

Research on receipt of quality treatment for persons with SMI shows mixed results. McGinty et al. (2015) reviewed the literature published between 2000 and 2013 on quality of care for persons with SMI who were being treated for cardiovascular disease, diabetes, dyslipidemia, and HIV/AIDS. Differing results were found in studies comparing quality of care for cardiovascular disease, cardiovascular risk factors, and HIV/AIDS for persons with and without SMI (McGinty et al. 2015). For example, among studies comparing quality-of-care measures for inpatient treatment of acute myocardial infarction, guideline adherence related to catherization, thrombolytic therapy, coronary artery bypass grafting, and angioplasty was less likely for persons with SMI as compared with the general population samples, while some studies showed no difference (McGinty et al. 2012; Petersen et al. 2003). Examinations of adherence to guidelines for treatment with beta-blocker medications also showed disparate results, with persons with SMI faring worse than those in the general population in some studies but with no differences noted in other studies (Petersen et al. 2003). Rates of adherence to national guidelines for hospital treatment of acute myocardial infarction, outpatient care and treatment of diabetes, treatment of dyslipidemia, and treatment of HIV/AIDS were lowest for persons insured by Medicaid and highest for veterans (McGinty et al. 2015).

A review and meta-analysis of 61, primarily U.S., studies that compared prescription rates for persons with and without mental illness demonstrated that persons with mental illness receive differential care (Mitchell et al. 2012). Persons with mental illness have lower odds of receiving a prescription for a condition when medically indicated. This includes medications for high cholesterol, beta-blockers, antiplatelet agents, anticoagulants, hypertension medications, and hormone replacement therapy for osteoporosis (hormone replacement therapy is no longer prescribed for osteoporosis) (Mitchell et al. 2012).

Quality Facilities

Persons with SMI are less likely than persons without SMI to be admitted to high-quality nursing homes (Temkin-Greener et al. 2018). With a sample of over 3.7 million admissions to more than 15,000 nursing homes across the country from 2012 to 2014, persons with SMI were more likely to be admitted to a nursing home with a lower staffing-quality rating than persons without a mental health diagnosis (Temkin-Greener et al. 2018). In an earlier study of 1.3 million nationwide nursing home admissions in 2007, a diagnosis of either schizophrenia or bipolar disorder was independently correlated with admission to a nursing home with greater total and health-related deficiencies as found by citations through government inspections (Li et al. 2011).

Psychiatrists can address health care access in their practice. First, psychiatrists must be attentive to the breadth of patients' health needs. Psychiatrists can conduct brief assessments to understand patient access to care, including screening and treatment. When health care coverage, primary care, specialty care, or other services are needed, psychiatrists should prioritize referrals to ensure patients have their needs met.

Factors Contributing to Health Service Disparities

Many different factors are associated with health service disparities among persons with SMI. Factors are categorized into three main groups: system-level, provider-level, and individual-level factors. Social determinants of health are further factors in undermining access to care.

System-Level Factors

Quality care involves ensuring access to care: services are timely, delivered without necessary delay, and affordable. Care coordination—providing recommended, evidence-based treatment across settings and systems—is an essential part of such care. Yet people with SMI routinely experience problems accessing affordable care and report receiving uncoordinated, substandard medical treatment. System-level factors such as health care delivery and coordination, organizational characteristics, and financing play a role in this poor-quality care.

Studies suggest that people with SMI report high levels of disappointment and frustration with their access to primary care and care coordination (Kaufman et al. 2012). Compared with the general population, people with SMI experience greater problems finding and obtaining services and are less likely to receive appropriate follow-up care (Bradford et al. 2008). Once they do receive treatment, the complexity of their physical and mental health problems means that they must seek treatment from various clinics and providers (e.g., help for their diabetes at a primary care clinic, help for their depression at a mental health center). Typically, there is little collaboration or coordination between these health care entities, resulting in fragmented and ineffective care.

Although the ACA and other policies have made great strides in integrating primary care and mental health services, primary care and behavioral health services largely continue to exist in completely separate systems (and facilities). Within these fragmented systems, organizations focus on their own area of expertise: primary care organizations and physicians only address physical health care needs, and mental health care organizations and mental health providers only address psychiatric symptoms (Pickett et al. 2015). Providers who do work in integrated care systems may rarely meet in person and may be hampered by limited information-sharing systems—that is, electronic health records that do not "talk" to one another and prohibit sharing of critical clinical data. The lack of communication and collaboration across systems and providers means that many people with SMI must try to navigate and coordinate care on their own. In a recent study of the health care needs of people with SMI, one project participant explained what it was like trying to navigate an uncoordinated system of care: "I go here, I go there, nobody has all my records, and the doctors all tell me different things. It's exhausting and I just don't know what to do" (Corrigan et al. 2017).

As an example, fragmentation of care is at play in low rates of metabolic screening. In a survey of primary care providers working in an urban safety net system, providers reported that difficulty collaborating with psychiatrists, difficulty arranging referral for psychiatric follow-up, and lack of access to qualified psychiatric follow-up were among the barriers to conducting metabolic screening and treatment (Mangurian et al. 2013). In a similar survey, Parameswaran et al. (2013) surveyed psychiatrists working in one of two urban areas and found that although most psychiatrists believe that they should conduct metabolic screening, they do not think they should prescribe medications for metabolic abnormalities. In addition, psychiatrists identified that difficulty arranging for referral for medical follow-up, wait times for medical follow-up, and difficulty collaborating with physicians providing medical follow-up are barriers to metabolic screening and monitoring abnormalities (Parameswaran et al. 2013).

Financing—no or low investment in medical care for people with SMI—also contributes to health service disparities (Liu et al. 2017). The federal and state governments are major funders of mental health services, with state funding varying considerably based on each state's economic and political forces. Low investment is seen across all levels of government, with federal, state, and city governments consistently underfunding or slashing services for vulnerable populations, including people with SMI. Medicaid, the insurer of so many with SMI, has low reimbursement for care management, peer services, and other team-based interventions that are important for care (Druss et al. 2018). In other cases, quality health care systems are less accessible to persons with SMI. For example, lower-quality nursing facilities are heavily reimbursed by Medicaid, the insurer of a large proportion of persons with SMI (Temkin-Greener et al. 2018). Low investment can occur at the organizational level: organizations may lack the financial resources to expand or enhance services to meet the complex physical health needs of people with SMI; leadership may not consider providing primary care to people with SMI a priority for their organization (Hoge et al. 2013).

Provider-Level Factors

Mental illness stigma—a reaction to people with mental illness that includes stereotypes, prejudice, and discrimination—plays a critical role in health service disparities. Knaak and colleagues (2017) note that stigma, and health care providers' negative interactions with people with SMI, appear to be the norm, not the exception. Providers have reported experiencing patients with SMI as difficult or annoying and may blame patients for their illness (Welch et al. 2015). People with SMI report high levels of physician disrespect and discrimination (Boydell et al. 2012). This includes having their physical illnesses ignored or dismissed because providers attribute symptoms to their mental illness, being talked down to and threatened, and receiving little or no information about their physical health problem or treatment options because providers mistakenly assume that they lack the cognitive capability to understand and make health care decisions (Welch et al. 2015).

Providers' stigmatizing is rooted in several sources. Limited knowledge and training about etiology and course of mental illness may cause physicians to feel anxious or fearful about treating people with SMI. Stereotypes about specific disorders may negatively impact care. People with personality disorders are often labeled by physicians as difficult, manipulative, and unworthy of care (Knaak et al. 2015). Welch and colleagues (2015) found that physicians reported more negative attitudes about patients with schizophrenia with bizarre affect than about patients with schizophrenia with normal affect and patients with depression. Physicians also were less likely to trust patients with schizophrenia with bizarre affect as competent reporters and were more likely to alert their colleagues about these patients, shaping their colleagues' expectations about these patients before interactions took place. Doctors and nurses are less likely to diagnose a patient with SMI who complains about physical symptoms with a physical health problem than a person without SMI (Graber et al. 2000). Physician anxiety and stereotypes have been found to result in clinical avoidance (i.e., rejecting people with SMI or referring them elsewhere), less effective or appropriate treatment, and poorer health outcomes (Knaak et al. 2017).

Primary care doctors often underdiagnose or misdiagnose chronic medical conditions among people with SMI, and often falsely believe that people with SMI cannot achieve health and wellness goals. Knaak and Patten (2016) found that provider pessimism about mental health recovery was significantly associated with feelings of helplessness among providers: it is not worth treating people with SMI because they never get better. Negative beliefs about the ability of people with SMI to modify risky health behaviors or achieve and maintain a healthy lifestyle negatively affect providers' treatment decisions, such as decisions about referring people with SMI to specialty care (Corrigan et al. 2014).

Individual-Level Factors

Mental illness symptoms and treatment often have negative consequences on physical health. Cognitive and social deficits associated with SMI may make it difficult for some people with SMI to seek care and communicate with their providers. Persons with SMI may have difficulty obtaining care, as well as understanding the best course of treatment and adhering to treatment plans. Persons with SMI have higher rates of low health literacy (i.e., low ability to understand basic health information and make appropriate health care decisions) as compared with the general population (Clausen et al. 2015).

Prior negative experiences with health care providers may prevent people with SMI from seeking care. Interactions with providers who belittle them and dismiss their health concerns make many people with SMI reluctant to access and use physical health care services (Hoge et al. 2013).

Social Determinants of Health

Social determinants of health, including race/ethnicity, financial means, housing, and geography, also impact the physical health and well-being of people with SMI. People with SMI have higher rates of unemployment and poverty than the general population (Corrigan et al. 2014; Liu et al. 2017). Financial instability is highly correlated with morbidity and mortality. Living in poverty, people with SMI lack the means to pay for health care, and few qualify for insurance, including public entitlements, that would cover their care (Zur et al. 2017). Living in poverty also means that people with SMI are more likely to live in geographic areas with few or no health care resources.

In addition, people with SMI are at greater risk for homelessness, which worsens their physical health problems (LeBrun-Harris et al. 2013). Compared with the general population, homeless people have higher rates of heart, liver, and kidney disease; diabetes; hepatitis C; and cancer (LeBrun-Harris et al. 2013). Homeless people are less likely than the general population to have a regular source of care or receive routine preventive services (Hwang et al. 2013). They also often delay seeking help until a health problem becomes debilitating (Hwang et al. 2013; LeBrun-Harris et al. 2013). Studies suggest that death rates for homeless people are at least twice as high as those for their same-age, housed peers (Hwang et al. 2009).

Persons with SMI are at heightened risk for involvement with the criminal justice system (Anderson et al. 2015), and inadequate health care is common in jails and prisons (Dumont et al. 2012). In addition, incarceration disrupts Medicaid and may result in a gap in coverage upon release. Individuals may also have difficulty obtaining employment once they return to the community, adding additional challenges to health and health care access (Zur et al. 2017).

The impact of these social determinants of health may be even greater among people with SMI who are members of racial and ethnic minority groups. African Americans and Latinos are more likely than whites to be living in poverty (Semega et al. 2020). African Americans are also disproportionately more likely than whites to be homeless (Henry et al. 2020). People from minority groups are more likely to lack insurance and access to government safety services (Lee et al. 2012). The lack of health services in minority neighborhoods hinders access to care (Druss and Bornemann 2010). Compared with whites, African Americans have greater difficulty accessing care and receive less intensive treatment for a wide range of illnesses (Snowden 2012). African Americans with SMI are significantly more likely than their white counterparts to experience problems finding and obtaining services, and are less likely to receive follow-up care, increasing their morbidity and mortality risks. African Americans have poorer relationships with providers than do whites, reporting frustrating interactions with physicians who do not ask about or respond to their concerns, and fail to provide them with basic information about their medical condition (Moore et al. 2012). They report higher levels of physician disrespect and discrimination and feel that prescribed treatment does not meet their needs (Boydell et al. 2012).

Case Vignette

James is a 50-year-old African American man who lives on the West Side of Chicago. After graduating from high school, James worked for nearly 20 years as an accounting assistant at a large manufacturing company. He married, had two daughters, and owned his own home. At age 35, he began experiencing psychotic symptoms. James told his wife that the devil was after him, and he set fire to their home to "drive the devil out." He was hospitalized and diagnosed with paranoid schizophrenia. Although the antipsychotic medication prescribed to James in the hospital helped him manage his symptoms and return to work, the side effects caused him to gain a great deal of weight. He became diabetic and developed pain in his legs and feet. His physician's office was more than an hour away—high crime rates had long ago forced medical providers out of his neighborhood. The physician recommended that James get more exercise and take walks after work, but gang activity on his block made that a dangerous, impossible activity.

One year after his first psychiatric hospitalization, the manufacturing company was sold. James lost his job and with it his health insurance. He was unable to afford his medication and experienced another episode of psychosis. Frightened by his behavior, his wife and daughters left, leaving James alone in the house. As his symptoms worsened, he began wandering late at night through the neighborhood, shouting and shaking his fists at unseen demons. One of his neighbors called the police; James was taken to jail, held overnight, and released to the streets. Now homeless, he became increasingly psychotic. He wandered the streets for another 6 months, straying far from his neighborhood and eventually ending up in a homeless encampment in a park along Lake Michigan on the north side of Chicago.

Unlike in his West Side neighborhood, health care was more widely available in the neighborhood near the park: the hospital was located five blocks away, and several clinics were available throughout this upper middle class, predominantly white neighborhood. An outreach team from one of the mental health clinics associated with the hospital worked in the encampment. An outreach worker was eventually able to persuade James to go with her to the emergency room and be evaluated. James was hospitalized and discharged after a 2-week stay. He was given a 10-day supply of medication and instructions to follow up with a psychiatrist at the mental health clinic. James tried to make an appointment, but there was a 3-month waiting list for people without insurance to see the psychiatrist.

Two weeks after his medication ran out, James's psychotic symptoms returned. He could not adhere to the rules of the shelter he was staying at after leaving the hospital, and he became homeless again. For the next 2 years, James cycled in and out of hospitals and homelessness. His physical health deteriorated: his diabetes worsened, he developed open sores on his feet, and his legs began to swell, making it difficult to walk. James's mental health symptoms made him suspicious of others, and he frequently refused the help offered to him by outreach workers. Finally, during a subzero cold spell, he agreed to go to a city warming station. He was hospitalized for hypothermia; once stabilized, he was transferred to a state psychiatric facility due to lack of insurance. A social worker was able to secure housing and psychiatric care for James at a large behavioral health organization.

James moved into his apartment and began receiving intensive outpatient services from the mental health team. His apartment was located on the West Side, a few blocks from his old home. His caseworker helped enroll him in Medicaid. Once again, the antipsychotic medication he was prescribed caused him to gain weight, and his diabetes worsened. An old sore on his foot became infected. The caseworker took James to the emergency room; the doctors treated the infection and instructed him to see a podiatrist.

The mental health care agency that provided James's intensive outpatient services had recently begun working with a large primary care organization. In the past, the caseworker would have told James that because this was a medical and not a mental health problem, she would not be able to help him find a podiatrist. However, because of her agency's partnership with the primary care organization, she was able to make an appointment for James with one of the organization's physicians, who in turn referred James to a podiatrist. The podiatrist gave James a treatment plan, which James found complicated and difficult to understand. He asked the nurse if she could explain it to his caseworker. The nurse met with James and his caseworker, and together, they rewrote the treatment plan in easy-to-follow instructions. James was able to adhere to the treatment plan and his foot was soon completely healed.

The caseworker continues to help James manage his mental health symptoms, and he has not been hospitalized for nearly a year. When he recently began to experience shortness of breath and found it difficult to climb the stairs to his apartment, his caseworker made another appointment for him with the physician. The physician diagnosed emphysema. The caseworker and physician were able to work together to find and refer James to an apartment in a building with an elevator. James recently moved into that apartment. He now has monthly regular appointments with the physician to monitor both his diabetes and his emphysema. The physician and caseworker meet regularly to review James's overall health and ensure that both his medical and mental health issues are addressed. As James reported: "I have come a long way. I now feel confident that I can get help with both my mental health and medical problems—I don't have to choose which one to fix."

Key Points

- Health service disparities contribute to poor health outcomes among persons with serious mental illness (SMI).

- There is considerable evidence that persons with SMI have inadequate access to quality health care and are less likely to receive quality health care services.

- Persons with SMI are more likely to be uninsured than persons without SMI, decreasing the likelihood of obtaining health care. They are also less likely to have a primary care provider and are more likely to report that they needed care or a prescription and were unable to get it. Persons with SMI are more likely to use the hospital than are others, and have higher rates of being hospitalized for medical problems that are preventable.

- Persons with SMI are not screened frequently enough for metabolic syndrome, cardiovascular disease risk factors, some cancers, blood-borne infections, and oral health. They are not prescribed medications at the same rate as persons without SMI for a host of conditions, including high cholesterol and hypertension.

- System, provider, and individual factors contribute to health care disparities.

- Social determinants of health, including being African American or Latino, financial and housing instability, poor neighborhood conditions, unemployment, homelessness, and criminal justice involvement, further contribute to health care disparities among persons with SMI.
    - At the systems level, persons with SMI often have difficulty navigating fragmented care systems. Lack of adequate investment in health care services for persons with SMI also contributes to disparities.

- At the provider level, mental illness stigma gets in the way of the highest-quality care. Persons with mental illness often report feeling disrespected or discriminated against by health care providers. Providers may experience persons with SMI as difficult or may be inadequately trained to treat persons with SMI, leading to differential treatment. Indeed, providers are less likely to diagnose a physical health problem in a patient with SMI with physical health complaints than in other people. Chronic conditions are often misdiagnosed or underdiagnosed, with physicians believing that persons with SMI will not improve or will not carry out healthy behaviors.

- At the individual level, persons with SMI may have cognitive problems that interfere with their ability to seek care, communicate with health care providers, or follow treatment plans. Further, they may have had negative experiences with health care providers that hold them back from obtaining health care.

References

Agency for Healthcare Research and Quality: Guide to Prevention Quality Indicators: Hospital Admission for Ambulatory Care Sensitive Conditions. Rockville, MD, Agency for Healthcare Research and Quality, 2001, pp 20–21

American Diabetes Association, American Psychiatric Association, American Association of Clinical Endocrinologists, North American Association for the Study of Obesity: Consensus development conference on antipsychotic drugs and obesity and diabetes. Diabetes Care 27(2):596–601, 2004

Anderson A, Von Esenwein S, Spaulding A, et al: Involvement in the criminal justice system among attendees of an urban mental health center. Health Justice 3:4, 2015

Baller JB, McGinty EE, Azrin ST, et al: Screening for cardiovascular risk factors in adults with serious mental illness: a review of the evidence. BMC Psychiatry 15:55, 2015

Bergamo C, Juarez-Colunga E, Capp R: Association of mental health disorders and Medicaid with ED admissions for ambulatory care-sensitive conditions. Am J Emerg Med 34(5):820–824, 2016

Boydell J, Morgan C, Dutta R, et al: Satisfaction with inpatient treatment for first episode psychosis among different ethnic groups: a report from the UK AESOP study. Int J Soc Psychiatry 58(1):98–105, 2012

Bradford DW, Kim MM, Braxton LE, et al: Access to medical care among persons with psychotic and major affective disorders. Psychiatr Serv 59(8):847–852, 2008

Chaplain S, Taylor M: Drug points: second-generation antipsychotics. Prescriber 25(21):12–21, 2014

Chwastiak L, Tsai J, Rosenheck R: Impact of health insurance status and a diagnosis of serious mental illness on whether chronically homeless individuals engage in primary care. Am J Public Health 102(12):e83–e89, 2012

Clausen W, Watanabe-Galloway S, Baerentzen MB, et al: Health literacy among people with serious mental illness. Community Ment Health J 52(4):399–405, 2015

Corrigan PW, Pickett SA, Batia K, et al: Peer navigators and integrated care to address ethnic health disparities. Soc Work Public Health 29(6):581–593, 2014

Corrigan P, Pickett S, Stellon E, et al: Peer navigators to promote engagement of homeless African Americans with serious mental illness in primary care. Psychiatry Res 255:101–103, 2017

De Hert M, Correll CU, Bobes J, et al: Physical illness in patients with severe mental disorder, I: prevalence, impact of medications and disparities in health care. World Psychiatry 10(1):52–77, 2011

Druss BG, Bornemann TH: Improving health and health care for persons with serious mental illness: the window for US federal policy change. JAMA 303(19):1972–1973, 2010

Druss BG, Chwastiak L, Kern J, et al: Psychiatry's role in improving the physical health of patients with serious mental illness: a report from the American Psychiatric Association. Psychiatr Serv 69(3):254–256, 2018

Dumont DM, Brockmann B, Dickman S, et al: Public health and the epidemic of incarceration. Annu Rev Public Health 33:325–339, 2012

Essock SM, Covell NH, Leckman-Westin E, et al: Identifying clinically questionable psychotropic prescribing practices for Medicaid recipients in New York State. Psychiatr Serv 60(12):1595–1602, 2009

Graber MA, Bergus G, Dawson JD, et al: Effect of a patient's psychiatric history on physicians' estimation of probability of disease. J Gen Intern Med 15(3):204–206, 2000

Henry M, Watt R, Mahathey A, et al: The 2019 Annual Homeless Assessment Report (AHAR) to Congress, Part 1: Point-in-Time Estimates of Homelessness. Washington, DC, U.S. Dept of Housing and Urban Development, January 2020. Available at: www.huduser.gov/portal/sites/default/files/pdf/2019-AHAR-Part-1.pdf. Accessed October 24, 2020.

Hoge MA, Stuart GW, Morris J, et al: Mental health and addiction workforce development: federal leadership is needed to address the growing crisis. Health Aff (Millwood) 32(11):2005–2012, 2013

Hughes E, Bassi S, Gilbody S, et al: Prevalence of HIV, hepatitis B, and hepatitis C in people with severe mental illness: a systematic review and meta-analysis. Lancet Psychiatry 3(1):40–48, 2016

Hwang SW, Wilkins R, Tjepkema M, et al: Mortality among residents of shelters, rooming houses and hotels in Canada. BMJ 339:b4036, 2009

Hwang SW, Chambers C, Chiu S, et al: A comprehensive assessment of health care utilization among homeless adults under a system of universal health insurance. Am J Public Health 103 (suppl 2):S294–S301, 2013

Institute of Medicine, Committee on Monitoring Access to Personal Health Care Services: Access to Health Care in America. Washington, DC, National Academy Press, 1993

Kaiser Family Foundation: The role of Medicaid for people with behavioral health conditions. 2012. Available at: https://kaiserfamilyfoundation.files.wordpress.com/2013/01/8383_bhc.pdf. Accessed April 28, 2019.

Kaiser Family Foundation: Facilitating access to mental health services: a look at Medicaid, private insurance, and the uninsured. 2017. Available at: http://files.kff.org/attachment/Fact-Sheet-Facilitating-Access-to-Mental-Health-Services-A-Look-at-Medicaid-Private-Insurance-and-the-Uninsured. Accessed April 28, 2019.

Kaiser Family Foundation: Key facts about the uninsured population. 2018. Available at: http://files.kff.org/attachment//fact-sheet-key-facts-about-the-uninsured-population. Accessed April 28, 2019.

Kaufman EA, McDonell MG, Cristofalo MA, Ries RK: Exploring barriers to primary care for patients with severe mental illness: frontline patient and provider accounts. Issues Ment Health Nurs 33(3):172–180, 2012

Kisely S, Lalloo R, Ford P: Oral disease contributes to illness burden and disparities. Med J Aust 208(4):155–156, 2018

Knaak S, Patten S: A grounded theory model for reducing stigma in health professionals in Canada. Acta Psychiatr Scand 134 (Suppl 446):53–62, 2016

Knaak S, Szeto ACH, Fitch K, et al: Stigma towards borderline personality disorder: effectiveness and generalizability of an anti-stigma program for healthcare providers. Borderline Personal Disord Emot Dysregul 2:9, 2015

Knaak S, Mantler E, Szeto A: Mental illness-related stigma in healthcare: barriers to access and care and evidence-based solutions. Healthc Manage Forum 30(2):111–116, 2017

LeBrun-Harris LA, Baggett TP, Jenkins DM, et al: Health status and health care experiences among homeless patients in federally supported health centers: findings from the 2009 patient survey. Health Serv Res 48(3):992–1016, 2013

Lee S, O'Neill A, Park J, et al: Health insurance moderates the association between immigrant length of stay and health status. J Immigr Minor 14(2):345–349, 2012

Li Y, Cai X, Cram P: Are patients with serious mental illness more likely to be admitted to nursing homes with more deficiencies in care? Med Care 49(4):397–405, 2011

Lin WC, Bharel M, Zhang J, et al: Frequent emergency department visits and hospitalizations among homeless people with Medicaid: implications for Medicaid expansion. Am J Public Health 105 (suppl 5):S716–S722, 2015

Liu NH, Daumit GL, Dua T, et al: Excess mortality in persons with severe mental disorders: a multilevel intervention framework and priorities for clinical practices, policy and research agendas. World Psychiatry 16(1):30–40, 2017

Mangurian C, Giwa F, Shumway M, et al: Primary care providers' views on metabolic monitoring of outpatients taking antipsychotic medication. Psychiatr Serv 64(6):597–599, 2013

Mangurian C, Newcomer JW, Modlin C, et al: Diabetes and cardiovascular care among people with severe mental illness: a literature review. J Gen Intern Med 31(9):1083–1091, 2016

Mangurian C, Cournos F, Schillinger D: Low rates of HIV testing among adults with severe mental illness receiving care in community mental health settings. Psychiatr Serv 68(5):443–448, 2017

McGinty EE, Blasco-Colmenares E, Zhang Y, et al: Post-myocardial-infarction quality of care among disabled Medicaid beneficiaries with and without serious mental illness. Gen Hosp Psychiatry 34(5):493–499, 2012

McGinty EE, Baller J, Azrin ST, et al: Quality of medical care for persons with serious mental illness: a comprehensive review. Schizophr Res 165(2–3):227–235, 2015

Medford-Davis LN, Shah R, Kennedy D, et al: The role of mental health disease in potentially preventable hospitalizations. Med Care 56(1):31–38, 2018

Mitchell AJ, Lord O, Malone D: Differences in the prescribing of medication for physical disorders in individuals with v. without mental illness: meta-analysis. Br J Psychiatry 201(6):435–443, 2012

Moore AD, Hamilton JB, Knafl GJ, et al: Patient satisfaction influenced by interpersonal treatment and communication in African American men: The North Carolina–Louisiana Prostate Cancer Project (PCaP). American Journal of Men's Health 6(5):409–419, 2012

Newcomer JW: Metabolic syndrome and mental illness. Am J Manag Care 13(7 suppl):S170–S177, 2007

Parameswaran SG, Chang C, Swenson AK, et al: Roles in and barriers to metabolic screening for people taking antipsychotic medications: a survey of psychiatrists. Schizophr Res 143(2–3):395–396, 2013

Petersen LA, Normand SLT, Druss BG, et al: Process of care and outcome after acute myocardial infarction for patients with mental illness in the VA health care system: are there disparities? Health Serv Res 38(1 Pt 1):41–63, 2003

Pickett SA, Luther S, Stellon E, et al: Making integrated care a reality: lessons learned from Heartland Health Outreach's integration implementation. Am J Psychiatr Rehabil 18(1):87–104, 2015

Schmidt EM, Behar S, Barrera A, et al: Potentially preventable medical hospitalizations and emergency department visits by the behavioral health population. J Behav Health Serv Res 45(3):370–388, 2018

Semega J, Kollar M, Shrider EA, et al: Income and poverty in the United States: 2019. Current Population Reports P60-270. Washington, DC, U.S. Census Bureau, 2020

Sherrill E, Gonzales G: Recent changes in health insurance coverage and access to care by mental health status, 2012–2015. JAMA Psychiatry 74(10):1076–1079, 2017

Snowden LR: Health and mental health policies' role in better understanding and closing African American-white American disparities in treatment access and quality of care. Am Psychol 67(7):524–531, 2012

Temkin-Greener H, Campbell L, Cai X, et al: Are post-acute patients with behavioral health disorders admitted to lower-quality nursing homes? Am J Geriatr Psychiatry 26(6):643–654, 2018

Trager E, Khalili M, Masson CL, et al: Hepatitis C screening rate among underserved adults with serious mental illness receiving care in California community mental health centers. Am J Public Health 106(4):740–742, 2016

Walker ER, McGee RE, Druss BG: Mortality in mental disorders and global disease burden implications: a systematic review and meta-analysis. JAMA Psychiatry 72(4):334–341, 2015

Welch LC, Litman HJ, Borba CPC, et al: Does a physician's attitude toward a patient with mental illness affect clinical management of diabetes? Results from a mixed-method study. Health Serv Res 50(4):998–1020, 2015

Xiang X: Serious psychological distress as a barrier to cancer screening among women. Womens Health Issues 25(1):49–55, 2015

Zur J, Musumeci M, Garfield R: Medicaid's role in financing behavioral health services for low-income individuals. Kaiser Family Foundation Issue Brief, June 2017. Available at: www.kff.org/medicaid/issue-brief/medicaids-role-in-financing-behavioral-health-services-for-low-income-individuals/. Accessed June 23, 2020.

CHAPTER 5

Consequences of and Life Choices Related to Living With a Serious Mental Illness

Andrea B. Bink, Ph.D.
Patrick W. Corrigan, Psy.D.

The purpose of this chapter is twofold. The first is to inform psychiatrists and other providers of the varied and complex factors that have been proposed to account for the disparity in health and longevity for people with serious mental illness (SMI). The second is to offer guidance about how to use the information presented in this chapter to address these factors in face-to-face interactions with this vulnerable group. We first review consequences of having an SMI that are contributory factors to poor health and premature death—namely, poverty, violent victimization, homelessness, criminal justice involvement, and inadequate or substandard health care. We then provide a brief overview of the life choices or modifiable health risks common among people with SMI that are directly linked to poor health and premature mortality. Specifically, we review smoking, unhealthy diet, lack of exercise and sedentary behavior, alcohol and drug use, and high-risk sexual behaviors. The reader should note that a more in-depth examination of many of these lifestyle factors is available in other chapters in this volume (see Chapters 3, 11, and 12).

Life Consequences

Along with the challenges of living with the illness itself, people with SMI face additional hardships (Table 5–1). For example, compared with others in the population, people with SMI are more likely to be of low income or live in poverty (Levinson et al. 2010); to be victims of violence, including domestic violence (Teplin et al. 2005; Trevillion et al. 2012); and to be involved in the criminal justice system (Hiday and Burns 2009). They are also overrepresented in the homeless population (Fazel et al. 2008). Furthermore, people with SMI typically suffer from a variety of comorbid medical conditions (Janssen et al. 2015), for which they receive substandard medical care (Lawrence and Kisely 2010).

Low Income and Poverty

Worldwide estimates suggest that people with SMI are significantly more likely to have no or low earnings than others in the general population (Levinson et al. 2010). The reasons for this disparity are complex, but several key factors have been implicated. Symptoms of SMI commonly emerge early in life (Kessler et al. 1995), often interrupting education efforts and derailing early career development. However, at all levels of educational attainment for people with mental illnesses, illness-related factors (e.g., symptoms, cognitive impairment, social cognitive skill deficits) and stigmatizing and unlawful discriminatory hiring practices often get in the way of obtaining and maintaining employment (Baron and Salzer 2002). Given the difficulty in obtaining and maintaining employment, a large number of people with SMI are not in the workforce (Marwaha and Johnson 2004).

Some researchers have suggested that low socioeconomic status is a fundamental cause of health inequalities and is largely responsible for population-level morbidity and mortality (Phelan et al. 2010). A large population study (Chetty et al. 2016) in the United States matching income data from tax records to Social Security Administration death records from 1999 to 2014 found a positive relationship between life expectancy and income. The data also revealed a 10- to 15-year gap in life expectancy between the top and bottom 1% of the income distribution, a disparity that

TABLE 5–1. Consequences and life choices related to living with serious mental illnesses

Possible health/mortality risk

Consequences

Low income	Cardiovascular disease
	Social isolation and chronic stress
Violent victimization	Homicide
Homelessness	Infectious disease
	Accidents and unintentional injury
	Poisoning
	Assault (physical, sexual)
	Suicide
Criminal justice involvement	Infectious disease
	Cardiovascular disease
	Suicide
	Drug overdose
	Homicide
	Cancer
	Motor vehicle accidents
Substandard medical care	**Provider level:**
	Underdiagnosed medical conditions
	Untreated medical conditions
	Nonstandard practice including:
	• Routine screenings
	• Routine procedures
	• Medications
	Surgical complications
	Stigma
	Lack of attention to lifestyle risks
	System level:
	Underfunding of mental health services
	Fractured systems of care
	Lack of provider coordination

TABLE 5–1. Consequences and life choices related to living with serious mental illnesses *(continued)*

Possible health/mortality risk

Consequences *(continued)*

Substandard medical care *(continued)*	**Patient level:**
	Symptoms:
	• Reduced pain perception
	• Cognitive impairment
	• Communication difficulties

Life choices

Smoking cigarettes	Respiratory disease
	Cardiovascular disease
	Metabolic disease
	Lung and other cancers
	Lowered immunity
	Increased inflammation
	Poor bone, oral, and eye health
	Reduced smell and taste
Unhealthy diet	Overweight and obesity
	• Hypertension
	• High cholesterol
	• Sleep apnea
	• Type 2 diabetes
	• Coronary heart disease
	• Stroke
	• Gallbladder disease
	• Osteoarthritis
	• Some cancers
Lack of exercise/ Sedentary behavior	Cardiovascular disease
	Cancer
	Type 2 diabetes
	Musculoskeletal stress

TABLE 5–1.   Consequences and life choices related to living with serious mental illnesses *(continued)*

Possible health/mortality risk

Life choices *(continued)*

Substance use (alcohol and drugs)	Infectious disease
	Cardiovascular disease
	Lowered respiratory function
	Kidney and liver damage
	Stroke
	Some cancers
	Suicide
	Accidental overdose
	Injury
High-risk sexual behaviors	Infectious disease
	Sexually transmitted disease

has been increasing over time. Morbidity among the poor is also high, particularly in the United States, where adults living in poverty have a five times greater risk of poor or fair health, are three times more likely to report limited mobility due to chronic illnesses, and are more likely to have coronary heart disease than those with greater means (Bravement and Egerter 2008). The rate of heart disease among people living in poverty is mirrored within the population of people with SMI, who, when compared with geographically matched populations, are 53% more likely to have cardiovascular disease, 78% more likely to develop cardiovascular disease, and 85% more likely to die of cardiovascular disease (Correll et al. 2017). Increased cardiovascular disease for people with mental illness could result from the cumulative effect of a lifetime of social isolation (Xia and Li 2018) and chronic stress affiliated with both living in poverty and living with a mental illness (Halaris 2013).

Violent Victimization and Domestic Violence

Violent victimization, including assault, sexual assault, and homicide, is a common occurrence for people with SMI. For example, the first large-scale epidemiological study to examine the violent victimization of people with SMI in the United States found the prevalence of past-year violence to be more than 11 times greater for people with SMI than for others in the general population (Teplin et al. 2005). Both men and women with SMI are more at risk of sexual assault than others of their respective genders in the population (Khalifeh et al. 2015; Teplin et al. 2005), and people with SMI are two to five times as likely as others in the general population to be victims of homicide (Crump et al. 2013).

Just as tragic as violent victimization by strangers are the high rates of intimate partner and/or domestic violence perpetrated against people with SMI. A systematic review and meta-analysis of 41 high-quality studies examining prevalence rates and odds ratios by gender and mental illness type found that both men and women with mental illnesses are more likely than others in the general public to be victims of intimate partner violence (Trevillion et al. 2012). For example, they found that women with depressive disorders are 2.77 times more likely to experience domestic violence than women without a mental illness. Although the rigorous inclusion criteria of the review discussed above precluded including findings from perpetrators other than partners, other reviews have reported domestic violence committed by ex-partners as well as distant and nuclear family members (Howard et al. 2010). Khalifeh et al. (2015) compared rates of domestic violence between psychiatric patients and others in the general public and found that nonpartner family violence was 28% higher for men and women with SMI than for others in the general public.

Trevillion et al. (2012) outlined several limitations and weaknesses of the research on domestic violence that affected their ability to report results and draw conclusions. For example, study characteristics varied widely by definition of domestic violence, instruments used to assess domestic violence, time period assessed, and type of violent behavior (sexual, physical, psychological, or a combination). They found a limited number of longitudinal studies and no or few high-quality studies by type of disorder (e.g., schizophrenia, nonaffective psychosis, bipolar disorder) and type of perpetrator (e.g., intimate partner, ex-partner, distant or nuclear family member). Methodological weaknesses included selection bias, use of nonprobability samples, and no information on sample representativeness and the impact of nonparticipation.

Homelessness

People with SMI are overrepresented among the homeless and in prisons and jails (Fazel et al. 2008; Hiday and Burns 2009). The media and many researchers widely implicate failures in community mental health care after deinstitutionalization as a causal factor for the large numbers of people with mental illnesses who are homeless and involved in the criminal justice system (Baron and Salzer 2002). However, other researchers argue that rather than the after-effects of deinstitutionalization, larger societal trends, such as an overall increase in incarceration rates as well as globalization, limited access to affordable housing, recent economic downturns, and changes in government supports, might be more to blame (Baron and Salzer 2002; Draine et al. 2002). In fact, Draine and colleagues (2002) assert that poverty moderates the relationship between SMI and problems such as criminal justice involvement, homelessness, and unemployment.

People who are homeless have mortality rates two to five times greater than the population averages (Fazel et al. 2014), and men with schizophrenia who are homeless have been found to die approximately 25 years earlier than others in the general population (Foster et al. 2012). Excess morbidity and mortality for the homeless population are associated with infectious diseases (hepatitis C, HIV) (Beijer et al. 2012), accidents and unintentional injuries, and suicide (Frencher et al. 2010). Frencher et al. (2010) found that depending on age group, people who are homeless seek medical care at a higher rate for injury-related causes such as falls, burns, and exposure (i.e., cold and heat); poisoning from medication or other substances; assault or violence; suicidality; and infection (tuberculosis) than do people of low socioeconomic status who are housed. Rates of physical and sexual assault have been reported to be roughly 27%–52% (Fazel et al. 2014). In one study, assaults accounted for 12% of hospitalizations for homeless people, a rate higher than those for low-socioeconomic comparison groups (Frencher et al. 2010).

It has been observed that estimates of the general homeless population are difficult to obtain, and there is a dearth of recent epidemiological studies. Research in this area is challenging because of methodological variations (e.g., definitions of homelessness, sampling methods) and complexities of the population (Foster et al. 2012). A systematic review and meta-regression analysis examining prevalence rates of mental illness in the homeless population in seven Western countries/regions (United States, United Kingdom, Australasia, mainland Europe) accounted for some methodological inconsistencies (Fazel et al. 2008). Studies in this review included a clear definition of homelessness, standardized measures and diagnostic criteria, and time frame restrictions for psychiatric disorders. Nonetheless, the review authors found a great deal of heterogeneity across studies. For example, prevalence rates for psychosis ranged from 2.8% to 42.3% (pooled 27%), and rates for depression ranged from 0% to 40.9% (pooled 11.4%).

Criminal Justice Involvement

People with SMI are disproportionately represented in the criminal justice system, a trend that has been increasing over time. According to Hiday and Burns (2009), people with SMI are more likely to be arrested than others in the general public and are more likely to be arrested for minor offenses (e.g., vagrancy, disorderly conduct, trespassing) than for serious violent or index crimes (e.g., sexual assault, homicide). People with SMI often stay in jail longer than other inmates. One reason for longer prison and jail stays is that the competency evaluation/restoration process can extend pretrial detention for people with SMI for a longer period than the sentence they would have received had they gone directly to trial.

According to Fazel and Baillargeon (2011), the prison population is rife with chronic medical conditions, sexually transmitted diseases, and communicable infectious diseases (e.g., HIV, tuberculosis, hepatitis B). In addition, there appear to be higher rates of hypertension, diabetes, asthma, arthritis, and some cancers. Health care in prison is generally poor, with not even the minimal adherence to standards of care and few standardized guidelines for treating common chronic conditions (Jacobi 2005). Prisoners are not routinely screened for common communicable diseases, and nonadherence to drug protocols has resulted in drug-resistant strains of some communicable diseases (Fazel and Baillargeon 2011; Jacobi 2005). As Jacobi (2005) pointed out, these practices affect not only the prisoner and the prison population but also the communities to which the prisoner returns after the prison term ends.

Inside prison, death by natural causes is surprisingly lower than is found among people who are not incarcerated (Fazel and Baillargeon 2011). However, risk of death is high upon release. Binswanger et al. (2007) found that the mortality rate for people released from prison was 3.5 times that for other community residents with similar demographics, with a much higher risk (12.7 times greater) within the first 2 weeks after release. Proposed reasons for the high rate of death after release are the stress associated with difficulties related to reentry (securing housing and employment and reestablishing with family) and difficulty accessing medical care after release (Binswanger et al. 2007; Fazel and Baillargeon 2011).

Substandard Medical Care

Many comorbid health conditions (e.g., cardiovascular disease) are found at a higher rate among people with SMI compared with the general population (Janssen et al. 2015). Yet medical comorbidities are often missed and/or go untreated, and people with SMI very often receive substandard or inadequate medical care (see Chapters 1 and 4). In their review of the inequalities in health care for people with SMI, Lawrence and Kisely (2010) described contributory factors at the patient, system, and provider levels. At the patient level, challenges of the illness (e.g., cognitive impairment, symptoms, communication difficulties), psychosocial stressors, and/or distrust of the medical system (or systems in general) can interfere with care. System-level factors include a segregation of mental health services from physical health services, which contributes to limited coordination between providers, no or poor continuity of care, and insufficient funding of mental health services.

At the provider level, there is confusion among practitioners (e.g., primary care physicians, psychiatrists) regarding who should be (or who is) managing the physical health of patients with SMI. However, above all, health care professionals endorse negative and stigmatizing attitudes toward patients with SMI. For example, patients with SMI describe a lack of empathy from physicians about common conditions such as weight gain resulting from medication side effects (Graham et al. 2013). It has been speculated that a causal factor implicated in underdiagnosing medical problems is that providers might attribute reports of physical symptoms to a mental illness presentation/symptoms instead of an actual medical condition that requires attention (Lawrence and Kisely 2010). In a study that might illuminate some of the more nuanced issues concerning problems with medical care for people with SMI, Daumit et al. (2016) found a stunning 142 incidents of surgical complications per 100 admissions among patients with SMI (mostly schizophrenia), compared with up to nearly 100 fewer complications found in other studies within the general hospital population. These incidents were associated with 30-day physical harm and death and included, but were not limited to, respiratory complications, integumentary events, dysrhythmia, aspiration, deep venous thrombosis or pulmonary embolus, and infections. The authors suggested several causal factors, including medication misuse or interactions, use of restraints, underlying medical conditions, provider inexperience with this population, delays in treatment due to misreading a report of physical symptoms as part of the psychiatric presentation, communication difficulties (both patient and provider), and stigmatizing attitudes.

Recommendations for Health Care Professionals

First and foremost, when treating or interacting with people with SMI, primary care physicians, psychiatrists, and other health care professionals should be minimally as respectful and nonjudgmental as they are to people without an SMI. Health care professionals should educate themselves about the many biases that might contribute to stigmatizing attitudes and behaviors that result in substandard health care (Lawrence and Kisely 2010). Moreover, once fully informed, health care professionals are uniquely positioned to advocate for appropriate and equitable health care for people with mental illnesses. Advocacy should be directed at the person, physician, system, and governmental levels (Lawrence and Kisely 2010; Suetani et al. 2015).

Simple screening and brief conversations to identify the services or treatment options that are most salient to the individual's health and overall well-being should be routine. For example, screening and monitoring for infectious or cardiovascular disease should be discussed and recommended to people who are currently or were recently living in poverty (Bravement and Egerter 2008), who are homeless (Beijer et al. 2012) or have had recent criminal justice involvement (Fazel and Baillargeon 2011), or who indicate that they have a history of substance use (Schulte and Hser 2014). In cases in which treatment itself might have an iatrogenic effect on physical health, health care professionals across disciplines should increase monitoring and offer patient education about how to ameliorate the negative health effects (Lawrence and Kisely 2010). For example, psychiatrists should inform patients receiving psychiatric medications in plain language that they should be closely monitored for cardiometabolic risks (Lawrence and Kisely 2010). Psychiatrists should alert primary care providers about new or existing medications, and if the patient is not currently linked with a primary care provider, the psychiatrist should have a mechanism for providing adequate monitoring (Lawrence and Kisely 2010).

Life Choices

As outlined in Table 5–1, many people with SMI tend to engage in an unhealthy lifestyle. Smoking and other substance use, unhealthy diet, sedentary behavior, lack of physical activity, and risky sexual practices are all common modifiable risk factors that contribute to premature mortality for people with SMI. Research examining unhealthy behaviors among people with SMI has determined that these behaviors and SMI tend to co-occur. For example, Prochaska et al. (2014) found an average of 5.2 unhealthy behaviors (smoking, poor diet, inadequate sleep, sedentary behavior, and marijuana use) among 693 participants in an inpatient facility who reported smoking prior to hospitalization.

In this section of the chapter, we briefly review these unhealthy behaviors, their prevalence among people with SMI, patterns of co-occurrence, and risks to health. The second half of this book will review these topics in greater depth, focusing on strategies that could assist people with SMI in related goals. Note that the unhealthy behaviors reviewed here are not unique to people with SMI, but the patterns of some of these behaviors tend to be more extreme for this population. It is also important to keep in mind that the context in which the person functions can have a differential effect on activating or reinforcing healthy behaviors. For example, as Phelan et al. (2010) explain, the consequences of social status for privileged groups situate them in contexts that promote health and are supportive of healthy lifestyle choices. However, a different picture emerges for marginalized groups. Living in poverty puts people in neighborhoods with high concentrations of tobacco retailers (U.S. Department of Health and Human Services 2014), limited places to purchase healthy foods, and few parks or safe outdoor spaces in which to safely engage in physical activities (Botchwey et al. 2015). Along with poverty and the other consequences of having a mental illness addressed in the first section of this chapter, additional contextual factors that are particular to living with a mental illness can impact health behaviors. Symptoms such as cognitive impairment and lack of motivation can make it challenging to manage the instruments of daily living associated with optimal health (e.g., food planning and preparation, taking medications, communicating with health care providers) (Lipskaya et al. 2011). Furthermore, people with SMI often function within the context of psychiatric facilities or services in which unhealthy behaviors might be part of the culture. Prochaska and colleagues (2017) describe an environment in psychiatric care that is, at times, permissive and historically promotive of smoking. Smoking in some institutions and geographic regions continues to be permitted indoors, and providers are reluctant to engage patients in smoking cessation for fear that quitting will exacerbate symptoms and interfere with treatment. However, meta-analytic results indicate that smoking cessation can lower symptoms (Taylor et al. 2014).

Smoking Cigarettes

According to the U.S. Surgeon General, smoking is harmful to almost every bodily organ and is associated with an elevated risk of respiratory, cardiovascular, and metabolic diseases as well as lung and other cancers (U.S. Department of Health and Human Services 2014). Smoking also lowers immune function, increases inflammation, and negatively affects bone, oral, and eye health. Differential trends in smoking have developed between the general population and people with SMI. Although there has been a steady decline in smoking overall, smoking among people with SMI has remained excessively high (De Leon and Diaz 2005). This is especially true for people with schizophrenia, who are, evidence suggests, 5.3 times more likely to be current smokers than others in the general population and 1.9 times more likely to currently smoke than people with other SMI (De Leon and Diaz 2005). Compared with others who smoke, people with SMI start smoking younger, are heavier smokers (≥ 30 cigarettes per day), and seem to have a more difficult time quitting (De Leon and Diaz 2005).

Unhealthy Diet

People with SMI tend to engage in unhealthy food consumption and disordered eating patterns. Literature reviews examining the dietary patterns of people with SMI (e.g., Teasdale et al. 2017) report food consumed as higher in saturated fat, sugar, and calories and lower in fiber, fruit, vegetable, and dairy content than food consumed by others in the general population (who also, by the way, rarely adhere to nutritional guidelines). Processed and convenience foods are often chosen over healthier options. Along with unhealthy food choices, Teasdale et al. (2017) described disordered eating behaviors such as fast-eating syndrome, continual snacking, emotional eating, binge eating, and other eating disorders.

One of the most serious health risks associated with the eating patterns described above is overweight and obesity, conditions that are more common for people with SMI than for others in the general population (Allison et al. 2009). Obesity is associated with hypertension, high cholesterol, sleep apnea, and chronic comorbidities such as type 2 diabetes, coronary heart disease, stroke, gallbladder disease, osteoarthritis, and some cancers (Centers for Disease Control and Prevention 2017). Weight gain is directly associated with antidepressants and antipsychotic medication (Allison et al. 2009) and secondary to other side effects such as insatiable hunger and dry mouth (Teasdale et al. 2017).

Lack of Exercise and Sedentary Behavior

Evidence suggests that people with SMI, particularly people with schizophrenia and major depression, are less likely to engage in physical activity compared with control subjects (Vancampfort et al. 2017). Studies have also found that along with physical activity, people with SMI are more prone to sedentary behavior (e.g., sitting for long periods of time) than control subjects (Vancampfort et al. 2017). Meta-analytic findings (Biswas et al. 2015) indicate that sedentary behavior has an adverse effect on health independently of physical activity. However, the negative health effects of sedentary behavior tend to be markedly worse at lower levels of physical activity.

Some of the barriers to engaging in physical activity are associated with other unhealthy behaviors. For example, smoking can interfere with exercise because of diminished cardiovascular fitness (Kobayashi et al. 2004). The self-stigma of being overweight and participating in group exercise has also been reported as a barrier (Graham et al. 2013). Soundy et al. (2014) found that participants with SMI reported that being overweight and their current fitness level were barriers to engaging in physical activity. Participants were also concerned about exercising in stressful, unsafe neighborhoods where they might be subject to harassment and violence. Other reported barriers were symptoms of illness such as lack of motivation, the sedative side effects of medication, and health limitations. Participants also described a culture of sedentary behavior in inpatient and outpatient settings, the limited opportunities for physical activities, and medical and mental health professionals prioritizing mental health symptoms over physical activity.

Substance Use (Alcohol and Drugs)

Another modifiable risk factor commonly associated with mortality and morbidity for people with SMI is substance use and substance use disorders (Temmingh et al. 2018). Estimates of substance use disorder among people with SMI range from 25% to 74% in developed countries and from 51% to 68% in developing countries (Temmingh et al. 2018). While the number of people with SMI who use substances is alarming, so is the rate of high-risk behavior associated with drug use. For example, a systematic review of 52 studies examining HIV risk behavior in people with SMI found that 20% reported a lifetime history of injecting drugs (4% in the past year) and needle sharing (mainly in the United States) (Meade and Sikkema 2005). They also found that one-third of people with a dual diagnosis (SMI and substance use disorder) had a history of injecting drugs.

According to the Schulte and Hser (2014), alcohol and drugs have negative health effects throughout the lifespan. Intravenous drug use and needle sharing can expose people to infectious diseases such as HIV and hepatitis C. Alcohol and drugs affect cardiovascular, kidney, liver, and respiratory functioning, and can lead to stroke, and some cancers. Other risk factors related to premature mortality for those who use substances are suicide, accidental overdose, and injury.

High-Risk Sexual Behaviors

People with SMI who are sexually active often engage in high-risk sexual behaviors to a greater degree than others in the general public and comparative demographic groups (Meade and Sikkema 2005). A review of the literature on self-reported high-risk sexual behavior of people with SMI found that of the sexually active participants (~60% past year and ~45% past 3 months), approximately half had multiple partners and did not use condoms (Meade and Sikkema 2005). Roughly a third reported a lifetime sexually transmitted disease. U.S. participants reported engaging more often in transactional sex (e.g., trading sex for money, shelter, or substances) than participants in other countries (~25% of participants compared with 5% outside the United States).

Risky sexual behaviors affect mortality and morbidity mainly through exposure to sexually transmitted (Chen et al. 2018) and blood-borne infectious diseases such as HIV, hepatitis B, and hepatitis C (Hughes et al. 2016). A recent meta-analysis showed that blood-borne viruses were higher than population averages for people with SMI, particularly in countries with low prevalence rates (Hughes et al. 2016). For example, comparative estimates of HIV prevalence in the United States is 0.6% for the general population and 6.0% for people with SMI.

Recommendations for Health Care Professionals

Health care professionals, particularly psychiatrists and primary care physicians, are best suited to introduce the education process about the dangers of the modifiable risk factors discussed above and to advocate for behavior change for people with mental illnesses. According to the AARC Tobacco-Free Lifestyle Roundtable (2014), two of the main identified barriers to initiating conversations about these issues with people with mental illnesses are time constraints and provider reluctance. To meet these challenges, brief (1- to 3-minute) intervention models such as the 5 A's model (ask, advise, assess, assist, and arrange) coupled with the 5 R's model (relevance, risks, rewards, roadblocks and repetition) provide practitioners with a simple road map to guide these interactions. The 5 A's/5 R's models are best suited for practitioners who provide services in integrated health systems that provide supports such as smoking cessation and nutrition education. The ultra-brief AAR model—ask, advise, refer—can be used by those who refer out to the community for these supports. Below is a brief illustration of how these models can be used to promote behavior change. The examples presented below have been modified from the *Clinician's Guide to Treating Tobacco Dependence* (AARC Tobacco-Free Lifestyle Roundtable 2014). Although specific to smoking cessation, the principles presented in this guide can be adapted for other modifiable health risks.

- **Ask** open-ended questions to elicit a higher level of detail about duration, frequency, intensity, and previous successful behavior-change attempts.
  - "Would you please tell me about your [modifiable risk behavior (e.g., diet, smoking, sexual activity)]?"
  - "What types of [substances (e.g., tobacco products, non-prescribed drugs, alcohol)/behaviors (e.g., risky sexual practices, exercise)] have you [used/engaged in] in the last year?"
  - "How long has it been since you tried to [change the behavior (e.g., change your diet, quit using substances, used a condom, start an exercise routine)]?"
- **Advise** using an approach tailored toward the individual and use the 5 R's at this stage.
  - Indicate the importance of behavior change.
  - For those who are reluctant to change, employ the 5 R's:
    - **Relevance**—Address the patient's specific situation and needs (e.g., recent cancer or diabetes diagnosis).
    - **Risks**—Outline risks important to the patient's health or lifestyle concerns.
    - **Rewards**—Emphasize the rewards of behavior change.
    - **Roadblocks**—Educate the patient to address their specific barriers to change.
    - **Repetition**—Repeat these messages and questions over time to demonstrate the importance of change.
- **Assess** the patient's willingness, confidence, and opportunity to change. In this stage, health care professionals should not automatically assume that a lack of willingness and confidence indicates a lack of willpower or motivation. Accordingly, care should be taken not to misinterpret lack of resources for a lack of willingness and confidence. Although a person might be willing to change a behavior and confident about doing so, in the abstract, the reality of their situation might preclude changing or make it very difficult to change. By way of example, those with limited finances who live in deprived neighborhoods might be willing and want to lose weight but also might be making their decision based on access to grocery stores selling fresh produce and safe places to exercise. If these are not readily available, the person might not seem willing to lose weight if no further assessment is done. In essence, the endorsement or lack of endorsement of willingness and confidence might be intertwined with what the person understands or does not understand about

the limits of their specific circumstance. Therefore, a skilled health care professional will ask relevant and sensitive questions to unravel the desire for change from the barriers.

- A 1–10 rating scale is helpful to uncover the importance of change to the person and their confidence to make a change. Questions such as "What is good/not good about [modifiable risk behavior]?" can help assess whether the person is interested in changing a behavior. Questions such as "Is there a grocery store in your neighborhood that sells different types of fruits and vegetables?" can help assess if the person lives in a situation or environment that is conducive to making a change.
- **Assist** the patient in finding an education or behavior change program, outline treatment options for change, and outline options to address the barriers uncovered in the assessment stage.
- **Arrange** a follow-up visit with the patient and/or refer to an educational or behavior change program. The clinician should schedule follow-up at regular intervals for those who are not referred out and sooner for those who are, to ensure patients are indeed linked with the program and that they are satisfied with the program's offerings. If they are not satisfied, the clinician should ask patients to return for assistance and repeat the process.

The very brief AAR model—ask, advise, refer—using the appropriate guidelines above can be used when time is limited or referral to the community is necessary.

Conclusion

People with SMI face multiple hardships and engage in unhealthy behaviors that contribute to a wide mortality gap and increased morbidity. The complexity and interrelatedness of these problems seem to suggest that solutions to these problems are also complex. Some researchers suggest that solutions need to be sought by addressing the broader societal trends that account for population level, health disparities and life consequences (Draine et al. 2002; Phelan et al. 2010). However, others assert that solutions should be sought at the provider-level with support by institutions and governmental policies to facilitate and drive these solutions (Suetani et al. 2015). One target for intervention is stigma within the medical and mental health care community. As Lawrence and Kisely (2010) pointed out,

"If there is one sector of society that should be able to recognize that the behaviours that are otherwise seen as signs of a difficult or negative person are actually symptoms of illness, it would be expected to be the healthcare sector" (p. 64). Furthermore, researchers suggest that rather than a narrow focus on clinical and functional outcomes, physical and mental health care should address broader aspects of recovery (Drake and Whitley 2014) and optimal health (Graham et al. 2013) that are identified by people with SMI as important. Practically, physical and mental health care should be empowering and should promote autonomy and agency (Drake and Whitley 2014), with the understanding that recovery is best accomplished within the context of everyday experiences (Graham et al. 2013).

Key Points

When interacting with and treating people with serious mental illnesses, primary care physicians, psychiatrists, and other health care professionals should

- Apply the same level of respect and standards of care as are applied to others in the community.
- Take a nonjudgmental stance in interactions and recommendations.
- Become educated about the biases in the health care field and work to change stigmatizing beliefs and behaviors.
- Advocate for better practices, higher standards, and more funding for mental health facilities.
- Screen for and monitor the resultant health effects related to the consequences and life choices outlined in this book chapter.
- Link patients with appropriate social services.
- Follow up until the person is linked and satisfied.
- Deliver the brief 5 A's/5 R's models when health-risk behaviors necessitate a change and appropriate supports are available within the professionals' institutions. Use the very brief AAR model when referring to supports in the community.

References

AARC Tobacco-Free Lifestyle Roundtable: Clinician's Guide to Treating Tobacco Dependence. Irving, TX, American Association for Respiratory Care, 2014. Available at: www.aarc.org/education/online-courses/clinicians-guide-treating-tobacco-dependence. Accessed July 6, 2020.

Allison DB, Newcomer JW, Dunn AL, et al: Obesity among those with mental disorders: a National Institute of Mental Health meeting report. Am J Prev Med 35(4):341–350, 2009

Baron RC, Salzer MS: Accounting for unemployment among people with mental illness. Behav Sci Law 20(6):585–599, 2002

Beijer U, Wolf A, Fazel S: Prevalence of tuberculosis, hepatitis C virus, and HIV in homeless people: a systematic review and meta-analysis. Lancet Infect Dis 12(11):859–870, 2012

Binswanger IA, Stern MF, Deyo RA, et al: Release from prison—a high risk of death for former inmates. N Engl J Med 356(2):157–165, 2007

Biswas A, Oh PI, Faulkner GE, et al: Sedentary time and its association with risk for disease incidence, mortality, and hospitalization in adults: a systematic review and meta-analysis. Ann Intern Med 162(2):123–132, 2015

Botchwey ND, Falkenstein R, Levin J, et al: The built environment and actual causes of death. Journal of Planning Literature 30(3):261–281, 2015

Bravement P, Egerter S: Overcoming obstacles to health. 2008. Available at: www.commissiononhealth.org/PDF/ObstaclesToHealth-Report.pdf. Accessed June 24, 2020.

Centers for Disease Control and Prevention: Adult obesity causes & consequences. 2017. Available at: www.cdc.gov/obesity/adult/causes.html. Accessed June 24, 2020.

Chen S-F, Chiang J-H, Hsu C-Y, et al: Schizophrenia is associated with an increased risk of sexually transmitted infections: a nationwide population-based cohort study in Taiwan. Schizophr Res 202:316–321, 2018

Chetty R, Stepner M, Abraham S, et al: The association between income and life expectancy in the United States, 2001–2014. JAMA 315(16):1750–1766, 2016

Correll CU, Solmi M, Veronese N, et al: Prevalence, incidence and mortality from cardiovascular disease in patients with pooled and specific severe mental illness: a large-scale meta-analysis of 3,211,768 patients and 113,383,368 controls. World Psychiatry 16(2):163–180, 2017

Crump C, Sundquist K, Winkleby MA, et al: Mental disorders and vulnerability to homicidal death: Swedish nationwide cohort study. BMJ 346:f557, 2013

Daumit GL, McGinty EE, Pronovost P, et al: Patient safety events and harms during medical and surgical hospitalizations for persons with serious mental illness. Psychiatr Serv 67(10):1068–1075, 2016

De Leon J, Diaz FJ: A meta-analysis of worldwide studies demonstrates an association between schizophrenia and tobacco smoking behaviors. Schizophr Res 76(2–3):135–157, 2005

Draine J, Salzer MS, Culhane DP, et al: Role of social disadvantage in crime, joblessness, and homelessness among persons with serious mental illness. Psychiatr Serv 53(5):565–573, 2002

Drake RE, Whitley R: Recovery and severe mental illness: description and analysis. Can J Psychiatry 59(5):236–242, 2014

Fazel S, Baillargeon J: The health of prisoners. Lancet 377(9769):956–965, 2011

Fazel S, Khosla V, Doll H, et al: The prevalence of mental disorders among the homeless in Western countries: systematic review and meta-regression analysis. PLoS Med 5(12):e225, 2008

Fazel S, Geddes JR, Kushel M: The health of homeless people in high-income countries: descriptive epidemiology, health consequences, and clinical and policy recommendations. Lancet 384(9953):1529–1540, 2014

Foster A, Gable J, Buckley J: Homelessness in schizophrenia. Psychiatr Clin North Am 35(3):717–734, 2012

Frencher SK, Benedicto CMB, Kendig TD, et al: A comparative analysis of serious injury and illness among homeless and housed low income residents of New York City. J Trauma 69(4 suppl):S191–S199, 2010

Graham C, Griffiths B, Tillotson S, et al: Healthy living? By whose standards? Engaging mental health service recipients to understand their perspectives of, and barriers to, healthy living. Psychiatr Rehabil J 36(3):215–218, 2013

Halaris A: Co-morbidity between cardiovascular pathology and depression: role of inflammation. Inflammation in Psychiatry 28:144–161, 2013

Hiday VA, Burns PJ: Mental illness and the criminal justice system, in A Handbook for the Study of Mental Health, 2nd Edition. Edited by Scheid TL, Brown TN. Cambridge, UK, Cambridge University Press, 2009, pp 478–498

Howard LM, Trevillion K, Khalifeh H, et al: Domestic violence and severe psychiatric disorders: prevalence and interventions. Psychol Med 40(6):881–893, 2010

Hughes E, Bassi S, Gilbody S, et al: Prevalence of HIV, hepatitis B, and hepatitis C in people with severe mental illness: a systematic review and meta-analysis. Lancet Psychiatry 3(1):40–48, 2016

Jacobi J: Prison health, public health: obligations and opportunities. Am J Law Med 31(4):447–478, 2005

Janssen EM, McGinty EE, Azrin ST, et al: Review of the evidence: prevalence of medical conditions in the United States population with serious mental illness. Gen Hosp Psychiatry 37(3):199–222, 2015

Kessler RC, Foster CL, Saunders WB, et al: Social consequences of psychiatric disorders, I: educational attainment. Am J Psychiatry 152(7):1026–1032, 1995

Khalifeh H, Moran P, Borschmann R, et al: Domestic and sexual violence against patients with severe mental illness. Psychol Med 45(4):875–886, 2015

Kobayashi Y, Takeuchi T, Hosoi T, et al: Effects of habitual smoking on cardiorespiratory responses to sub-maximal exercise. J Physiol Anthropol Appl Human Sci 23(5):163–169, 2004

Lawrence D, Kisely S: Review: inequalities in healthcare provision for people with severe mental illness. J Psychopharmacol 24(4 suppl):61–68, 2010

Levinson D, Lakoma MD, Petukhova M, et al: Associations of serious mental illness with earnings: results from the WHO World Mental Health Surveys. Br J Psychiatry 197(2):114–121, 2010

Lipskaya L, Jarus T, Kotler M: Influence of cognition and symptoms of schizophrenia on IADL performance. Scand J Occup Ther 18(3):180–187, 2011

Marwaha S, Johnson S: Schizophrenia and employment: a review. Soc Psychiatry Psychiatr Epidemiol 39(5):337–349, 2004

Meade CS, Sikkema KJ: HIV risk behavior among adults with severe mental illness: a systematic review. Clin Psychol Rev 25(4):433–457, 2005

Phelan JC, Link BG, Tehranifar P: Social conditions as fundamental causes of health inequalities: theory, evidence, and policy implications. J Health Soc Behav 51 Suppl:S28–S40, 2010

Prochaska JJ, Fromont SC, Delucchi K, et al: Multiple risk-behavior profiles of smokers with serious mental illness and motivation for change. Health Psychol 33(12):1518–1529, 2014

Prochaska JJ, Das S, Young-Wolff KC: Smoking, mental illness, and public health. Annu Rev Public Health 38:165–185, 2017

Schulte MT, Hser YI: Substance use and associated health conditions throughout the lifespan. Public Health Rev 35(2), 2014

Soundy A, Freeman P, Stubbs B, et al: The transcending benefits of physical activity for individuals with schizophrenia: a systematic review and meta-ethnography. Psychiatry Res 220(1–2):11–19, 2014

Suetani S, Whiteford HA, McGrath JJ: An urgent call to address the deadly consequences of serious mental disorders. JAMA Psychiatry 72(12):1166–1167, 2015

Taylor G, McNeill A, Girling A, et al: Change in mental health after smoking cessation: systematic review and meta-analysis. BMJ 348:g1151, 2014

Teasdale SB, Samaras K, Wade T, et al: A review of the nutritional challenges experienced by people living with severe mental illness: a role for dietitians in addressing physical health gaps. J Hum Nutr Diet 30(5):545–553, 2017

Temmingh HS, Williams T, Siegfried N, et al: Risperidone versus other antipsychotics for people with severe mental illness and co-occurring substance misuse. Cochrane Database Syst Rev 1(1):CD011057, 2018

Teplin LA, McClelland GM, Abram KM, et al: Crime victimization in adults with severe mental illness: comparison with the National Crime Victimization Survey. Arch Gen Psychiatry 62(8):911–921, 2005

Trevillion K, Oram S, Feder G, et al: Experiences of domestic violence and mental disorders: a systematic review and meta-analysis. PLoS One 7(12):e51740, 2012

U.S. Department of Health and Human Services: The health consequences of smoking—50 years of progress: a report of the Surgeon General. 2014. Available at: www.cdc.gov/tobacco/data_statistics/sgr/50th-anniversary/index.htm. Accessed June 24, 2020.

Vancampfort D, Firth J, Schuch FB, et al: Sedentary behavior and physical activity levels in people with schizophrenia, bipolar disorder and major depressive disorder: a global systematic review and meta-analysis. World Psychiatry 16(3):308–315, 2017

Xia N, Li H: Loneliness, social isolation, and cardiovascular health. Antioxid Redox Signal 28(9):837–851, 2018

CHAPTER 6

Impact of Medication Effects on Physical Health

Marc De Hert, M.D., Ph.D.
Johan Detraux, M.Psy.
Davy Vancampfort, Ph.D.

Although many nonmedical factors, including an unhealthy lifestyle and disparities in health care, contribute to the poor physical health of people with serious mental illness (SMI), including schizophrenia, bipolar disorder, and major depressive disorder (MDD), the use of psychotropic medication (antipsychotics, antidepressants, and mood stabilizers) is an important risk factor for physical complications and disorders.

Nutritional and Metabolic Diseases

Metabolic Syndrome

Metabolic syndrome is characterized by the simultaneous occurrence of metabolic abnormalities, including abdominal obesity, glucose intolerance or insulin resistance, dyslipidemia (i.e., higher levels of triglycerides and decreased high-density lipoprotein [HDL] cholesterol levels), and hypertension (De Hert et al. 2011a, 2011b). Several meta-analyses (Vancampfort et al. 2013a, 2013b, 2014, 2015) showed that compared with matched general population control subjects, people with SMI have a significantly increased risk for developing metabolic syndrome (relative risk [RR]=1.58, 95% confidence interval [CI]: 1.35–1.86; $P<0.001$) and all its components, except for hypertension ($P=0.07$). Approximately one-third (32.6%, 95% CI: 30.8%–34.4%) of this population has metabolic syndrome, with no statistically significant differences in prevalence of metabolic syndrome across schizophrenia (33.4%), bipolar disorder (31.7%), and MDD (31.3%) diagnostic subgroups (Vancampfort et al. 2015). Within the schizophrenia subgroup, prevalence of metabolic syndrome is significantly ($P<0.001$) higher in individuals with multi-episode schizophrenia (34.2%), compared with persons in their first episode (13.7%) or those who are antipsychotic-naive (10.2%), even after correction for age (Vancampfort et al. 2013b). Although metabolic abnormalities, such as higher levels of triglycerides and impaired glucose tolerance, may already be present in antipsychotic-naive patients with psychosis, compared with healthy control subjects (Misiak et al. 2017) (reflecting potential disease-specific mechanisms), it appears that a cumulative long-term effect of poor health behaviors and psychotropic medication use places people with SMI at the greatest risk for metabolic syndrome, independent of psychiatric disease.

Patients with schizophrenia taking antipsychotic medications are at significantly ($P<0.001$) higher risk of developing metabolic syndrome, when compared with those who are antipsychotic-naive. Risk of metabolic syndrome also differs significantly across commonly used antipsychotic medications, with clozapine (prevalence rate=47.2%), quetiapine (prevalence rate=37.3%), and olanzapine (prevalence rate=36.2%) being associated with the highest risk, and aripiprazole (prevalence rate=19.4%) and amisulpride (prevalence rate=22.8%) being associated with the lowest risk (Vancampfort et al. 2015). Although no relationship was found between antidepressant use and metabolic syndrome prevalence in patients with MDD, the use of antipsychotics in these patients, as well as in bipolar disorder patients, seems to be a significant moderator for increased prevalence of metabolic syndrome (Vancampfort et al. 2013a, 2014).

Obesity

Compared with the general population, people with SMI are at increased risk for being overweight and obese (Correll et al. 2015; De Hert et al. 2011a, 2011b; Mazereel et al. 2020; Vancampfort et al. 2015). The likelihood of being obese is increased 2.8- to 4.4-fold in patients with schizophrenia and 1.2- to 1.7-fold in those with MDD or bipolar disorder, compared with matched general population control subjects (Correll et al. 2015). Overall, the proportion of patients with SMI and abdominal obesity lies between 50% and 63%, depending on the employed criteria. Although lifestyle factors such as diet and lack of physical activity do contribute to obesity in these patients, weight gain also seems to be mediated by psychotropic medication (Vancampfort et al. 2015).

Weight gain—commonly assessed as body weight change, change in body mass index, or clinically relevant ($\geq 7\%$) weight change from baseline—is a well-established side effect of antipsychotics during both the acute and maintenance phases of treatment of patients with SMI (Correll et al. 2015). There is, however, a hierarchy for risk of weight gain among antipsychotics that has been confirmed in different reviews and meta-analyses (De Hert et al. 2011a, 2011b). Weight gain is greatest with the second-generation antipsychotics (SGAs) clozapine and olanzapine, while quetiapine, risperidone, paliperidone, and iloperidone have an intermediate risk. Aripiprazole, amisulpride, ziprasidone, asenapine, and lurasidone have less or little effect on body weight. Among the first-generation antipsychotics (FGAs), the so-called low-potency agents, such as chlorpromazine and thioridazine, have higher weight gain potential than the high-potency drugs, such as haloperidol (Correll et al. 2015; De Hert et al. 2011a, 2011b). No antipsychotic, however, should be considered truly weight neutral, because virtually all antipsychotics are associated with weight gain after prolonged use, compared with placebo (De Hert et al. 2011b). There are, however, marked individual variations in weight gain, irrespective of the prescribed antipsychotic: some subjects lose weight, whereas others maintain or gain weight with the same agent. Although (partial) nonadherence can be a confounder, this observation, together with the results from monozygotic twin and sibling studies, suggests that genetic factors play an important role in medication-induced weight gain, with estimates as high as 60%–80% for antipsychotic-related weight gain (Zai et al. 2018).

Relative to adults, youth seem to be at higher risk for antipsychotic-induced weight gain. In children and adolescents (<18 years old), roughly the same hierarchy for risk of weight gain with these agents has been identified (with olanzapine having the highest risk, risperidone showing an intermediate risk, and aripiprazole having the least effect on body weight), but with weight gain occurring at a higher rate. Antipsychotic-naive and first-episode patients also are more vulnerable to weight gain, as these subgroups show more robust increases in weight gain with duration of antipsychotic use. Once again, olanzapine seems to induce significantly more long-term (>12 weeks) weight gain in these patients, compared with other antipsychotic medications (Correll et al. 2015).

Generally, weight gain with antipsychotics is rapid during the first few weeks, slows gradually, and often reaches a plateau within 1 year. Results indicate that the first year of antipsychotic treatment is a critical period for weight gain and other metabolic abnormalities, as initial rapid weight gain is a good indicator for long-term weight gain and obesity (Pérez-Iglesias et al. 2014). Switching subjects to metabolically more neutral compounds may result in weight loss in some, but not all, cases.

Although the drug is currently off-label and additional high-quality evidence is needed, recent meta-analytical evidence shows that metformin might decrease weight in adults, adolescents, and children treated with SGAs (de Silva et al. 2016).

Long-term use (>6 months) and polypharmacy of antidepressants, such as the tricyclic antidepressant (TCA) amitriptyline, the tetracyclic mirtazapine, and the selective serotonin reuptake inhibitor (SSRI) paroxetine, as well as mood stabilizers, such as lithium and valproate, have been associated with weight gain (Galling et al. 2015; Wang et al. 2018). However, weight gain is generally more modest or mild with antidepressants and mood stabilizers, compared with antipsychotics, and differences between antidepressants are modest (Correll et al. 2015). Bupropion is more likely to cause weight loss than gain (Patel et al. 2016).

Clinical and animal study data suggest that increased appetite and food intake, as well as delayed satiety signaling, are key behavior changes induced by antipsychotics. A decrease in caloric expenditure due to the sedative effects, and an increased intake of caloric beverages due to dry mouth/throat induced by certain antidepressants, may contribute to antidepressant-induced weight gain. Antagonism at the serotonergic $5\text{-}HT_{2C}$ and histaminergic H_1 receptors has been identified as the key mechanism contributing to antipsychotic-induced weight gain. Among antipsychotics, clozapine and olanzapine, which have the highest weight gain/obesity risk, also have the highest affinities for $5\text{-}HT_{2C}$ and H_1 receptors. H_1 antagonism has been identified as the strongest predictor of weight gain with antidepressants (Salvi et al. 2016).

Case Vignette 1[1]

A 33-year-old man with two prior hospitalizations for mania presented to the emergency department (ED) with decreased need for sleep, grandiosity,

---

[1]Adapted from case described in Kimmel RJ, Levy MR: "Profound Hypertriglyceridemia and Weight Gain in the First Week Following Initiation of Olanzapine: A Case Report With Implications for Lipid Monitoring Guidelines." *Psychosomatics* 54(4):392–394, 2013.

irritability, increased rate of speech, auditory hallucinations, and a delusion that he could fly. Labs in the ED were entirely normal, and the patient was not obese. The patient was given 10 mg of olanzapine orally in the ED and was hospitalized involuntarily. Fasting labs were drawn the first morning on the psychiatry unit, and on the basis of ongoing mania and psychosis, the patient's olanzapine was increased to 10 mg PO bid. He also agreed to take lamotrigine, which was started at 25 mg. The plan was to use olanzapine for several months and then taper off that medication when the lamotrigine was at a dose more likely to be effective for bipolar maintenance. On day 7, nursing staff noted that the patient had gained 6 kg since admission. Fasting labs drawn in the morning on day 8 revealed significant and abrupt triglyceride changes (from 130 mg/dL on day 1 to 810 mg/dL on day 8). To make sure that this was not a lab error, repeat fasting labs were done on day 9. With the lipid abnormalities confirmed (1,041 mg/dL on day 9) and apparently worsening daily, the olanzapine was immediately discontinued. On day 10, fasting labs showed improvement (739 mg/dL on day 9), and aripiprazole 10 mg was started for ongoing hypomanic symptoms. The patient was discharged 2 days later, with hypomania resolved (triglyceride levels were 627 mg/dL on day 12), taking aripiprazole 15 mg, clonazepam 1 mg bid, and lamotrigine 25 mg. An outpatient titration schedule for lamotrigine was planned.

Dyslipidemia

Compared with general population control subjects, people with SMI have a significantly increased risk for elevated triglycerides (RR=1.49, 95% CI: 1.28–1.73; $P<0.001$) and decreased HDL cholesterol (RR=1.33, 95% CI: 1.15–1.54; $P<0.001$) (Vancampfort et al. 2015). Moreover, in multiepisode patients with schizophrenia, compared with first-episode and untreated patients with schizophrenia, metabolic syndrome criteria are significantly ($P<0.001$) more commonly met for elevated triglycerides (39% vs. 10.5% and 23.3%) and low HDL cholesterol (41.7% vs. 16% and 24.2%) (Vancampfort et al. 2013b). A statistically significant ($P=0.008$) higher risk for hypertriglyceridemia was also found in patients with MDD compared with age- and gender-matched general population control subjects (Vancampfort et al. 2014).

Antipsychotics have been associated with lipid abnormalities (De Hert et al. 2011a, 2011b). Adverse effects on triglycerides and cholesterol can occur early and may even precede weight gain, pointing to weight-independent molecular effects, in addition to weight-related ones (De Hert et al. 2011b). Clozapine, olanzapine, and risperidone have all been associated with a higher risk for dyslipidemia compared with FGAs (Buhagiar and Jabbar 2019).

Although some antidepressants have been associated with weight gain, which is a risk factor for lipid abnormalities, data on adverse lipid effects of these medications remain scarce. At this moment, results show that most antidepressants have not been associated with dyslipidemia. Moreover, a direct weight-independent effect on serum cholesterol has not been consistently reported (Correll et al. 2015).

Among mood stabilizers, lithium has not been associated with relevant lipid abnormalities, although lithium-induced hypothyroidism can lead to weight gain and changes in lipid profile. Valproate has been associated with reductions in total and low-density lipoprotein cholesterol in patients with schizophrenia and bipolar disorder, despite its association with weight gain, increased triglycerides and glucose, and insulin abnormalities (Correll et al. 2015).

Cardiovascular Diseases

Cardiovascular diseases (CVDs) are a group of diseases that involve both the heart and blood vessels, thereby including coronary heart disease (CHD), among several other conditions. *Coronary heart disease*, also known as ischemic heart disease or coronary artery disease, is a common term for the buildup of a waxy substance, called *plaque*, in the heart's arteries, leading to the failure of coronary circulation to supply adequate blood to cardiac muscle and surrounding tissue—a phenomenon that can result in a myocardial infarction (MI). The main risk factors for CHD are dyslipidemia, diabetes, arterial hypertension, obesity, smoking, and a sedentary lifestyle, as well as stress, older age, male gender, and a family history of CHD (De Hert et al. 2011a, 2011b).

It is well documented that the presence of conventional cardiovascular risk factors at a young age is predictive of long-term CVDs. Moreover, the adverse effects of these risk factors on cardiovascular health are already present in childhood. Obesity during this early life stage is associated with vascular damage, subclinical indicators of atherosclerosis, and impaired cardiac function (Devlin and Panagiotopoulos 2015). A recent study (Hagen et al. 2017) revealed that duration of antipsychotic medication and cumulative exposure to antipsychotics are correlated with advanced glycation end products. These are considered metabolic biomarkers of increased oxidative stress, and the accumulation of these products has been shown to be associated with the development and progression of CVDs. Thus, children who develop cardiometabolic adverse effects with SGA treatment may be at risk for early and late cardiovascular damage.

Coronary Heart Disease

According to the most comprehensive meta-analysis of CVD risk in people with SMI conducted to date, which involved studies totaling 3,211,768 patients and 113,383,368 control subjects, SMI patients as a group have a statistically significantly increased risk of CHD versus control groups (a 51% higher risk in cross-sectional studies and a 54% higher risk in longitudinal studies) (Correll et al. 2017).

The use of antipsychotic medication may increase the risk of CHD. In addition to obesity and other cardiometabolic-related mechanisms, a direct effect of antipsychotics on cardiovascular risk may exist. Among antidepressants, the incidence rates of cardiovascular adverse drug reactions are higher during treatment with monoamine oxidase inhibitors (MAOIs), TCAs (even with therapeutic doses), and serotonin-norepinephrine reuptake inhibitors (SNRIs) (with the exception of mirtazapine) than during treatment with SSRIs (with the exception of citalopram) (Spindelegger et al. 2015; Wang et al. 2018).

Myocardial Infarction

For rare adverse events, such as MI, observational studies are still the main source of evidence. Although recent meta-analyses of observational studies suggest that antipsychotic use might be a potential risk factor of MI (with more pronounced MI risk in short-term users [≤2 months] and in people with schizophrenia)],[2] the association between antipsychotics and MI remains controversial because of heterogeneous clinical settings and methodological limitations (Correll et al. 2015; Huang et al. 2017). Moreover, the higher MI risk observed in antipsychotic users with schizophrenia could partly be explained by the unhealthy lifestyle (e.g., smoking, lack of physical activity, an unhealthy diet) of these patients. Only a few studies provided data on individual drugs, suggesting that amisulpride, haloperidol, chlorpromazine, and aripiprazole might be worse than other antipsychotic drugs. Mechanisms of MI risk and exposure to antipsychotics remain unclear. Potential pharmacological mechanisms include affinity of antipsychotics to dopamine D_3 and serotonin 5-HT_{2A} receptors (Huang et al. 2017).

According to a meta-analysis of 14 observational studies, reporting data on more than 800,000 participants, including 85,941 MI case patients, antidepressant use is associated with a twofold increased risk of MI (RR=2.03, 95% CI: 1.30–3.18; $P<0.01$). TCA use in particular seems to be associated with an increased MI risk, while the use of SSRIs may decrease this risk (Undela et al. 2015). Differences in outcome have also been found between

---

[2]Dose-response relationships between antipsychotic use and the risk of MI could not be investigated in these meta-analyses because of insufficient data and therefore need further investigation.

patients who received antidepressants after acute MI and those who did not. Antidepressant use after acute MI seems to be associated with increased mortality 1 year after discharge. Nevertheless, the role of antidepressant use in the development of MI continues to be debated because of the inconsistency of results across studies. Differences in study design and the problem of confounding (specifically depression) might explain the contradictory results published in the literature on this topic.

QTc Prolongation

Some psychotropic drugs have been associated with QTc prolongation, predisposing the patient to life-threatening ventricular arrhythmias, such as torsades de pointes (TdP). Although QTc remains the best marker for risk of TdP, the association between QTc and TdP is neither linear nor straightforward. TdP can occur at therapeutic doses of antipsychotics and antidepressants and with a QTc interval <500 milliseconds, and not all medications that have demonstrated QTc prolongation have been associated with the development of TdP. While it is clear that antipsychotics with a greater risk of QTc prolongation/TdP include thioridazine (greatest risk), sertindole, and ziprasidone, whereas aripiprazole appears safest, it remains difficult to rank other antipsychotics for this risk (Beach et al. 2018; Correll et al. 2015; Salvo et al. 2016). With the exception of citalopram, SSRIs are associated with a clinically insignificant dose-dependent increase in the QTc interval compared with placebo (Beach et al. 2018; Correll et al. 2015; Wang et al. 2018). SSRI-associated TdP at therapeutic concentrations is a very rare event: very few cases have been reported. TCAs, MAOIs, and SNRIs prolong the QTc interval to a greater extent than SSRIs (Wang et al. 2018).

Case Vignette 2[3]

A 40-year-old woman presented at the ED after two syncopal episodes. During the first episode, she lost consciousness, fell down some stairs, and awakened later with a scalp laceration. She continued to have spells of light-headedness and drove to her mother's house, where she had another syncopal episode. Physical examination at the ED revealed nothing unusual except for a minor scalp laceration. A 12-lead electrocardiogram (ECG),

---

[3]Adapted from case described in Deshmukh A, Ulveling K, Alla V, et al.: "Prolonged QTc Interval and Torsades de Pointes Induced by Citalopram." *Texas Heart Institute Journal* 39(1):68–70, 2012.

however, showed a prolonged QTc of 535 milliseconds. The patient had multiple episodes of TdP during her hospitalization. Although most of these were asymptomatic, she had a recurrence of syncope in the ED during one such episode. The patient had a long-standing history of depression, which had been treated with fluoxetine. Four weeks before the current presentation, her therapy had been switched to citalopram 40 mg twice daily because of worsening symptoms of depression. She was not taking any other prescribed medications. There was no family history of sudden cardiac or unexplained deaths. Citalopram therapy was discontinued, and a 12-lead ECG was performed daily to evaluate the QTc interval. The QTc interval improved appropriately upon discontinuation of citalopram. She was started on 15 mg/day of mirtazapine for depression. Upon follow-up 6 months later, the patient's QTc interval remained within the normal range and she had experienced no further syncopal episodes.

Sudden Cardiac Death

Sudden cardiac death (SCD), typically defined as death due to a cardiac cause within a short time (minutes to hours) after the symptoms initially appear, is reported to be two to four times as likely among patients with schizophrenia compared with individuals from the general population (Correll et al. 2015). Although reasons for this increased risk remain unclear, age, smoking, underlying CHD, metabolic profile, and a higher prevalence of electrocardiographic abnormalities seem to be relevant factors. The use of psychotropic medications may aggravate this risk. The association between SCD and specific psychotropic drugs has been explained by a lengthening of ventricular repolarization (QTc prolongation), predisposing the patient to life-threatening ventricular tachyarrhythmias (i.e., TdP) (Correll et al. 2015).

Patients using FGAs or SGAs have an increased risk of SCD, compared with nonusers with or without a psychiatric illness, with ratios ranging from 1.5 to 5.8, depending on the type of antipsychotic and restrictiveness of the SCD definition (Correll et al. 2015). In a meta-analysis of observational studies of SCD, higher odds ratios (ORs) were found with thioridazine (OR=4.58), clozapine (OR=3.67), risperidone (OR=3.04), haloperidol (OR=2.97), olanzapine (OR=2.04), and quetiapine (OR=1.72) (Salvo et al. 2016). Although other mechanisms may also be involved, the increased risk of SCD associated with the use of some antipsychotics seems to be related to the mean *hERG* (human ether-à-go-go-related gene) potassium channel blockade potency of these agents (Salvo et al. 2016). An increased risk among patients receiving higher doses of TCAs has been found, suggesting that such doses should be used cautiously, particularly in elderly patients or in patients with preexisting CVD (Correll et al. 2015).

Myocarditis and Cardiomyopathy

Early myocarditis and later cardiomyopathy are most commonly associated with the use of clozapine. Myocarditis is a potentially life-threatening risk of clozapine treatment, occurring often early during therapy (within the first 2–8 weeks, with incidence ranging from <0.1% to 1.0% and rates as high as 3% with more systematic monitoring) (Correll et al. 2015; Curto et al. 2016). Rapid dose titration, concomitant sodium valproate administration (which may inhibit clozapine metabolism), and older age are risk factors for clozapine-associated myocarditis. Although discontinuation of clozapine leads to cardiac functional recovery, mortality is still high (with a mortality rate between 10% and 30%). The role of rechallenging a patient with clozapine after myocarditis remains controversial (Curto et al. 2016). The mechanism of clozapine-induced myocarditis has not been well established.

Case Vignette 3[4]

A man in his late 20s who had been treated for schizophrenia for more than 10 years was admitted to the hospital because of severe auditory hallucinations and delusions that had not responded to antipsychotics, including olanzapine (15 mg), blonanserin (24 mg), and aripiprazole (30 mg). Clozapine was started at 12.5 mg (day 1), and the dosage was increased gradually: 12.5 mg for 4 days, 25 mg for 3 days, 50 mg for 4 days, 75 mg for 4 days, 100 mg for 1 day, and 50 mg for 1 day. Coadministration of sodium valproate (600 mg) and cross-tapering blonanserin (8–16 mg) and flunitrazepam (1 mg) was carried out. The patient's psychiatric symptoms improved markedly. On day 15, the patient developed high-grade fever (39.3°C), tachycardia with pulse 112 beats per minute, leukocytosis (9,500 cells/µL), and elevated C-reactive protein (4.40 mg/dL). On day 17, the clozapine was discontinued because of suspected clozapine-induced myocarditis, and on day 18 the patient was moved to the intensive care unit. Normal angiocardiographic findings excluded coronary diseases. Chest X-ray and cardiac magnetic resonance imaging equally showed no abnormalities. Viral infections were excluded. Myocarditis improved rapidly after clozapine cessation, and the patient was returned to the psychiatric ward on day 24 and discharged from the hospital on day 67. However, his auditory hallucinations and delusions were exacerbated after discharge, and he was readmitted on day 77. After receiving an explanation of the risks, benefits, and alternative therapies, the patient consented to clozapine retrial from day 89 with a gradual increase in dosage of 12.5–37.5 mg every 1–2 weeks up to 275 mg on day 220. Olanzapine (20 mg) and flunitrazepam (2 mg) were also administered on the day of retrial and were tapered off over 3–6

---

[4]Adapted from case described in Otsuka Y, Idemoto K, Hosoda Y, et al.: "Clozapine-Induced Myocarditis: Follow-up for 3.5 Years After Successful Retrial." *Journal of General and Family Medicine* 20(3):114–117, 2019.

weeks. The clozapine dosage on day 240 (day of discharge) was 200 mg. After discharge, clozapine was administered at 150–300 mg, and there has been no recurrence of myocarditis for 3.5 years. Successful rechallenge was likely the result of slower titration and cessation of sodium valproate.

Hypertension

According to meta-analytic data, people with SMI, compared with matched general population control subjects, do not seem to have a significantly increased risk for hypertension ($P=0.07$) (Vancampfort et al. 2014, 2015).

There is little information in the literature on the appearance of hypertension due to antipsychotics, and future studies should clarify the existing diverse results. The largest existing cohort study, comprising 284,234 individuals, showed that persons within 1 year of exposure to SGAs showed a small heightened risk of essential hypertension (hazard ratio=1.16, $P<0.0001$), compared with those using antidepressants. The possible increased risk in hypertension after antipsychotic treatment probably can be attributed to antipsychotic-induced weight gain/obesity and to the anti-dopaminergic effect of these agents, because all five dopamine receptor subtypes (D_1, D_2, D_3, D_4, and D_5) regulate blood pressure (Alves et al. 2019).

Among antidepressants, TCAs (mainly attributed to the anticholinergic effects of these agents) and SNRIs (particularly venlafaxine) show a significantly higher risk for hypertension (Correll et al. 2015; Wang et al. 2018). Hypertension associated with SSRIs seems to be very rare (Wang et al. 2018). Generally, mood stabilizers do not affect blood pressure, unless chronic renal failure induced by lithium affects volume distribution (Correll et al. 2015).

Endocrine System Diseases
Diabetes Mellitus

Evidence suggests that the prevalence of type 2 diabetes mellitus (DM) in people with schizophrenia, bipolar disorder, and schizoaffective disorder is two- to threefold higher than in the general population. Moreover, the age at onset of DM in individuals with an SMI seems to be about 10–20 years earlier than in the general population (Correll et al. 2015).

A causative link, albeit of uncertain magnitude, seems to exist between antipsychotics and DM, with DM affecting about 12% of people receiving these medications. Specifically, olanzapine and clozapine, and to a lesser extent (followed in ranking) asenapine, paliperidone, quetiapine, and risperidone, were shown to be associated with an increased risk of glucose dysregulation or DM in people with schizophrenia or bipolar disorder

(Correll et al. 2015; De Hert et al. 2011a; Zhang et al. 2017). Ziprasidone, lurasidone, and aripiprazole are associated with minimal glucose changes, compared with other antipsychotics or placebo (Zhang et al. 2017).

Antipsychotic-induced cardiometabolic abnormalities that are associated with an increased risk of DM (e.g., obesity, hyperglycemia, dyslipidemia) tend to appear faster and to a greater extent in children and adolescents than in adults (Correll et al. 2015; De Hert et al. 2011b; Pisano et al. 2016). Although the occurrence of new-onset DM in antipsychotic-exposed youth remains limited, SGA-treated children nevertheless have a two- to threefold increased risk of developing DM, compared with SGA-naive children. This risk increases with higher cumulative doses (particularly with olanzapine), longer treatment duration, and adjunctive antidepressant use, and it seems to remain high for a certain period of time after discontinuation (Pisano et al. 2016).

The potential mechanisms for antipsychotic-induced DM include 1) antipsychotic-induced insulin resistance through weight gain/obesity, 2) insulin resistance due to direct effects of antipsychotics, and 3) antipsychotic-induced β-cell dysfunction and apoptosis (Chen et al. 2017). Antipsychotics thus appear to contribute to insulin resistance and DM both indirectly, by inducing weight gain, and directly, by promoting insulin resistance and β-cell deterioration. Muscarinic M_3 receptors play a crucial role in the regulation of insulin secretion through both peripheral and central cholinergic pathways. Olanzapine and clozapine, the SGAs with the highest risk to induce DM, also possess the highest M_3 receptor–binding affinity (Chen et al. 2017; Correll et al. 2015).

Although a recent meta-analysis (Salvi et al. 2017) demonstrated the association between antidepressant use and new-onset DM (RR=1.27, 95% CI: 1.19–1.35; $P<0.001$), it still remains a matter of debate whether this association is causal or not. Depression itself is a well-acknowledged risk factor for DM, and improvement in depression has a favorable effect on glycemic control that is weight independent (Roopan and Larsen 2017). Although it is unclear whether single antidepressants exert a different effect on the risk of DM (Salvi et al. 2017), short-term use of SSRIs in general stabilizes or lowers blood glucose levels (with a possible risk of hypoglycemia), while TCAs are associated with hyperglycemia and worsening of glycemic control (Roopan and Larsen 2017). Particularly long-term use of antidepressants with high or moderate daily doses has been associated with an increased risk of DM. Although several reports suggest that the concurrent use of (certain) antidepressants is associated with an increased risk of glucose dysregulation or DM, others do not (Correll et al. 2015).

Not only antipsychotics but also antidepressants have been associated with an increased risk of type 2 DM in youth. Recent evidence seems to suggest that in antipsychotic-treated youth, concomitant SSRI/SNRI use is associated with an even higher risk of type-2 DM, which markedly intensifies with increasing duration of SSRI/SNRI use and cumulative SSRI/SNRI dose (Correll and Galling 2017).

Several reasons have been postulated to explain the possible association between antidepressant exposure and the risk of DM, including antidepressant-induced weight gain, altered glucose metabolism through insulin resistance and inhibition of insulin secretion, and hyperglycemia, particularly with antidepressants that have high affinity for norepinephrine reuptake transporter, serotonin 5-HT_{2C} receptor, and histamine H_1 receptor.

Case Vignette 4[5]

Mr. X is a 48-year-old man with a diagnosis of treatment-resistant paranoid schizophrenia. Various medications were trialed, but clozapine (up to 400 mg/day) proved to be the most effective treatment for symptom control. The patient, however, developed rapid loss of glycemic control within days of starting the medication, meaning it was unlikely to have been caused by intermediate factors such as increased appetite, weight gain, or insulin resistance. He was not taking any other medication likely to cause hyperglycemia. Clozapine produced a linear dose-related increase in glycemic levels during the first 2 months of treatment, which from 400 mg onward seemed to reach a plateau. Given the lack of any effective symptom management with other antipsychotic medication and the complexity of the clinical presentation, it was decided to continue clozapine, but to manage the hyperglycemia while continuing with the medication. To do this, the Maudsley Prescribing Guidelines' recommendations for treatment of antipsychotic-related diabetes were followed, and a collaboration was started with a clinical pharmacist specializing in mental health and with endocrinologists, who oversaw the individual's treatment. This approach required vigorous baseline and follow-up monitoring of glucose levels and hemoglobin A1c values, a slower clozapine titration schedule, and full control of glycemic levels before every dose increase of clozapine. Insulin and long-acting exenatide—a glucagon-like peptide-1 (GLP-1) agonist that requires a weekly injection—were added to his existing metformin.

Diabetic Ketoacidosis

Although diabetic ketoacidosis (DKA), a potentially fatal condition, is a rare complication of DM, its incidence is approximately 10 times higher in patients with schizophrenia exposed to SGAs compared with the general

---

[5]Adapted from case described in Porras-Segovia A, Krivoy A, Horowitz M, et al.: "Rapid-Onset Clozapine-Induced Loss of Glycaemic Control: Case Report." *BJPsych Open* 3(3):138–140, 2017.

population. Physical symptoms include increased thirst (polydipsia) and urination (polyuria), excessive appetite (polyphagia), nausea, abdominal pain and vomiting, dehydration, Kussmaul breathing, acetone ("fruity apple-like") breath, weakness or lethargy, confusion, and altered consciousness (Correll et al. 2015). While the underlying mechanisms are not well understood, antipsychotic-related DKA can occur soon after treatment onset and in the absence of weight gain (over one-third of cases present with either no weight gain or even weight loss) (Guenette et al. 2013). Although at least half of the reports involve individuals on polypharmacy, complicating the risk attribution to a specific antipsychotic, the greatest number of DKA cases has been observed with clozapine and olanzapine. However, cases have also been reported with quetiapine, risperidone, and even aripiprazole (Guenette et al. 2013), although order or channeling effects (i.e., shifting high-risk patients to lower-risk agents) cannot be excluded.

Musculoskeletal Diseases

Osteoporosis

Schizophrenia, bipolar disorder, and MDD are associated with lower bone mineral density (BMD) and higher prevalence of osteoporosis, as well as increased fracture risk, compared with the general population (Correll et al. 2015; De Hert et al. 2016a). The etiology of BMD loss in these patients is complex and multifactorial. Risk factors related to the patients' lifestyle (e.g., smoking, reduced physical activity, alcohol abuse, vitamin D and calcium deficiency, polydipsia), as well as the use of psychotropic medication, are likely to be involved (De Hert et al. 2016a; Schweiger et al. 2018).

Most meta-analyses, reviews, and individual studies have found that antipsychotic use is associated with an increased risk of fracture in people with schizophrenia (ORs between 1.2 and 2.6) (Lee et al. 2017). Several side effects of antipsychotics, including sedation, somnolence, extrapyramidal symptoms, and orthostatic hypotension, may lead to an elevated risk of fracture. In addition, an elevated serum prolactin level has been considered to be one of the causal factors of bone fracture. Although long-standing raised prolactin levels induced by antipsychotics can have an impact directly (on human osteoblasts) or indirectly (in the presence of hypogonadism) on the rate of bone metabolism and have been found to be associated with decreased BMD in both female and male subjects, to date, clinical data remain limited and inconsistent, precluding definitive conclusions concerning the relationship between hyperprolactinemia, antipsychotics, and osteoporosis. Moreover, increased prolactin levels also have been found in both male and female antipsychotic-naive patients with schizophrenia or related disorders, compared with control subjects, making the interpretation of research data even more complicated (De Hert et al. 2016a; González-Blanco et al. 2016). Compared with SGAs, a higher fracture risk was found for FGAs in several meta-analyses, possibly due to their higher risk of extrapyramidal symptoms causing gait disturbances and impairing mobility and balance, which are risk factors for falls (and, thus, fractures), particularly in older adults. However, other studies found no significant differences between FGAs and SGAs or confirmed that fracture risk exists among both FGAs and SGAs (Lee et al. 2017). Moreover, it is also unclear whether individual antipsychotics differ in the risk of falls or fractures.

Although the relationship between the use of antidepressant medication and the development of osteoporosis and resultant fracture remains controversial, most reviews, meta-analyses, and large-scale studies suggest that antidepressants, especially those with serotonergic properties such as SSRIs, are associated with decreased BMD and increased fracture risk, particularly in older adults and with increasing dose (Correll et al. 2015; Schweiger et al. 2018; Zhou et al. 2018). The effect of SSRIs on bone formation and resorption appears to be governed by the activation of a number of 5-HT receptors on osteoblasts (decreasing the proliferation of osteoblasts) and osteoclasts (increasing bone resorption) via endocrine, autocrine/paracrine, and neuronal pathways (Correll et al. 2015).

The current evidence suggests that anticonvulsant mood stabilizers (e.g., carbamazepine, valproate), particularly in the setting of polypharmacy, chronic use, or high doses, can have a detrimental effect on bone health through a reduction in serum vitamin D and impaired calcium absorption. There is insufficient evidence to suggest a negative impact of lithium on bone health. Moreover, a recent systematic review and meta-analysis even suggests that lithium may be associated with a reduced fracture risk (Liu et al. 2019).

Childhood and adolescence are critical periods for healthy bone formation, and impaired bone acquisition during this time can lead to longstanding reduction in BMD. Compared with the rather well-established relationship in the elderly population, in youth the association between SSRI use and decreased BMD is less clear, with conflicting evidence (Calarge et al. 2017). However, in light of the evidence indicating that longer treatment duration with SSRIs may be more problematic in terms of bone health, it is reasonable to attempt to limit duration of this treatment where possible in this vulnerable population. Most anticonvulsant mood stabilizers (lamotrigine is an exception) exert a negative impact on bone health in youth. Although available evidence suggests a likely negative effect, studies examining the effects of antipsychotics on bone health in youth are scarce.

Respiratory Tract Diseases

One century ago, respiratory diseases such as pneumonia and tuberculosis accounted for the majority of deaths among people with SMI who lived in institutions. Although health care quality has improved globally since then, findings suggest that these diseases are still a vital clinical concern requiring close attention in people with SMI. Today, respiratory diseases (i.e., pneumonia, chronic obstructive pulmonary disease, chronic bronchitis, pleural empyema) are still more prevalent in these individuals, compared with the general population, and among the most common causes of death. In addition, use of psychotropic medication is a risk factor for respiratory tract diseases (Haga et al. 2018).

Pneumonia

A dose-dependent increased risk for pneumonia is associated with current use of SGAs in patients with schizophrenia (Haga et al. 2018) and bipolar disorder (Yang et al. 2013). Similarly, in elderly patients without an SMI, current use of SGAs and FGAs seems to be associated with a dose-dependent increase in the risk for pneumonia (Correll et al. 2015). A recent analysis showed that the use of SGAs (OR=2.7, 95% CI: 1.0–17.7; P=0.046), as well as large doses (total chlorpromazine equivalent dose ≥600 mg) of antipsychotics (OR=2.6, 95%CI: 1.7–4.0; P<0.001), more than advanced age and smoking habit, is a significant risk factor for pneumonia in people with schizophrenia (Haga et al. 2018). In patients with schizophrenia and those with bipolar disorder, the current use of clozapine in particular is associated with an elevated and dose-dependent risk of pneumonia compared with no current use of antipsychotics; this risk is generally lower for olanzapine, quetiapine, and risperidone (Kuo et al. 2013; Yang et al. 2013).

No increased risk of pneumonia with antidepressants has been found in most studies (Correll et al. 2015). There also seems to be no significant association between mood stabilizers and pneumonia, and lithium even has a dose-dependent protective effect. However, the combination of mood stabilizers and SGAs or FGAs can be associated with an increased risk. Among drug combinations, olanzapine plus carbamazepine seems to have the highest risk (adjusted risk ratio [ARR]=11.88, P<0.01), followed by clozapine plus valproic acid (ARR=4.80, P<0.001) (Yang et al. 2013; Yuo).

Although further research is needed to elucidate the pathogenesis of medication-induced pneumonia, as for clozapine and olanzapine, sedation induced by H_1 antagonism (as well as the additive sedating effect by carbamazepine or valproic acid) could facilitate aspiration pneumonia. M_1 antagonism, contributing to aspiration pneumonia through swallowing problems such as esophageal dilatation and hypomotility, may further be involved. Finally, clozapine-induced sialorrhea also can lead to aspiration pneumonia (Haga et al. 2018; Yang et al. 2013).

Neoplasms

The relationship between cancer and schizophrenia still is an area of controversy. Although people with schizophrenia generally show higher rates of smoking, substance use, obesity, and an unhealthy diet, as well as lower rates of physical activity (all independent risk factors for the development of cancer), lower overall incidence cancer rates than those in the general population have been reported (Kisely et al. 2016; Xu et al. 2017). It therefore has been suggested that some of the etiological factors predisposing to schizophrenia are protective against the development of cancer. However, most cancers accumulate with age, and people with SMI die on average 10–20 years earlier than the general population (De Hert et al. 2011a). Moreover, gender and type of cancer are two important confounding factors contributing to the heterogeneity that require adjustment in cancer incidence meta-analyses (Li et al. 2018). All these factors explain why findings remain inconclusive, with meta-analyses documenting increased (Catalá-López et al. 2014; Zhuo et al. 2017), decreased (Xu et al. 2017), and no difference (Catalá-López et al. 2014) in cancer risk in patients with schizophrenia, compared with the general population. In general, patients with schizophrenia seem to have a lower incidence of many types of cancer (including prostate cancer and malignant melanoma) but are possibly at higher risk of breast cancer. No association has been found, or the data have been inconsistent, for several other types of cancer, such as brain cancer, colorectal cancer, or lung cancer (Catalá-López et al. 2014).

Breast Cancer

According to the GLOBOCAN 2018 estimates of cancer incidence and mortality, produced by the International Agency for Research on Cancer, breast cancer is the most commonly diagnosed cancer among females (accounting for almost one in four cancer cases among women) in all regions of the world (except in East Africa, where cervical cancer dominates), as well as the leading cause of cancer death in most countries. Given that women with schizophrenia have lower parity and higher frequencies of other known breast cancer risk factors (obesity, DM, unhealthy lifestyle behaviors, including alcohol dependence and smoking), one would anticipate higher breast cancer rates in this population. However, because the data are conflicting, at present, there is still no consensus on breast cancer incidence in patients with schizophrenia. Although all recent meta-analyses (e.g., Catalá-López et al. 2014) showed that the risk of patients with schizophrenia having breast cancer is higher than that of patients without schizophrenia or the general population, a substantial between-study variance is present in these analyses, making it possible that a future meta-analysis will show a decreased breast cancer risk in women with schizophrenia compared with the general population.

Increasing experimental and epidemiological data point to the influence of prolactin in mammary carcinogenesis (De Hert et al. 2016b), raising questions about the possible relationship between prolactin-raising antipsychotics and breast cancer risk. The current evidence base, however, is very limited. The majority of studies focused on patients treated with FGAs and did not find an increased breast cancer risk (De Hert et al. 2016b). An exception is the cohort study by Wang et al. (2002), in which 52,819 women taking antipsychotic dopamine antagonists were compared with 55,289 women who were not taking antipsychotics. The authors found that compared with nonusers, women who used antipsychotic dopamine antagonists had a 16% greater risk (adjusted hazard ratio=1.16, 95% CI: 1.07–1.26) of developing breast cancer, with a direct dose-response relationship. The authors noted that the magnitude of the observed risk, although statistically significant, was small in absolute terms (1,239 cases of breast cancer in the user group vs. 1,228 cases in the nonuser group). Furthermore, it was estimated that there was less than a 14% chance that a dopamine antagonist user who developed breast cancer did so on the basis of her antipsychotic use. The authors therefore concluded that their findings "do not warrant changes in patients' antipsychotic medication regimens." Among SGAs, there has been concern that risperidone, amisulpride, and paliperidone, which have been associated with hyperprolactinemia, may increase the risk of breast cancer. However, so far, results of studies involving humans generally do not suggest a clinically important association between the use of (prolactin-raising) antipsychotics and risk of breast cancer (De Hert et al. 2016b). Moreover, several reports described mechanisms of cancer protection with (prolactin-raising) antipsychotics (or antidepressants) or demonstrated the feasibility of antipsychotics (i.e., the prolactin-elevating antipsychotic olanzapine) without safety concerns in the management of chemotherapy-induced nausea and vomiting in patients with breast cancer (De Hert et al. 2016b). Finally, as for the potential mechanisms underlying the association with slightly increased breast cancer risk in women with schizophrenia that has been found in certain studies, many other factors may be involved, such as nulliparity, obesity, DM, and unhealthy lifestyle behaviors (alcohol dependence, smoking, low physical activity) (De Hert et al. 2016b). Despite this, analyses stratified by estrogen receptor status (Wang et al. 2016) showed that when a relationship was found, the observed slightly increased risk was specific to estrogen receptor + breast cancer types and was seen only with long-term use (a cumulative exposure of 10,000 mg olanzapine equivalents) of prolactin-raising antipsychotics.

There have also long been concerns that SSRIs may promote breast cancer by increasing prolactin levels. Epidemiological studies that specifically evaluated the effect of SSRIs on cancer risk, however, yielded conflicting results. Some recent studies showed that continuous use of SSRIs might be associated with lower survival in cancer patients. SSRIs may, for example, affect cancer outcomes by interfering with tamoxifen metabolism through inhibition of the cytochrome P450 2D6 enzyme (Busby et al. 2018). Other studies or meta-analyses have found no significantly increased risk for breast or other types of cancer after SSRI exposure or even have demonstrated a possible protective effect of SSRIs against cancers of the breast (and colon or liver) (Boursi et al. 2018). Also, no increased risk of subsequent breast cancer was observed in women who concurrently used tamoxifen and antidepressants, including paroxetine (Haque et al. 2015). Moreover, positive findings must be interpreted with caution because they are particularly vulnerable to confounding by indication (i.e., depression), meaning that SSRI users already have a higher underlying risk of mortality than nonusers.

Other Physical Diseases
Kidney Diseases

Lithium treatment can be associated with severe renal side effects. It causes three types of renal impairment: acute kidney injury, nephrogenic diabetes insipidus, and chronic kidney disease (CKD) (Alsady et al. 2016; Shine et al. 2015). Acute kidney injury has been described in lithium intoxication. Because the toxic concentrations for lithium (≥ 1.5 mEq/L or mmol/L) are close to the therapeutic range (0.8–1.2 mEq/L or mmol/L), lithium toxicity can occur at doses close to those that produce therapeutic concentrations, particularly in patients who are abnormally sensitive to lithium. Within days to weeks following administration of lithium at therapeutic doses, up to 40% of patients exhibit some degree of polyuria, occasionally leading to nephrogenic diabetes insipidus, which is characterized by polyuria, dehydration, thirst, and compensatory polydipsia (Alsady et al. 2016). According to the International Group for The Study of Lithium Treated Patients, approximately 25% of patients on medium-term lithium therapy (<15 years), as well as most patients on long-term lithium treatment (>15 years), develop some form of chronic lithium nephropathy (Kampf 2018). However, this condition manifests primarily as impaired urinary concentration with or without polyuria, which generally has little clinical relevance. Although an earlier meta-analysis (which included very short-term studies) reported that lithium use does not cause CKD, a more recent analysis by the same research group showed that lithium appears to have the ability to cause at least stage 3 CKD (Shine et al. 2015). Kidney failure or end-stage renal disease (stage 5) due to the use of lithium, however, remains an uncommon complication (Aiff et al. 2015; Davis et al. 2018; Shine et al. 2015). End-stage renal failure only starts appearing in some patients after continuous treatment for more than 15–20 years. As of this writing, there is no evidence to regard renal tumor development as a side effect of long-term lithium use (Alsady et al. 2016; Kessing et al. 2015).

Polypharmacy and medical morbidities, which are quite common in the elderly, as well as the use of higher maintenance doses than those recommended and inadequate lithium monitoring, are all precipitating factors for acute lithium toxicity, which increases the long-term risk of CKD. Despite concerns regarding the vulnerability of older adults to lithium toxicity, there is no compelling evidence to suggest that lithium should be avoided in these patients when the above-mentioned risk factors are taken into account. Identification of the potential causal effect of lithium remains difficult because bipolar disorder itself is associated with CKD independent of drug treatment. DM and CVDs (potentially leading to end-stage renal failure) are increased in patients with bipolar disorder, compared with the general population, and as such can be confounding factors. Moreover, lithium seems to have paradoxical effects on the kidney: whereas long-term exposure to higher doses of lithium may be nephrotoxic, short-term low doses of lithium may have a kidney-protective effect (Alsady et al. 2016).

The use of antipsychotics or antidepressants seems not to be associated with CKD.

Case Vignette 5[6]

An 18-year-old woman with borderline personality, anxiety disorder, and depression was referred to our hospital with nephrotic syndrome and acute kidney injury with anuria. Her current medication, included lithium carbonate, amitriptyline, quetiapine, and zolpidem. She had been receiving lithium treatment for 2 years. Her serum lithium levels and renal functions had been repeatedly within the normal range. On initial examination, serum lithium value was 1.88 mmol/L. Fractional excretion of urea was 9%, suggesting the prerenal etiology of acute kidney injury. A percutaneous kidney biopsy was performed and revealed minimal change disease. Lithium

---

[6]Adapted from case described in Zieg J, Simankova N, Hradsky O, et al.: "Nephrotic Syndrome and Acute Kidney Injury in a Patient Treated With Lithium Carbonate." *Australas Psychiatry* 22(6):591–592, 2014.

therapy was discontinued, and symptomatic management with fluid restriction and electrolyte and albumin infusions along with diuretics was initiated. Serum lithium levels were regularly assessed. The patient finally went into full remission 31 days after lithium treatment discontinuation. This was the first time that lithium was not detected in the serum of the patient.

Diseases of the Endocrine System

Lithium is also associated with hypothyroidism (Shine et al. 2015). According to the International Group for The Study of Lithium Treated Patients, approximately 10%–20% of patients receiving lithium treatment have latent/subclinical hypothyroidism (i.e., a greater than normal increase in thyroid-stimulating hormone production) (Bschor et a. 2018).

Hematological Diseases

Leukocytopenia and Agranulocytosis

Antipsychotics, antidepressants (e.g., clomipramine and imipramine), and mood stabilizers (especially carbamazepine) have been associated with leukocytopenia and agranulocytosis.

A recent meta-analysis (reporting data on more than 450,000 people, collected over four decades) suggested that 3.9% of patients exposed to clozapine will develop mild neutropenia (with an absolute neutrophil count [ANC] of <1,500/μL) (Myles et al. 2018). The incidence of clozapine-associated severe neutropenia (with an ANC of <500/μL) was 0.7%. Most cases of severe clozapine-associated neutropenia occur during the first 12 months of treatment. The risk for severe neutropenia drops to negligible levels thereafter. Death from clozapine-associated neutropenia is rare, occurring in only 1 in 7,700 people exposed (Myles et al. 2018). These results have been confirmed by another, more recent meta-analysis (Li et al. 2020). There is a widespread assumption that clozapine has specific, causal, and clinically important hematological risks that do not apply to other antipsychotic medications. However, a recent meta-analysis of data from controlled trials suggests there is no statistically significant increased relative risk of neutropenia associated with clozapine compared with other antipsychotic medications (Myles et al. 2019).

Clinical Guidelines

Given that the individual components of metabolic syndrome are critical in predicting the morbidity and mortality of CVDs, DM, cancer, and other related diseases, they should be checked at baseline and measured regularly thereafter (Maj et al. 2020, 2021).

Clinicians should monitor the weight of every patient at every visit. However, assessment of central/abdominal adiposity, by measuring waist circumference, has a stronger correlation with insulin resistance and better predicts future DM and CVDs than total body weight or body mass index. This assessment can easily be done with a simple and inexpensive waist tape measure.

Because the cost for measuring is low and hypertension is a risk factor for CVDs, blood pressure ought to be assessed routinely. Importantly, at least two separate, independent measurements are required for the diagnosis of elevated blood pressure/hypertension. Moreover, out-of-office measurements are recommended to confirm this diagnosis.

Finger prick tests should be carried out at baseline and after 3 months to capture early cases of hyperglycemia and then, at a minimum, yearly. Ideally, blood glucose measurement should be conducted in the fasting state because this is the most sensitive measurement for the detection of developing glucose abnormalities. Conventional tests for screening hyperglycemia are the fasting plasma glucose test, the oral glucose tolerance test, and the glycosylated hemoglobin (HbA1c) test.

Lipid parameters, especially triglycerides and HDL cholesterol, should also be assessed at baseline and at 3 months, with 12-month assessments thereafter. More frequent screening is unnecessary, unless in case of abnormal values. Fasting is not routinely required for the determination of a lipid profile.

Clinicians who provide care to people with SMI should understand the clinical features of DM and be able to identify potential life-threatening episodes. The clinician should check whether patients have significant risk factors (i.e., family history, body mass index ≥25, waist circumference above critical values).

Whatever psychotropic medication a psychiatrist is intending to prescribe, patients should be asked about heart risks, such as family history of early cardiac death (i.e., <50 years in men and <55 years in women) or sudden death, personal history of a heart murmur, previous prescription of cardiac medications or antihypertensives, or whether they have ever had an episode of simple syncope. A baseline ECG is especially important in patients with clinical risk factors for arrhythmias—that is, those with a family history of early cardiac death, personal history of a heart murmur, hypertension or DM, tachycardia at rest, and irregular heartbeats and fainting spells, particularly upon exertion. As a general rule, every patient should have an ECG performed before psychotropic drugs that have been associated with QTc prolongation are prescribed. A routine ECG during the administration of these drugs also is recommended. Antipsychotics or antidepressants known to be associated with QTc prolongation should not be prescribed for SMI patients with known heart disease, a personal history of syncope, a family history of SCD at an early age (especially if both parents had SCD), or congenital long QT syndrome. Withdrawal of any offending drugs and correction of electrolyte abnormalities are recommended in patients presenting with TdP.

Because regular lithium level monitoring may protect against acute and chronic renal failure, it should be mandatory in long-term lithium-treated patients. Patients treated with clozapine need special monitoring.

If DM or another severe physical illness has been diagnosed, patients with SMI should be referred to specialist services, including diabetology, endocrinology, and cardiology, to receive the appropriate health care.

Key Points

- Patients with SMI are at increased risk for physical diseases and related premature mortality.

- Besides mental illness–related factors, disparities in health care access and utilization, and unhealthy lifestyle, psychotropic medications can contribute to the emergence or aggravation of physical diseases.

- In general, adverse effects on physical health are greatest with antipsychotics, followed by mood stabilizers and antidepressants. However, effects vary greatly among individual agents, and interactions with underlying host factors are relevant.

- Higher dosages, polypharmacy, and the treatment of vulnerable (e.g., old or young) people seem to be associated with a greater effect on most physical diseases.

- The screening, assessment, and management of physical health aspects in patients with SMI remain poor, even in developed countries. One important reason for this is that most psychiatrists remain focused on their own specialty. Doctors who pursue a career in psychiatry, however, not only should be educated and trained to recognize physical illness, but also should take the lead responsibility to properly monitor the physical health of these vulnerable patients, at least for the first 12 months or until the patient's condition has stabilized. Thereafter, primary care providers should assume that responsibility, unless there are particular reasons for remaining with secondary care.

References

Aiff H, Attman PO, Aurell M, et al: Effects of 10 to 30 years of lithium treatment on kidney function. J Psychopharmacol 29(5):608–614, 2015

Alsady M, Baumgarten R, Deen PM, et al: Lithium in the kidney: friend and foe? J Am Soc Nephrol 27(6):1587–1595, 2016

Alves BB, Oliveira GP, Moreira Neto MG, et al: Use of atypical antipsychotics and risk of hypertension: a case report and review literature. SAGE Open Med Case Rep 7:2050313X19841825, 2019

Beach SR, Celano CM, Sugrue AM, et al: QT prolongation, torsades de pointes, and psychotropic medications: a 5-year update. Psychosomatics 59(2):105–122, 2018

Boursi B, Lurie I, Haynes K, et al: Chronic therapy with selective serotonin reuptake inhibitors and survival in newly diagnosed cancer patients. Eur J Cancer Care (Engl) 27(1):1–7, 2018

Bschor T, Bauer M, Albrecht J: The effects of lithium on thyroid function. International Group for the Study of Lithium-Treated Patients, 2018. Available at: www.igsli.org/general-information-on-lithium/adverse-effects-of-lithium-salts.html. Accessed 27 October 2020.

Buhagiar K, Jabbar F: Association of first- vs. second-generation antipsychotics with lipid abnormalities in individuals with severe mental illness: a systematic review and meta-analysis. Clin Drug Investig 39(3):253–273, 2019

Busby J, Mills K, Zhang SD, et al: Selective serotonin reuptake inhibitor use and breast cancer survival: a population-based cohort study. Breast Cancer Res 20:4, 2018

Calarge CA, Mills JA, Janz KF, et al: The effect of depression, generalized anxiety, and selective serotonin reuptake inhibitors on change in bone metabolism in adolescents and emerging adults. J Bone Miner Res 32(12):2367–2374, 2017

Catalá-López F, Suárez-Pinilla M, Suárez-Pinilla P, et al: Inverse and direct cancer comorbidity in people with central nervous system disorders: a meta-analysis of cancer incidence in 577,013 participants of 50 observational studies. Psychother Psychosom 83(2):89–105, 2014

Chen J, Huang XF, Shao R, et al: Molecular mechanisms of antipsychotic drug-induced diabetes. Front Neurosci 11:643, 2017

Correll CU, Galling B: Polypharmacy in youth treated with antipsychotics: do antidepressants or stimulants add to the risk for type 2 diabetes? J Am Acad Child Adolesc Psychiatry 56(8):634–635, 2017

Correll CU, Detraux J, De Lepeleire J, et al: Effects of antipsychotics, antidepressants and mood stabilizers on risk for physical diseases in people with schizophrenia, depression and bipolar disorder. World Psychiatry 14(2):119–136, 2015

Correll CU, Solmi M, Veronese N, et al: Prevalence, incidence and mortality from cardiovascular disease in patients with pooled and specific severe mental illness: a large-scale meta-analysis of 3,211,768 patients and 113,383,368 controls. World Psychiatry 16(2):163–180, 2017

Curto M, Girardi N, Lionetto L, et al: Systematic review of clozapine cardiotoxicity. Curr Psychiatry Rep 18(7):68, 2016

Davis J, Desmond M, Berk M: Lithium and nephrotoxicity: a literature review of approaches to clinical management and risk stratification. BMC Nephrol 19(1):305, 2018

De Hert M, Correll CU, Bobes J, et al: Physical illness in patients with severe mental disorders, I: prevalence, impact of medications and disparities in health care. World Psychiatry 10(1):52–77, 2011a

De Hert M, Detraux J, van Winkel R, et al: Metabolic and cardiovascular adverse effects associated with antipsychotic drugs. Nat Rev Endocrinol 8(2):114–126, 2011b

De Hert M, Detraux J, Stubbs B: Relationship between antipsychotic medication, serum prolactin levels and osteoporosis/osteoporotic fractures in patients with schizophrenia: a critical literature review. Expert Opin Drug Saf 15(6):809–823, 2016a

De Hert M, Peuskens J, Sabbe T, et al: Relationship between prolactin, breast cancer risk, and antipsychotics in patients with schizophrenia: a critical review. Acta Psychiatr Scand 133(1):5–22, 2016b

de Silva VA, Suraweera C, Ratnatunga SS, et al: Metformin in prevention and treatment of antipsychotic induced weight gain: a systematic review and meta-analysis. BMC Psychiatry 16(1):341, 2016

Devlin AM, Panagiotopoulos C: Metabolic side effects and pharmacogenetics of second-generation antipsychotics in children. Pharmacogenomics 16(9):981–996, 2015

Galling B, Calsina Ferrer A, Abi Zeid Daou M, et al: Safety and tolerability of antidepressant co-treatment in acute major depressive disorder: results from a systematic review and exploratory meta-analysis. Expert Opin Drug Saf 14(10):1587–1608, 2015

González-Blanco L, Greenhalgh AMD, Garcia-Rizo C, et al: Prolactin concentrations in antipsychotic-naïve patients with schizophrenia and related disorders: a meta-analysis. Schizophr Res 174(1–3):156–160, 2016

Guenette MD, Hahn M, Cohn TA, et al: Atypical antipsychotics and diabetic keto-acidosis: a review. Psychopharmacology (Berl) 226(1):1–12, 2013

Haga T, Ito K, Sakashita K, et al: Risk factors for pneumonia in patients with schizophrenia. Neuropsychopharmacol Rep 38(4):204–209, 2018

Hagen JM, Sutterland AL, Koeter MW, et al: Advanced glycation end products in recent-onset psychosis indicate early onset of cardiovascular risk. J Clin Psychiatry 78(9):1395–1401, 2017

Haque R, Shi J, Schottinger JE, et al: Tamoxifen and antidepressant drug interaction in a cohort of 16,887 breast cancer survivors. J Natl Cancer Inst 108(3):djv337, 2015

Huang KL, Fang CJ, Hsu CC, et al: Myocardial infarction risk and antipsychotics use revisited: a meta-analysis of 10 observational studies. J Psychopharmacol 31(12):1544–1555, 2017

Kampf D: Lithium and kidney function, in Adverse Effects of Lithium Salts. International Group for the Study of Lithium Treated Patients, 2018. Available at: www.igsli.org/general-information-on-lithium/adverse-effects-of-lithium-salts.html. Accessed June 25, 2020.

Kessing LV, Gerds TA, Feldt-Rasmussen B, et al: Lithium and renal and upper urinary tract tumors—results from a nationwide population-based study. Bipolar Disord 17(8):805–813, 2015

Kisely S, Forsyth S, Lawrence D: Why do psychiatric patients have higher cancer mortality rates when cancer incidence is the same or lower? Aust N Z J Psychiatry 50(3):254–263, 2016

Kuo CJ, Yang SY, Liao YT, et al: Second-generation antipsychotic medications and risk of pneumonia in schizophrenia. Schizophr Bull 39:648–657, 2013

Lee SH, Hsu WT, Lai CC, et al: Use of antipsychotics increases the risk of fracture: a systematic review and meta-analysis. Osteoporos Int 28(4):1167–1178, 2017

Li H, Li J, Yu X, et al: The incidence rate of cancer in patients with schizophrenia: a meta-analysis of cohort studies. Schizophr Res 195:519–528, 2018

Li XH, Zhong XM, Lu L, et al: The prevalence of agranulocytosis and related death in clozapine-treated patients: a comprehensive meta-analysis of observational studies. Psychol Med 50(4):583–594, 2020

Liu B, Wu Q, Zhang S, et al: Lithium use and risk of fracture: a systematic review and meta-analysis of observational studies. Osteoporos Int 30(2):257–266, 2019

Maj M, Stein DJ, Parker G, et al: The clinical characterization of the adult patient with depression aimed at personalization of management. World Psychiatry 19(3):269–293, 2020

Maj M, van Os J, De Hert M, et al: The clinical characterization of the adult patient with primary psychosis aimed at personalization of management. World Psychiatry 20(1), 2021

Mazereel V, Detraux J, Vancampfort D, et al: Impact of psychotropic medication effects on obesity and the metabolic syndrome in people with serious mental illness. Front Endocrinol October 9, 2020

Misiak B, Stanczykiewicz B, Łaczmanski Ł, et al: Lipid profile disturbances in antipsychotic-naive patients with first-episode non-affective psychosis: a systematic review and meta-analysis. Schizophr Res 190:18–27, 2017

Myles N, Myles H, Xia S, et al: Meta-analysis examining the epidemiology of clozapine-associated neutropenia. Acta Psychiatr Scand 138(2):101–109, 2018

Myles N, Myles H, Xia S, et al: A meta-analysis of controlled studies comparing the association between clozapine and other antipsychotic medications and the development of neutropenia. Aust N Z J Psychiatry 53(5):403–412, 2019

Patel K, Allen S, Haque MN, et al: Bupropion: a systematic review and meta-analysis of effectiveness as an antidepressant. Ther Adv Psychopharmacol 6(2):99–144, 2016

Pérez-Iglesias R, Martínez-García O, Pardo-Garcia G, et al: Course of weight gain and metabolic abnormalities in first treated episode of psychosis: the first year is a critical period for development of cardiovascular risk factors. Int J Neuropsychopharmacol 17(1):41–51, 2014

Pisano S, Catone G, Veltri S, et al: Update on the safety of second generation antipsychotics in youths: a call for collaboration among paediatricians and child psychiatrists. Ital J Pediatr 42(1):51, 2016

Roopan S, Larsen ER: Use of antidepressants in patients with depression and comorbid diabetes mellitus: a systematic review. Acta Neuropsychiatr 29(3):127–139, 2017

Salvi V, Mencacci C, Barone-Adesi F: H1-histamine receptor affinity predicts weight gain with antidepressants. Eur Neuropsychopharmacol 26(10):1673–1677, 2016

Salvi V, Grua I, Cerveri G, et al: The risk of new-onset diabetes in antidepressant users—a systematic review and meta-analysis. PLoS One 12(7):e0182088, 2017

Salvo F, Pariente A, Shakir S, et al: Sudden cardiac and sudden unexpected death related to antipsychotics: a meta-analysis of observational studies. Clin Pharmacol Ther 99(3):306–314, 2016

Schweiger JU, Schweiger U, Hüppe M, et al: The use of antidepressive agents and bone mineral density in women: a meta-analysis. Int J Environ Res Public Health 15(7):1373, 2018

Shine B, McKnight RF, Leaver L, et al: Long-term effects of lithium on renal, thyroid, and parathyroid function: a retrospective analysis of laboratory data. Lancet 386(9992):461–468, 2015

Spindelegger CJ, Papageorgiou K, Grohmann R, et al: Cardiovascular adverse reactions during antidepressant treatment: a drug surveillance report of German-speaking countries between 1993 and 2010. Int J Neuropsychopharmacol 18(4):pyu080, 2015

Undela K, Parthasarathi G, John SS: Impact of antidepressants use on risk of myocardial infarction: a systematic review and meta-analysis. Indian J Pharmacol 47(3):256–262, 2015

Vancampfort D, Vansteelandt K, Correll CU, et al: Metabolic syndrome and metabolic abnormalities in bipolar disorder: a meta-analysis of prevalence rates and moderators. Am J Psychiatry 170(3):265–274, 2013a

Vancampfort D, Wampers M, Mitchell AJ, et al: A meta-analysis of cardio-metabolic abnormalities in drug naïve, first-episode and multi-episode patients with schizophrenia versus general population controls. World Psychiatry 12(3):240–250, 2013b

Vancampfort D, Correll CU, Wampers M, et al: Metabolic syndrome and metabolic abnormalities in patients with major depressive disorder: a meta-analysis of prevalences and moderating variables. Psychol Med 44(10):2017–2028, 2014

Vancampfort D, Stubbs B, Mitchell AJ, et al: Risk of metabolic syndrome and its components in people with schizophrenia and related psychotic disorders, bipolar disorder and major depressive disorder: a systematic review and meta-analysis. World Psychiatry 14(3):339–347, 2015

Wang M, Wu X, Chai F, et al: Plasma prolactin and breast cancer risk: a meta-analysis. Sci Rep 6:25998, 2016

Wang PS, Walker AM, Tsuang MT, et al: Dopamine antagonists and the development of breast cancer. Arch Gen Psychiatry 59(12):1147–1154, 2002

Wang SM, Han C, Bahk WM, et al: Addressing the side effects of contemporary antidepressant drugs: a comprehensive review. Chonnam Med J 54(2):101–112, 2018

Xu D, Chen G, Kong L, et al: Lower risk of liver cancer in patients with schizophrenia: a systematic review and meta-analysis of cohort studies. Oncotarget 8(60):102328–102335, 2017

Yang SY, Liao YT, Liu HC, et al: Antipsychotic drugs, mood stabilizers, and risk of pneumonia in bipolar disorder: a nationwide case-control study. J Clin Psychiatry 74(1):e79–e86, 2013

Zai CC, Tiwari AK, Zai GC, et al: New findings in pharmacogenetics of schizophrenia. Curr Opin Psychiatry 31(3):200–212, 2018

Zhang Y, Liu Y, Su Y, et al: The metabolic side effects of 12 antipsychotic drugs used for the treatment of schizophrenia on glucose: a network meta-analysis. BMC Psychiatry 17(1):373, 2017

Zhou C, Fang L, Chen Y, et al: Effect of selective serotonin reuptake inhibitors on bone mineral density: a systematic review and meta-analysis. Osteoporos Int 29(6):1243–1251, 2018

Zhuo C, Tao R, Jiang R, et al: Cancer mortality in patients with schizophrenia: systematic review and meta-analysis. Br J Psychiatry 211(1):7–13, 2017

CHAPTER 7

Role of Medical Homes in Primary Care

Evelyn T. Chang, M.D., M.S.H.S.
Alexander S. Young, M.D., M.S.H.S.

In this chapter we discuss challenges to delivery of high-quality medical care to people with serious mental illness (SMI) and approaches that organizations can adopt to improve their care. There clearly are problems with traditional medical care models of delivering primary care to people with SMI. We review these problems and present alternative care models, such as the patient-centered medical home (PCMH). Although PCMH models are a promising way to integrate mental health care and primary care, they can be challenging to implement. Also, for PCMH models to be successful for people with SMI, it may be helpful to augment them with an interdisciplinary team or enrich them as a specialty medical

This work was supported by award SDP12-177 from the U.S. Department of Veterans Affairs (VA) Health Services Research and Development Service, Quality Enhancement Research Initiative; and by the VA VISN22 Mental Illness Research, Education and Clinical Center. The contents do not necessarily represent the views of affiliated institutions, the VA, or the U.S. government.

home. Although improving health care for people with SMI is not easy, we can draw on substantial experience and proven approaches that offer value to individuals with these disorders and the organizations that provide care for them.

Traditional medical care models may not be effective for many people with SMI. By *traditional medical care models*, we mean health care organized so that there are separate providers for primary care and for mental health, both of whom may or may not communicate with each other. People with SMI tend to have low levels of primary care utilization despite a need for routine preventive and chronic care (Druss and Walker 2011). This even occurs in integrated delivery systems with fewer barriers to access such as the Veterans Health Administration (Chwastiak et al. 2008), though disparities are smaller. Furthermore, the quality of care delivered to people with mental health conditions is clearly worse than that delivered in the general population (Druss et al. 2001).

Traditional medical models may be problematic for several reasons. Primary care providers typically have little training and experience in the treatment of SMI, and individuals with SMI experience stigma in interactions with their primary care providers at levels similar to those they experience in interactions with the general population (Institute of Medicine 2006; Lester et al. 2005). Poor primary care continuity, lack of empathy, and difficulties communicating with providers can impede building a trusting relationship between the patient and provider (Kaufman et al. 2012; Lester et al. 2005). People with SMI often have ongoing psychiatric symptoms and cognitive deficits, impaired social skills, socioeconomic disadvantages, lifestyle instability, and increased rates of substance use disorders, which limit their ability to perform self-care and adhere to recommended treatment (Dimatteo et al. 2002; Kaufman et al. 2012). Qualitative studies have found that lack of timely access to primary care or mental health care can result in higher rates of emergency department (ED) visits (Kaufman et al. 2012). Finally, coordinating and communicating between primary care and mental health care, even in integrated delivery systems, are necessary but challenging (Chang et al. 2014; Croghan and Brown 2010).

A variety of care models and interventions have been proposed or implemented with the goal of improving health outcomes among people with SMI (Collins et al. 2010; Gerrity et al. 2014). One approach is to physically co-locate mental health and primary care, either in the mental health setting (Pirraglia et al. 2011) or in the primary care setting (Pomerantz et al. 2010). Another is to fully integrate care with joint treatment planning (Collins et al. 2010). Each of these is intuitively appealing. However, these models either have not been well studied or have failed to produce substantial improvement in outcomes when formally studied (Bradford et al. 2013).

Another strategy is to have mental health providers provide guideline-concordant preventive screening and routine medical care under the supervision of an internist (World Health Organization 2018) or be identified as primary care providers themselves. These types of approaches would require mental health providers to receive considerable training and thus have rarely been implemented (Moran 2015). There is also research supporting a small number of care models that include care management (Druss et al. 2010). An understudied, yet critical, component is coordination of medical care, mental health care, and addiction care in a complex population with high levels of need in each domain and treatments that frequently interact.

Patient-Centered Medical Home Models

The PCMH is a team-based approach to primary care that emphasizes a longitudinal relationship with a primary care provider for continuous and comprehensive care; whole-person orientation, including acute, chronic, preventive, and end-of-life care; coordinated care across all health care settings and the community; enhanced access with open access and multiple communication options; and commitment to quality and safety (Table 7–1) (American Academy of Family Physicians et al. 2007). Practices that meet a set of standards may apply for certification from the National Committee for Quality Assurance (NCQA), which can provide public recognition and financial incentives (Table 7–2). Transforming a typical medical practice to a PCMH can be challenging and often requires additional resources (Rosland et al. 2013). Thus far, the PCMH has been linked to improvements in patient experience, reduced clinician burnout, decreases in ED and hospitalization rates, and cost savings (Jabbarpour et al. 2017; Nelson et al. 2014; Reid et al. 2009, 2010). People were more likely to receive preventive screenings and care for chronic health conditions through a PCMH (Jabbarpour et al. 2017).

The PCMH model may be able to address barriers to accessing and receiving high-quality primary care for patients with SMI. Most importantly, patients are impaneled to one provider, so patients are able to build a trusting relationship with one provider over time (Grumbach and Olayiwola 2015). The whole-person orientation includes a comprehensive screening for psychiatric symptoms, which may lead to more accurate psychiatric diagnosis and treatment. Providers are often trained in patient-centered communication techniques, such as motivational interviewing, to explore the patient's perspectives of illness and shared decision making. The model also includes timely access to primary care, which may decrease the number

TABLE 7–1. Features of the patient-centered medical home as defined by the Agency for Healthcare Research and Quality

Patient-centered: A partnership among practitioners, patients, and their families ensures that decisions respect patients' wants, needs, and preferences, and that patients have the education and support they need to make decisions and participate in their own care.

Comprehensive: A team of care providers is wholly accountable for a patient's physical and mental health care needs, including prevention and wellness, acute care, and chronic care.

Coordinated: Care is organized across all elements of the broader health care system, including specialty care, hospitals, home health care, community services and supports.

Accessible: Patients are able to access services with shorter waiting times, "after hours" care, 24/7 electronic or telephone access, and strong communication through health IT [information technology] innovations.

Committed to quality and safety: Clinicians and staff enhance quality improvement to ensure that patients and families make informed decisions about their health.

Source. Reprinted from the Primary Care Collaborative: "Defining the Medical Home: A Patient-Centered Philosophy That Drives Primary Care Excellence." 2020. Available at: www.pcpcc.org/about/medical-home. Accessed June 26, 2020.

of urgent care or ED visits. Finally, it involves care coordination with medical home "neighbors," which includes specialty mental health settings. Mental health clinicians, in fact, can serve as a member of the PCMH team.

PCMH models represent a promising way to integrate mental health into primary care (Croghan and Brown 2010). The PCMH is an extension of the chronic care model, a primary care–based approach to practice redesign (Bradford et al. 2013). The goal of the chronic care model is to improve health care quality through interventions at the community and health system level (i.e., self-management support, delivery system support, clinical information support) that result in productive interactions between an activated patient and a proactive clinical team (Wagner et al. 2001). Similarly, PCMHs utilize decision support tools, care coordination, self-management support, and clinical information sharing to provide high-quality, coordinated, and cost-effective care. These features usually require health information technology in order to identify patients with certain conditions and track their outcomes over time (Piette et al. 2011). Thus far, evidence has shown that the most successful models of integrating mental health into primary care use the principles of the chronic care model (Bower et al. 2006). These integrated models, also called *collaborative care*

TABLE 7–2. National Committee for Quality Assurance patient-centered medical home criteria

Team-based care and practice organization

Knowing and managing your patients

Patient-centered access and continuity

Care management and support

Care coordination and care transitions

Performance measurement and quality improvement

Source. Adapted from Jabbarpour et al. 2018.

models, have been shown to be effective and cost-effective, particularly for patients with mild to moderate depression and anxiety (Bower et al. 2006).

Evidence of PCMH model effect on people with mental health conditions is growing. Among people with mental health conditions, PCMHs seem to facilitate increased access to mental health services (Jones et al. 2015) and mental health recovery (Sklar et al. 2015). PCMHs also may reduce ED visits (Hearld et al. 2019) and improve care coordination after hospitalizations (Domino et al. 2016) in people with SMI.

It has become increasingly clear that mental health should be integrated into PCMHs. According to Croghan and Brown (2010), "Because mental health and substance use problems are among the most common conditions seen in primary care settings and frequently co-occur with other medical problems, PCPs [primary care providers] are often in the best position to identify, diagnose, and treat them. These facts alone make it clear that the PCMH will not reach its full potential without adequately addressing patients' mental health needs" (p. 13). In fact, the American Academy of Family Physicians and a number of family medicine and primary care organizations endorsed a set of joint principles that outlined a blueprint of how to incorporate behavioral health into PCMH (Baird et al. 2014).

Challenges to Patient-Centered Medical Homes

Although the importance of mental health in PCMHs is recognized, implementation can be challenging. In a survey of primary care practices certified as PCMHs by the NCQA, fewer than half had a mental health provider (often social workers in those that did) (Kessler et al. 2014). Practices were also less likely to have care coordination procedures and referrals for mental health and substance use services compared with other medical subspecialties (Kessler et al. 2014). A little more than half (54%) used evidence-based health behavior protocols for mental health and substance use disorders (Kessler et al. 2014). Main barriers to integrating mental health into PCMHs included lack of reimbursement for mental health care that is provided in primary care (91% of practices), limited time (92%), and limited expertise (74%). Lack of access to psychiatrists in the community remains a prevalent problem. Also, despite practice redesign and PCMH features, people with SMI still do not seem to utilize medical homes as much as the general population (Lichstein et al. 2014). Furthermore, primary care providers may be uncomfortable managing people with psychiatric symptoms and need further training to deliver mental health treatment in PCMHs (Croghan and Brown 2010; Lester et al. 2005). As a result, the effect of the PCMH on preventive care and health care quality may be limited among people with SMI (Alakeson et al. 2010). Other models beyond the PCMH may be needed for people with SMI.

Augmentation of Patient-Centered Medical Homes

Medical homes can be augmented with interdisciplinary team members for complex, high-need patients. This has been referred to as "intensive primary care" (Chang et al. 2017; Edwards et al. 2017). In this model, the primary care provider offers comprehensive and longitudinal care for the patient but uses an interdisciplinary team for time-limited intensive case management. Members of these interdisciplinary intensive primary care teams thought to be critical include social workers and mental health clinicians (Chang et al. 2017). There is also emerging experience suggesting that peer support specialists may have roles in assisting patients with health care navigation, education, and coaching. Features of intensive primary care include comprehensive patient assessment and evaluation, preventive home visits, health coaching, transitional care management posthospitalization, caregiver education and support, advanced care planning, and medication management. Rigorous evaluations have shown that intensive primary care teams may increase patient engagement in outpatient care and trust in their health care providers and support PCMH teams at no greater cost to the health care system (Yoon et al. 2018; Zulman et al. 2019).

Medical Care Management

There have been studies of the use of medical care management to improve medical care in people with SMI. Care management includes ongoing monitoring of basic health indicators and proactive provision of preventive services, based on established medical guidelines. One study examined a medical care management program at a Veterans Affairs medical center and found that compared with usual care, care management increased use of primary care, improved 15 of 17 preventive measures, and improved health at no additional total cost (Druss et al. 2001). Another study compared care management with usual care for homeless people with SMI and found that those treated in integrated care were more rapidly enrolled in primary care, received more preventive services, made more primary care visits, and made fewer ED visits (McGuire et al. 2009). Another study, called Primary Care Access, Referral, and Evaluation (PCARE), a controlled trial of medical care management at a large urban mental health clinic, found an increase in preventive services from 22% to 59%; substantial improvements in cardiometabolic treatments, cardiovascular risk, and health-related quality of life; and a significant reduction in total treatment costs (Druss et al. 2010, 2011). A systematic review of this area (Gerrity et al. 2014) concluded that medical care management improves both mental health outcomes and use of preventive medical services by adults with SMI.

Specialty Medical Homes

Specialty medical homes may be an alternative to PCMH models (Alakeson et al. 2010; Perrin et al. 2018; Young et al. 2018). These medical homes have a structure and features similar to those of the PCMH (Table 7–1), such as continuity with a single provider, comprehensive care, supports for access, and coordinated care. In addition, specialty medical homes generally include increased primary care provider training, additional resources to meet the patients' needs (i.e., specialists as part of the health care team, more time to spend with patients or decreased panel sizes), and joint treatment planning. These models, however, are newer enhancements of the PCMH and have not been studied as extensively as traditional PCMH models.

In one type of specialty medical home, the primary care provider and mental health provider are part of an interdisciplinary team that formulates treatment plans together. In the Veterans Health Administration, this type of team has been widely deployed for homeless veterans, many of whom have SMIs and substance use disorders (Gabrielian et al. 2014). The core PCMH team includes a primary care provider with expertise in homeless populations, mental health provider, nurse care manager, and social worker who offer intensive management. Team members meet regularly to discuss clinical cases. Thus far, observational studies suggest that this model can successfully engage homeless people in primary care and mental health care

(O'Toole et al. 2016). Participants report better experiences with this model than the usual PCMH model, particularly in their ability to communicate with providers, the extent to which providers pay attention to mental health, and courteousness of the staff (Jones et al. 2019). They also received more preventive screenings and have improved outcomes of chronic medical conditions and decreased hospitalizations and ED visits compared with homeless people in the usual PCMH model (O'Toole et al. 2016, 2018).

In another type of specialty medical home, a primary care provider and nurse care manager are trained to manage both the chronic medical conditions *and* the chronic, stable SMIs under the supervision of a psychiatrist (Young et al. 2018). This model emphasizes a recovery-oriented approach, and people with stable mental health symptoms experience primary care that is tailored to their mental health needs (Chang et al. 2019). The primary care provider is trained in motivational interviewing and has weekly case conferences with the supervising psychiatrist. The nurse care manager performs proactive care management through population registries and dashboards. Additionally, the nurse care manager provides case management for people who are highly complex.

Case Study

A community-based health center has been having difficulty providing effective services to high-risk, high-need patients because of serious mental health and addiction issues in many patients. The staff have heard that it is possible to develop specialized, evidence-based, collaborative care services for patients with SMI. They engage a consulting psychiatrist and begin to transform one of their teams into a PCMH for SMI. The psychiatrist begins discussions with center leadership and weekly meetings with the SMI team. A registry of patients is developed. Patients are selected to transfer to the team based on having demonstrated high medical need and known psychosis, bipolar disorder, or persistent major depression. The psychiatrist uses the established collaborative care model to provide services. Services are billed using collaborative care model or behavioral health integration CPT codes at federally qualified health centers and rural health clinics, for payers that allow such codes (Medicare and some commercial payers and Medicaid plans). Patients are tracked for progress using the registry. The psychiatrist meets weekly with the primary care physician and nurse to consult regarding patients and review the registry for complex patients. The psychiatrist is also available between meetings. Patient psychiatric outcomes are monitored using validated rating scales. The psychiatrist coordinates care with other mental health providers and organizations; recommends changes in treatment, including medications; and trains and supervises clinic staff in the provision of behavioral activation, motivational interviewing, and other focused treatment strategies.

Key Points

- Many different care models have been implemented for people with serious mental illness (SMI).
  - Patient-centered medical home (PCMH) models may offer more helpful features for people with mental health conditions than traditional medical models, particularly continuity with a single provider, comprehensiveness, and improved access. This form of care has been linked to increased preventive screenings, improved patient experiences, improved health care quality, and decreased health care costs.
  - Augmented PCMH models or specialty medical homes may be beneficial for people with SMI.
- Future research could focus on adaptations of these care models and on how to match people with appropriate care models and interventions, given the reality of costs and constrained resources.
  - Little is known about which types of people benefit from a PCMH versus a specialty medical home.
  - Some attributes of the specialty medical home could be feasible in a PCMH, such as mental health integration with regular interdisciplinary treatment planning.
  - Strategies to engage people with mental health conditions to ensure access to and use of primary care could be investigated for feasibility and potential dissemination to a PCMH.
  - Use of virtual modalities such as live video telehealth could increase mental health care capacity for medical homes given the limited number and distribution of mental health providers.
- Enough evidence exists that we can implement effective care models and practices to improve medical care for people with SMI.
  - Evidence-based practices exist for mental health assessments and management within primary care and care coordination between primary care and mental health providers.
  - Implementation strategies can train primary care providers in the assessment and management of mental health conditions.

- Implementation approaches can train mental health providers in preventive screenings and management of chronic medical conditions and provide strategies for integrating mental health within primary care.

References

Alakeson V, Frank RG, Katz RE: Specialty care medical homes for people with severe, persistent mental disorders. Health Aff (Millwood) 29(5):867–873, 2010

American Academy of Family Physicians, American Academy of Pediatrics, American College of Physicians, American Osteopathic Association: Joint principles of the patient-Centered medical home. March 2007. Available at: www.aafp.org/dam/AAFP/documents/practice_management/pcmh/initiatives/PCMHJoint.pdf. Accessed June 26, 2020.

Baird M, Blount A, Brungardt S, et al: Joint principles: integrating behavioral health care into the patient-centered medical home. Ann Fam Med 12(2):183–185, 2014

Bower P, Gilbody S, Richards D, et al: Collaborative care for depression in primary care. Making sense of a complex intervention: systematic review and meta-regression. Br J Psychiatry 189:484–493, 2006

Bradford DW, Cunningham NT, Slubicki MN, et al: An evidence synthesis of care models to improve general medical outcomes for individuals with serious mental illness: a systematic review. J Clin Psychiatry 74(8):e754–e764, 2013

Chang ET, Wells KB, Young AS, et al: The anatomy of primary care and mental health clinician communication: a quality improvement case study. J Gen Intern Med 29 (suppl 2):S598–S606, 2014

Chang ET, Raja PV, Stockdale SE, et al: What are the key elements for implementing intensive primary care? A multisite Veterans Health Administration case study. Healthc (Amst) 6(4):231–237, 2017

Chang ET, Vinzon M, Cohen AN, et al: Effective models urgently needed to improve physical care for people with serious mental illnesses. Health Serv Insights 12:1178632919837628, 2019

Chwastiak LA, Rosenheck RA, Kazis LE: Utilization of primary care by veterans with psychiatric illness in the national Department of Veterans Affairs health care system. J Gen Intern Med 23(11):1835–1840, 2008

Collins C, Hewson DL, Munger R, et al: Evolving Models of Behavioral Health Integration in Primary Care. New York, Milbank Memorial Fund, 2010

Croghan TW, Brown JD: Integrating Mental Health Treatment Into the Patient Centered Medical Home (AHRQ Publ No 10-0084-EF). Rockville, MD, Agency for Healthcare Research and Quality, June 2010

Dimatteo MR, Giordani PJ, Lepper HS, et al: Patient adherence and medical treatment outcomes: a meta-analysis. Med Care 40(9):794–811, 2002

Domino ME, Jackson C, Beadles CA, et al: Do primary care medical homes facilitate care transitions after psychiatric discharge for patients with multiple chronic conditions? Gen Hosp Psychiatry 39:59–65, 2016

Druss BG, Walker ER: Mental Disorders and Medical Comorbidity (Research Synthesis Report No 21). Robert Wood Johnson Foundation, 2011. Available at: www.rwjf.org/content/dam/farm/reports/issue_briefs/2011/rwjf69438/subassets/rwjf69438_1. Accessed June 26, 2020.

Druss BG, Bradford WD, Rosenheck RA, et al: Quality of medical care and excess mortality in older patients with mental disorders. Arch Gen Psychiatry 58(6):565–572, 2001

Druss BG, Von Esenwein SA, Compton MT, et al: A randomized trial of medical care management for community mental health settings: the Primary Care Access, Referral, and Evaluation (PCARE) study. Am J Psychiatry 167(2):151–159, 2010

Druss BG, Von Esenwein SA, Compton MT, et al: Budget impact and sustainability of medical care management for persons with serious mental illnesses. Am J Psychiatry 168(11):1171–1178, 2011

Edwards ST, Peterson K, Chan B, et al: Effectiveness of intensive primary care interventions: a systematic review. J Gen Intern Med 32(12):1377–1386, 2017

Gabrielian S, Gordon A, Gelberg L, et al: Primary care medical services for homeless veterans. Fed Pract 31(10):10–19, 2014

Gerrity M, Zoller E, Pinson N, et al: Integrating Primary Care Into Behavioral Health Settings: What Works for Individuals With Serious Mental Illness. New York, Milbank Memorial Fund, 2014

Grumbach K, Olayiwola JN: Patient empanelment: the importance of understanding who is at home in the medical home. J Am Board Fam Med 28(2):170–172, 2015

Hearld KR, Hearld LR, Landry AY, et al: Evidence that patient-centered medical homes are effective in reducing emergency department admissions for patients with depression. Health Serv Manage Res 32(1):26–35, 2019

Institute of Medicine: Improving the Quality of Health Care for Mental and Substance-Use Conditions. Washington, DC, National Academies Press, 2006

Jabbarpour Y, DeMarchis E, Bazemore A, et al: The Impact of Primary Care Practice Transformation on Cost, Quality, and Utilization: A Systematic Review of Research Published in 2016. Washington, DC, Patient-Centered Primary Care Collaborative and Robert Graham Center, 2017

Jabbarpour Y, Coffman M, Habib A, et al: Advanced Primary Care: A Key Contributor to Successful ACOs. Patient-Centered Primary Care Collaborative, August 2018. Table 4: Comparison NCQA 2017 PCMH and CPC + Requirements: Summary Table. Available at: www.pcpcc.org/sites/default/files/resources/PCPCC%202018%20Evidence%20Report.pdf. Accessed June 26, 2020.

Jones AL, Cochran SD, Leibowitz A, et al: Usual primary care provider characteristics of a patient-centered medical home and mental health service use. J Gen Intern Med 30(12):1828–1836, 2015

Jones AL, Hausmann LRM, Kertesz SG, et al: Providing positive primary care experiences for homeless veterans through tailored medical homes: the Veterans Health Administration's Homeless Patient Aligned Care Teams. Med Care 57(4):270–278, 2019

Kaufman EA, Mcdonell MG, Cristofalo MA, et al: Exploring barriers to primary care for patients with severe mental illness: frontline patient and provider accounts. Issues Ment Health Nurs 33(3):172–180, 2012

Kessler R, Miller BF, Kelly M, et al: Mental health, substance abuse, and health behavior services in patient-centered medical homes. J Am Board Fam Med 27(5):637–644, 2014

Lester H, Tritter JQ, Sorohan H: Patients' and health professionals' views on primary care for people with serious mental illness: focus group study. BMJ 330(7500):1122, 2005

Lichstein JC, Domino ME, Beadles CA, et al: Use of medical homes by patients with comorbid physical and severe mental illness. Med Care 52 (suppl 3):S85–S91, 2014

McGuire J, Gelberg L, Blue-Howells J, et al: Access to primary care for homeless veterans with serious mental illness or substance abuse: a follow-up evaluation of co-located primary care and homeless social services. Adm Policy Ment Health 36(4):255–264, 2009

Moran M: Board approves statement on role in reducing physical health disparities. Psychiatric News, September 2015

Nelson KM, Helfrich C, Sun H, et al: Implementation of the patient-centered medical home in the Veterans Health Administration: associations with patient satisfaction, quality of care, staff burnout, and hospital and emergency department use. JAMA Intern Med 174(8):1350–1358, 2014

O'Toole TP, Johnson EE, Aiello R, et al: Tailoring care to vulnerable populations by incorporating social determinants of health: the Veterans Health Administration's "Homeless Patient Aligned Care Team" program. Prev Chronic Dis 13:E44, 2016

O'Toole TP, Johnson EE, Borgia M, et al: Population-tailored care for homeless veterans and acute care use, cost, and satisfaction: a prospective quasi-experimental trial. Prev Chronic Dis 15:E23, 2018

Perrin J, Reimann B, Capobianco J, et al: A model of enhanced primary care for patients with severe mental illness. N C Med J 79(4):240–244, 2018

Piette JD, Holtz B, Beard AJ, et al: Improving chronic illness care for veterans within the framework of the patient-centered medical home: experiences from the Ann Arbor Patient-Aligned Care Team Laboratory. Transl Behav Med 1(4):615–623, 2011

Pirraglia PA, Kilbourne AM, Lai Z, et al: Colocated general medical care and preventable hospital admissions for veterans with serious mental illness. Psychiatr Serv 62(5):554–557, 2011

Pomerantz A, Shiner B, Watts B, et al: The White River model of colocated collaborative care: a platform for mental and behavioral health care in the medical home. Fam Syst Health 28(2):114–129, 2010

Reid RJ, Fishman PA, Yu O, et al: Patient-centered medical home demonstration: a prospective, quasi-experimental, before and after evaluation. Am J Manag Care 15(9):e71–e87, 2009

Reid RJ, Coleman K, Johnson EA, et al: The Group Health medical home at year two: cost savings, higher patient satisfaction, and less burnout for providers. Health Aff (Millwood) 29(5):835–843, 2010

Rosland AM, Nelson K, Sun H, et al: The patient-centered medical home in the Veterans Health Administration. Am J Manag Care 19(7):e263–e272, 2013

Sklar M, Aarons GA, O'Connell M, et al: Mental health recovery in the patient-centered medical home. Am J Public Health 105(9):1926–1934, 2015

Wagner E, Austin B, Davis C, et al: Improving chronic illness care: translating evidence into action. Health Aff (Millwood) 20(6):64–78, 2001

World Health Organization: Management of Physical Health Conditions in Adults With Severe Mental Disorders. Geneva, World Health Organization, 2018

Yoon J, Chang E, Rubenstein LV, et al: Impact of primary care intensive management on high-risk veterans' costs and utilization: a randomized quality improvement trial. Ann Intern Med 168(12):846–854, 2018

Young AS, Cohen AN, Chang ET, et al: A clustered controlled trial of the implementation and effectiveness of a medical home to improve health care of people with serious mental illness: study protocol. BMC Health Serv Res 18(1):428, 2018

Zulman DM, Chang ET, Wong A, et al: Effects of intensive primary care on high-need patient experiences: survey findings from a Veterans Affairs randomized quality improvement trial. J Gen Intern Med 34 (suppl 1):75–81, 2019

CHAPTER 8

Shared Decision Making

Karina J. Powell, Ph.D.
Patrick W. Corrigan, Psy.D.

Shared decision making represents a paradigm shift away from paternalistic medical models and toward patient involvement in their own medical care. This approach is characterized by bidirectional exchange of information followed by dynamic interactional deliberation to achieve mutual agreement regarding treatment decisions (Charles et al. 1999). This model recognizes and draws on the extensive medical proficiency of providers, while also respecting the patient's expertise regarding one's own personal values, preferences, and goals in the negotiation of treatment options.

In this chapter, we review the origins of shared decision making emerging from ethical considerations and behavioral psychology, before exploring a theoretical model of shared decision making in a medical context. We then review available tools and resources for implementing and supporting this model within psychiatric practice.

A Brief History

Though the term *shared decision making* seem to have entered the medical lexicon in the early 1980s (President's Commission 1982), the conceptual foundations of mutual participation between provider and patient were first described decades prior (Szasz and Hollender 1956). This initial conceptualization of a collaborative approach to medical decision making deviated from the traditional provider-directed approach that had long been the cornerstone of medicine. Although the former approach was slow to gain traction, a number of factors came together to highlight the value of this shared health care approach in medical encounters. Amid increasing dissatisfaction with the concept of the "compliant patient," demands for patient autonomy and mutual participation increased (Brody 1980). The 1982 President's Commission for the Study of Ethical Problems in Medicine and Biomedical and Behavioral Research (President's Commission 1982) popularized the term *shared decision making* and outlined the provider's ethical responsibility to respect the autonomy and values of the individual through acknowledging self-determination and the right of the individual to engage in one's own medical decision making. As medical advancements permitted a shift from a primary focus on acute care to the provision of more long-term services for chronic conditions, the value of a shared approach to medical decision making gained support (Charles et al. 1997; Entwistle 2009; Gionfriddo et al. 2013). With a growing number of medical interventions and management options, weighing risks, benefits, and trade-offs became an increasingly complex task, compounded by psychological factors and an ethical obligation to consider individual preferences, values, and life plans (Entwistle 2009). Wennberg (1984) drew attention to the unwarranted variation in patient outcomes, attributing these differences to provider styles, furthering the rationale for shared decision making to enter common practice. He argued that "greater efforts are needed to base clinical choices more solidly on sound estimates of outcome probabilities and on values that correspond closely to patient preferences" (Wennberg 1984, p. 25).

Although the 1982 brief set forth an "appropriate ideal for patient-professional relationships" (President's Commission 1982, p. 30), a formal framework in which to employ shared decision making had yet to be developed. Charles and colleagues (1997) sought to consolidate the definition of shared decision making and establish a framework for engaging patients in health care that included the involvement of both provider and patient, the bidirectional exchange of information, and mutual understanding and consensus about preferred treatment. From this, shared decision making expanded to affect overarching care delivery, impacting not only individual patient outcomes but health care culture and policy as well (Frosch et al. 2011; Institute of Medicine 2001; Makoul and Clayman 2006).

Foundations and Ethics of Shared Decision Making

A multiyear research project conducted by the Picker Institute identified eight indicators of quality care: 1) provider respect for and consideration of patient values, preferences, and needs; 2) integrated care; 3) education and information exchange between patient and provider; 4) physical comfort achieved through health care; 5) emotional support and understanding of medical fear and anxiety; 6) involvement of the patient's support system; 7) continuity of care; and 8) overall access to care (Gerteis et al. 1993). These quality-of-care indicators highlight the importance of patient empowerment and active participation in medical decision making. Empowerment promotes self-directed engagement in care, improving health outcomes through enhancing intrinsic motivation rather than relying on external directives (Anderson and Funnell 2010). Self-determination theory provides a foundation for understanding behavior and psychological drive. Underlying this theory is the universal, innate psychological desire of the individual to satisfy the need for competence, autonomy, and relatedness (Ryan and Deci 2000).

An Evolution of Perspectives

As outlined in Figure 8–1, we provide a list of principles that represent treatment relations and decisional responsibility from relatively patriarchal notions that people failing treatment are resisting, to more partnership-centric perspectives like collaboration, encouraging the current evolution of self-determination. People who did not participate in services were believed to be *resisting* care in service of a psychodynamic process. Though these ideas may seem out of date, there are still practitioners who view working through treatment resistance as important to care (Shapiro 2009), including services for people with psychosis (Plakun 2008).

Compliance was meant as more of an objective indicator representing whether the person had taken medications or otherwise participated in the treatment as prescribed (Vuckovich 2010). Diminishing symptoms are the fundamental concern for this categorical (i.e., yes or no) approach, motivated by fears that treatment failure can lead to forms of irreversible tragedy like suicide. Concerns about compliance led researchers into a useful search for unbiased and sensitive measures of whether the person was participating in treatment as dictated by one's providers (Velligan et al. 2010). For some, compliance suggests the need for patients to concede to treatment, regardless of its impact on self-determination. Hence, strategies meant to serve compliance have included inpatient and outpatient commitment, more benign coercion (e.g., exercise of a guardian's authority), diminished personal control (e.g., committed injections of antipsychotic medication), and benevolent trickery (e.g., not sharing the full range of side effects) (Szasz 2007).

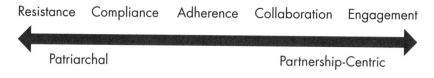

FIGURE 8–1. Progression of clinical treatment relationships and decisional responsibility.

Adherence evolved out of compliance; patients had to have active participation in treatment decisions, which was partly meant to reflect an ethical perspective, that by virtue of their humanity, patients were due agency over their lives (Rudnick 2008). However, this view also took into account recognition of years of behavioral science research; people will retreat from social exchanges where a specific behavior is forced on them (Miller and Quick 2010), resulting in an attitudinal rebound or a "don't tell me what to think" phenomenon. Adherence is a call to providers to open the floor for the active participation of patients in their own care. Providers might still dominate in developing and guiding treatment goals, but the process seeks to involve patients where possible.

Collaboration, as the natural evolution through resistance, compliance, and adherence (Corrigan et al. 1990), is the point at which shared decision making enters the relationship. Collaboration recognizes the expertise of both the provider and patient. The provider brings expertise in medicine, such as health conditions, disease course, biological processes, and available treatment options, including their risks, benefits, and side effects. Patients are experts on themselves, their own illness, and the context of their life. Their expertise also includes personal medical history, current symptoms, level of comfort with medical intervention, personal values, life goals, self-knowledge, core values, and environmental context. Collaboration elevates patients to equal status with the provider and establishes a relationship of mutual respect through which the most effective plan may be instituted.

Collaboration segued to *engagement*, which seems to be the standard in current discussions about health beliefs and decisions. The move from compliance and adherence to collaboration and engagement reflected a primary shift from outcome to process. Compliance posed outcomes as the essential value, whereas collaboration and engagement recognize the process, the environmental context, and the nature of the interactions as equally important.

The provider-patient relationship should be characterized by respect, compassion, and reciprocity in support of collaboration and engagement, encouraging self-determined health care decisions that foster well-being and growth for the empowered patient. Shared decision making is a facet of the larger concept of person-centered care that 1) identifies and builds on individual strengths and competencies in the context of environmental resources and opportunities, 2) empowers the patient to engage in self-management of medical conditions, 3) seeks collaboration and active participation, 4) recognizes degree of risk present in self-determined disease management, and 5) emphasizes the value of the patient and provider roles and partnership in medical collaboration (Charles et al. 1997; Davidson et al. 2015). In support of this, the U.S. Preventive Services Task Force suggested use of shared decision making in accordance with the ethical obligation of health care providers to protect and reinforce patient autonomy and self-determination (Sheridan et al. 2004).

Application and integration of these principles into psychiatric practice not only improves rapport but also enhances patient ownership of their own treatment. Making room in the treatment process for an approach that emphasizes collaboration and engagement empowers patients to be active participants, more comfortably sharing concerns, preferences, and other considerations that can be jointly explored and addressed throughout the course of treatment. It is important to not lose sight of the impact of the patient's contextual self—that is, the patient is the only person who is present with himself or herself every minute of every day. The patient will be the person responsible for daily management of one's care, which makes up the vast majority of the treatment process (i.e., all but the 15–60 minutes that the patient might spend in the medical office). A treatment plan that excludes the patient in the decision-making process has an increased likelihood of deteriorating once the patient leaves the psychiatrist's office, particularly if the patient has concerns or input about the plan that he or she has not had a welcoming opportunity to discuss with the provider.

Conceptual Challenges

While the cornerstones of shared decision making include understanding and collaboration, this approach does not preclude disagreement. When ideological differences become immovable barriers in achieving a mutually agreeable decision, calling on developed skills and competencies in deliberation and conflict negotiation is essential to moving the discussion forward (Towle and Godolphin 1999). Providers must cultivate an environment of comfort and compassion that encourages active patient participation (Charles et al. 1997; Towle and Godolphin 1999). Even the most well-intentioned providers may lose sight of patient self-determination and edge patients out of the decision-making process. Disproportionate concerns about treatment adherence may rob the patient of the "dignity to fail"

(Corrigan 2011) or "dignity of risk" (Townsend 2010). Attempting to make life "risk free" robs people of important prospects; for example, people do not land a better job if they do not pursue the opportunity despite the incumbent risk. The absence of clear results and uncertainty are part of what makes the pursuit of life goals a risk. Many meaningful achievements come the hard way: falling flat, picking oneself up, and moving forward. Despite this component of respect for autonomy, self-determination is not meant as carte blanche for the pursuit of goals and assumption of risk. Expecting all goals to be achievable without impact on others or regardless of real-world demands is unrealistic, and it remains the patient's responsibility to identify one's goals in the context of external pressures. Therefore, self-determination should be viewed in terms of personal responsibility and the limits experienced by most adults.

A Model of Shared Decision Making

A widely regarded model of shared decision making was developed by Charles and colleagues (1999), who describe three stages—information exchange, deliberation, and decision making—through which four core characteristics of the approach are established: 1) the provider and patient are both active participants in the decision-making process, 2) provider and patient engage in a two-way exchange of information, 3) the decision-making process is embodied by bidirectional expression of treatment preferences, and 4) consensus is achieved regarding treatment implementation (Charles et al. 1997, 1999).

Any interaction between provider and patient has two experts in the room. In the *information exchange* stage of shared decision making, these two entities share knowledge consistent with their expertise (Charles et al. 1999). This interface includes discussion of preferred roles and expectations for the patient-provider relationship to better define how the decision-making process should proceed. Available treatment options and potential outcomes are considered in the context of the knowledge of all key players in the relationship.

The *deliberation* stage of shared decision making involves interactional discussion of treatment options between provider and patient (Charles et al. 1999). The bidirectional nature of this part of the decision-making process emphasizes the investment of both parties—the patient because of personal health outcomes and the provider because of concern for the patient's well-being. Deliberation in the decision-making process involves each party articulating and negotiating treatment preferences in the context of individual values and beliefs. Decades of paternalistic medical models reinforced a power differential between provider and patient that may result in the patient's hesitation to participate. This hesitancy may be exacerbated by the provider having more familiarity with disease process and treatment outcomes, causing the patient to feel intimidated and disengage or recuse himself or herself from treatment discussions. Additionally, the patient may be concerned and anxious about the diagnosis, treatments, or prognosis, further contributing to one's withdrawal from decision making.

An added layer of complexity in this stage may arise from the inclusion of individuals beyond patient and provider. The patient may choose to involve friends or family in the deliberation process, or a provider may elect to consult with colleagues. There is variability in locus of decision making for patients of different ethnic backgrounds (Levine and Zuckerman 1999). For example, Western biomedical ethics presumes individual agency, potentially leading to the mistaken assumption that such an approach is the general preference of all patients. For some patients (whether because of age, culture, other demographics, or personal preference), family-centered decision making may be the most suitable approach. In these instances, family input should be viewed not as an impediment or barrier, but rather as valued participation that expands on the patient's expertise and autonomy.

The final stage of shared decision making is *deciding* on the preferred treatment to implement (Charles et al. 1999). Both information exchange and deliberation processes are the foundation of understanding and negotiation from which a joint decision may be reached. While the ideal scenario would result in the final treatment decision emerging clearly and unanimously, this is not always the case. These three stages are not necessarily linear in nature; for example, disagreement at the third stage may require revisiting the informational stage to share additional data (e.g., a particular side effect of a treatment, available experimental treatment options, additional patient concerns about outcomes, a patient's religious limitations) or the deliberation stage to continue negotiation and conflict resolution in the context of this new information, making the process iterative as needed.

In a meta-analytic review of shared decision-making components outlined in the research literature, Makoul and Clayman (2006) distilled essential and ideal elements of this integrative approach. Elements considered *essential* to engaging in shared decision making include clear communication of the problem, medical decision to be made, and available treatment options; consideration of individual patient preferences and desire to follow through when evaluating treatment plan viability; frequent verification of understanding of all parties involved; and mutual agreement and arranging of follow-up points of contact to track outcomes and revisit the treatment plan as needed. The *ideal* elements summarized by Makoul and Clayman

(2006) are considered to potentially enhance engagement in shared decision making but may not be essential to all encounters or situations. These ideal elements include delivery of unbiased information (i.e., if the patient desires the provider's opinion in the information exchange stage, unbiased information may not be essential to the shared decision-making process), clear defining and understanding of expectations for roles between patient and provider (i.e., in some circumstances, this information may not be known or be possible to clearly articulate during the interaction and may emerge later or not at all), and presentation of evidence regarding treatment options (i.e., this should be included when relevant evidence is available, but since adequate evidence may not be available in all circumstances, it is considered an ideal rather than essential element).

Impact of Shared Decision Making

Research has shown shared decision making to contribute to several positive outcomes, comprising affective-cognitive and interpersonal outcomes as well as patient and medical outcomes (Shay and Lafata 2015). Shared decision making has been associated with patient reports of a greater sense of personal control and empowerment in managing medical decisions (Brody et al. 1989; Johnson et al. 2012) and lower levels of persisting concern regarding illness and symptoms (Brody et al. 1989). Of benefit to patient-provider relationships is the establishment of improved interpersonal trust and greater satisfaction with perceived emotional support (Ommen et al. 2011; Sheridan et al. 2004). Shared decision making can improve patient knowledge of medical conditions, and treatment options, risks, and benefits (Sheridan et al. 2004). These educational gains lay the groundwork for improved understanding of relevant medical information and increased engagement in treatment discussions and deliberation between patient and provider.

Although shared decision making can be a more time-consuming process, such an approach improves both the process and resultant decision itself. Surveys suggest that most patients prefer to be active participants in medical decision making, though internalization of the historical patient-provider authority differential and hesitation about alienating providers may impede participation (Frosch et al. 2012). Despite these roadblocks to encouraging equal participation, shared decision-making research has demonstrated greater patient satisfaction with the decision-making process, decreased decisional conflict between patient and provider, increased patient confidence in decisions, increased patient satisfaction with decisions, and less decisional regret (Shay and Lafata 2015). Increased patient participation directly improves outcomes, including greater symptom improvement, greater improvements in overall medical condition, and improved self-care (Brody et al. 1989; Lim et al. 2012). Additionally, shared decision making has been shown to result in increased treatment engagement and adherence and greater reported satisfaction with care (Loh et al. 2007; Shay and Lafata 2015).

These improvements in relationship quality, decisional process factors, patient engagement and empowerment, and medical outcomes have been demonstrated across a broad range of chronic mental health and medical conditions, including schizophrenia, depression, cancer, diabetes, asthma, epilepsy, acquired injury, heart disease, and HIV (Shay and Lafata 2015). Chronic medical conditions and serious mental illnesses are potentially impacted by the cumulative consequences of treatment decisions and are therefore optimal for a shared decision-making approach in which the patient's long-term goals, preferences, and values can be weighed against the risks, benefits, and potential outcomes of treatment options (Gionfriddo et al. 2013). An ongoing, collaborative relationship between patient and provider is essential in this context. Though much of the research on shared decision making has been conducted on the management of chronic conditions, establishing such a partnership between provider and patient also holds utility in treatment of acute conditions, given that incorporating the necessary elements of shared decision making into medical practice regardless of disease chronicity has the potential to improve patient outcomes (Gionfriddo et al. 2013; Makoul and Clayman 2006).

Tools and Interventions to Support Shared Decision Making

As clinicians and researchers have increasingly recognized the benefits of shared decision making, resources designed to support such a process have proliferated in recent years. These include interventions to improve patient empowerment, communication, and comfort with engaging in the medical encounter; provider-targeted training to further enhance professional competencies and knowledge of available resources; and decision support tools that provide exploration of personal goals and values in addition to comprehensive and unbiased medical diagnosis and treatment information.

Patient Activation Interventions

Self-management programs aim to educate patients about their condition, promote the adoption of self-care skills, and enhance self-confidence to manage one's condition (Newman et al. 2004). Focusing on developing these capabilities improves patient activation, empowering individuals to overcome perceived status and knowledge asymmetries and play active roles in their health care. In one such intervention, developed by Greenfield and colleagues (1985), patients work with advocates to review their medical record, enhance information-seeking skills through learning about the medical care process, identify relevant medical decision points to discuss with their provider, and engage in a behavior change strategy intended to improve patient interactions with their provider. Patients receiving this service demonstrate increased engagement in discussions with their provider about treatment options and self-management, fewer perceived limitations in functional ability resulting from their condition, and increased desire for involvement in medical decision making (Williams et al. 2005).

An extensive intervention approach developed for improving activation and empowerment in mental health care comprised three 30-minute patient training sessions emphasizing health-related decision making, appointment preparation, and formulating questions about health information (Alegría et al. 2008). Conducting three sessions interposed by psychiatry appointments allowed opportunities for the patients to practice using both real and hypothetical content, engage in problem solving in preparation for future appointments, and receive feedback. Patients valued learning how to interact with psychiatrists and ask relevant questions in a way that maintained respect for the psychiatrist's knowledge and expertise. Participation in these sessions resulted in increased self-reported activation, appointment attendance, and treatment retention (Alegría et al. 2008). The quality of interaction between physician and patient and the degree of perceived fairness in the consultation process were associated with increased patient activation (Alexander et al. 2012).

Solomon and colleagues (2012) utilized an interactive, multimedia approach through an internet-based health information system to provide 24-hour access to educational modules covering medical information, self-management skills and guidelines, and treatment and intervention options. The complexity and the pace of information were tailored to the level of health literacy of the individual based on patient preference. A built-in option allowed online communication with providers through a secure message function, allowing patients to engage in meaningful discussions about their care and improving access to information. Evidence suggests that these types of interventions, whether delivered face-to-face or via telephone or the internet, can be effective at improving self-management knowledge and skills and patient activation (Légaré et al. 2018; Solomon et al. 2012).

Provider Training

Some providers may find it challenging to adjust to a changing relationship dynamic and increased exchange of information with patients (Alegría et al.

2008). Perspective must be maintained regarding the benefits of patient engagement, and providers should be receptive to increased participation, regardless of the nature of past relationships and patient behavior (Légaré et al. 2018). Interventions directed at modifying provider perspectives, skills, and values have yielded fruitful results in terms of adoption of shared decision making in clinical practice. For example, Loh and colleagues (2007) offered an intervention to physicians that utilized interactive and didactic modules to advance skills for involving patients in medical care and decision making. Physicians completed training modules that included lectures, content quizzes, role-playing, and video examples aimed at enhancing skills to encourage patient involvement. Additionally, targeted decision aids and informational brochures were provided for physicians to disseminate to patients during the decision-making process. This intervention resulted in improved patient satisfaction with care and increased patient participation in decision making.

Decision Support Tools

Decision support tools for a broad range of conditions and treatment options have become widely available to complement patient interactions with health care providers (Légaré et al. 2013). These tools differ from general health education materials in their specificity to the decision being considered. Decision support tools may include paper-based materials (e.g., brochures, comprehensive informational packets), websites and other online resources, interactive electronic checklists or questionnaires, and visual aids, models, or videos. These can aid shared decision making by offering patients unbiased health care information explicit to the disease management choices under deliberation. In many circumstances, treatment decisions do not involve an objectively "best" choice but rather are sensitive to individual preferences. Decision support tools often help patients explore and clarify personal preferences and weigh the value they place on treatment risks, benefits, and outcomes.

Decision support tools have been designed for use before, during, and after provider consultation to improve knowledge and patient engagement (Légaré et al. 2013). Despite their versatile nature and support of patient activation, adoption of these tools in routine practice has been low (Elwyn et al. 2008). Lack of robust design, limited knowledge of available decision support tools, and accuracy of information in the context of fast-paced developments in medicine have historically been barriers to implementation. Electronic decision support tools are gaining traction because they can directly link to available evidence, be regularly updated with newly released information, and be centralized for more effective use in clinical encounters. Although electronic versions vary greatly in content and structure, many include disease, symptom, and other medical information; a comprehensive list of treatment options, including risks and benefits; and a component (e.g., quiz, checklist of items) aimed at eliciting thoughts about personal goals, values, preferences, and environmental context to help guide the decision-making process to meet the needs of the individual. The Ottawa Hospital Research Institute (2020) maintains a comprehensive list of decision support tools available for an A-to-Z catalogue of medical conditions. Each tool is scored using the quality criteria established by the International Patient Decision Aids Standards (IPDAS) Collaboration (Elwyn et al. 2006). The IPDAS Collaboration was established in 2003 and comprises over 100 stakeholders (i.e., researchers, practitioners, patients, and policy makers) from 14 countries. Its work has helped institute a metric by which to gauge the reliability of health information and decisional utility of over 500 patient decision support tools that have been developed to date. Their 64-item criteria checklist is divided among three domains: clinical content (e.g., "Does the patient decision aid present probabilities of outcomes in an unbiased and understandable way?," "Does the patient decision aid include methods for clarifying and expressing patients' values?"), development process (e.g., "Does the patient decision aid have a systematic development process?"), and effectiveness (e.g., "Does the patient decision aid ensure decision making is informed and values based?") (International Patient Decision Aids Standards Collaboration 2005). This standardization offers a mechanism through which decision support tools can be graded for the unbiased presentation of accurate plain-language information with reference citations, clarification and elicitation of patient values regarding positive and negative features of decision options, ease of navigation and use, and utility in leading to a high-quality decision.

Case Vignette

A few years ago, Matt began feeling more tearful and depressed than usual. He found himself arguing more frequently with his husband and felt they were growing apart. Matt went to see a psychiatrist and during the intake session expressed concern about taking psychotropic medications. The psychiatrist informed him that the most effective mode of treatment for him was an antidepressant, and he was prescribed escitalopram. Matt felt that his concerns had been dismissed, but he did not feel he had had any input in making the decision. Matt took the escitalopram for about 6 weeks, and over that time he frequently suffered from insomnia and felt fatigued. When he told his psychiatrist about these side effects, he once again felt his concerns were dismissed. Feeling like a bystander in his own medical treatment, Matt discontinued the escitalopram and skipped all follow-up sessions with his psychiatrist.

Recently, Matt and his husband divorced, and he felt like his world was falling apart. He felt depressed and lost interest in activities he had once enjoyed. He struggled to get out of bed and go into work most days and often called in sick. He was afraid his employer would fire him if he kept calling in sick. He felt irritable and fatigued, yet he struggled to sleep at night. He felt isolated, hopeless, and ineffective both at work and in his personal life, and these feelings compounded his already persistent sense of worthlessness. Matt disliked the idea of returning to a psychiatrist because of his previous experience. However, he felt he had little choice, so he scheduled an appointment with a different psychiatrist.

During his intake session, the psychiatrist actively listened and openly invited Matt to share his thoughts and concerns about treatment. Matt quickly felt like an active participant and felt comfortable sharing his previous experience and the reasons he discontinued his medication years ago. Through active listening, his psychiatrist provided a safe environment to have an open dialogue, and Matt felt she took the time to understand his needs and desires. At the end of the intake, she told Matt that she believed the best treatment for his acute depressive symptoms was an antidepressant. She informed Matt that his concerns were important to her, and they developed a plan together to monitor and report any side effects that he might experience. Matt began taking bupropion, and he once again felt his insomnia worsen. He felt comfortable calling his psychiatrist's office, and she suggested taking the medication earlier in the day, an adjustment that addressed his insomnia and lessened his daytime fatigue. After a few weeks, he felt his depressive symptoms improve significantly. At a follow-up visit, he asked his psychiatrist about additional long-term treatment options to better manage his depression with minimal use of medication. After discussing additional options, they both agreed to add weekly psychotherapy to Matt's regimen, which he found tremendously helpful in developing better coping mechanisms and self-care behaviors.

In this interaction, the psychiatrist was able to establish trust and collaboration in the provider-patient relationship through a shared decision-making approach. She was able to 1) communicate clearly and deliver unbiased information, 2) openly consider Matt's individual preferences, 3) verify understanding of information and comfort in expressing opinions, 4) achieve mutual agreement regarding treatment, and 5) track outcomes and revisit the treatment plan as needed.

Key Points

- Decisions about treatment options, diagnostic tests, medications, and behaviors are commonplace in medicine and are shaped by the patient-provider relationship.

- Often viewed as the ideological balance between paternalistic and informed choice medical models, shared decision making supports equal participation of the provider and patient in medical decision making. Shared decision making is a key component of patient-centered care and has firmly rooted ties to self-determination and patient empowerment.

- In any given medical interaction, there are two experts in the room who possess information vital for service provision—the provider (the expert regarding medical knowledge and treatment options) and the patient (the expert on the patient's own personal values, preferences, goals, behaviors, and medical history).

- Though shared decision making relies on both key parties, providers play a fundamental role in instituting an approach to decision making that is participatory and collaborative. The provider must be prepared to initiate and facilitate conversation about shared decision making and employ the personal and professional skills necessary to support the process.

- The provider is ultimately responsible for creating a comfortable environment that encourages patient engagement, improves treatment adherence and outcomes, strengthens the patient-provider relationship, and reduces decisional conflict and regret.

- Decision support tools have become broadly available to assist in implementing shared decision making in clinical practice. Use of decision support tools results in improved patient knowledge regarding treatment options and outcomes, increased accuracy of perceived outcome risk probabilities, reduced decisional conflict and regret, and greater coherence between personal values and chosen treatment options.

- Decisional aids also have the potential to improve the patient-provider interaction, increasing patient activation and reducing the overall consultation time.

References

Alegría M, Polo A, Gao S, et al: Evaluation of a patient activation and empowerment intervention in mental health care. Med Care 46(3):247–256, 2008

Alexander JA, Hearld LR, Mittler JN, et al: Patient–physician role relationships and patient activation among individuals with chronic illness. Health Serv Res 47 (3 Pt 1):1201–1223, 2012

Anderson RM, Funnell MM: Patient empowerment: myths and misconceptions. Patient Educ Couns 79(3):277–282, 2010

Brody DS: The patient's role in clinical decision-making. Ann Intern Med 93(5):718–722, 1980

Brody DS, Miller SM, Lerman CE, et al: Patient perception of involvement in medical care. J Gen Intern Med 4(6):506–511, 1989

Charles C, Gafni A, Whelan T: Shared decision-making in the medical encounter: what does it mean? (or it takes at least two to tango). Soc Sci Med 44(5):681–692, 1997

Charles C, Gafni A, Whelan T: Decision-making in the physician–patient encounter: revisiting the shared treatment decision-making model. Soc Sci Med 49(5):651–661, 1999

Corrigan PW: The dignity to fail. Psychiatr Serv 62(3):241, 2011

Corrigan PW, Liberman RP, Engel JD: From noncompliance to collaboration in the treatment of schizophrenia. Psychiatr Serv 41(11):1203–1211, 1990

Davidson L, Tondora J, Miller R, et al: Person-centered care, in Person-Centered Care for Mental Illness: The Evolution of Adherence and Self-Determination. Edited by Corrigan PW. Washington, DC, American Psychological Association, 2015, pp 81–102

Elwyn G, O'Connor A, Stacey D, et al; International Patient Decision Aids Standards (IPDAS) Collaboration: Developing a quality criteria framework for patient decision aid: online international Delphi consensus process. BMJ 333(7565):417–419, 2006

Elwyn G, Légaré F, van der Weijden T, et al: Arduous implementation: does the Normalisation Process Model explain why it's so difficult to embed decision support technologies for patients in routine clinical practice. Implement Sci 3(1):57–66, 2008

Entwistle V: Patient involvement in decision-making: the importance of a broad conceptualization, in Shared Decision-Making in Healthcare: Achieving Evidence-Based Patient Choice. Edited by Edwards A, Elwyn G. New York, Oxford University Press, 2009, pp 17–22

Frosch DL, Moulton BW, Wexler RM, et al: Shared decision making in the United States: policy and implementation activity on multiple fronts. Z Evid Fortbild Qual Gesundhwes 105(4):305–312, 2011

Frosch DL, May SG, Rendle KA, et al: Authoritarian physicians and patients' fear of being labeled 'difficult' among key obstacles to shared decision making. Health Aff (Millwood) 31(5):1030–1038, 2012

Gerteis M, Edgman-Levitan S, Daley J, et al: Introduction: medicine and health from the patient's perspective, in Through the Patient's Eyes: Understanding and Promoting Patient-Centered Care. San Francisco, CA, Jossey-Bass, 1993, pp 1–15

Gionfriddo MR, Leppin AL, Brito JP, et al: Shared decision-making and comparative effectiveness research for patients with chronic conditions: an urgent synergy for better health. J Comp Eff Res 2(6):595–603, 2013

Greenfield S, Kaplan S, Ware JE Jr: Expanding patient involvement in care: effects on patient outcomes. Ann Intern Med 102(4):520–528, 1985

Institute of Medicine, Committee on Quality of Health Care in America: Crossing the Quality Chasm: A New Health System for the 21st Century. Washington, DC, National Academy Press, 2001

International Patient Decision Aids Standards Collaboration: Criteria for judging the quality of patient decision aids. 2005. Available at: http://ipdas.ohri.ca/IPDAS_checklist.pdf. Accessed June 30, 2020.

Johnson MO, Sevelius JM, Dilworth SE: Preliminary support for the construct of health care empowerment in the context of treatment for human immunodeficiency virus. Patient Prefer Adherence 6:395–404, 2012

Légaré F, Moumjid-Ferdjaoui N, Drolet R, et al: Core competencies for shared decision making training programs: insights from an international, interdisciplinary working group. J Contin Educ Health Prof 33(4):267–273, 2013

Légaré F, Adekpedjou R, Stacey D, et al: Interventions for increasing the use of shared decision making by healthcare professionals. Cochrane Database Syst Rev 7(7):CD006732, 2018

Levine C, Zuckerman C: The trouble with families: toward an ethic of accommodation. Ann Intern Med 130(2):148–152, 1999

Lim JW, Baik OM, Ashing-Giwa KT: Cultural health beliefs and health behaviors in Asian American breast cancer survivors: a mixed-methods approach. Oncol Nurs Forum 39(4):388–397, 2012

Loh A, Simon D, Wills CE, et al: The effects of a shared decision-making intervention in primary care of depression: a cluster-randomized controlled trial. Patient Educ Couns 67(3):324–332, 2007

Makoul G, Clayman ML: An integrative model of shared decision making in medical encounters. Patient Educ Couns 60(3):301–312, 2006

Miller CH, Quick BL: Sensation seeking and psychological reactance as health risk predictors for an emerging adult population. Health Commun 25(3):266–275, 2010

Newman S, Steed L, Mulligan K: Self-management interventions for chronic illness. Lancet 364(9444):1523–1537, 2004

Ommen O, Thuem S, Pfaff H, et al: The relationship between social support, shared decision-making and patient's trust in doctors: a cross-sectional survey of 2,197 inpatients using the Cologne Patient Questionnaire. Int J Public Health 56(3):319–327, 2011

Ottawa Hospital Research Institute: Alphabetical list of decision aids by health topic. 2020. Available at: https://decisionaid.ohri.ca/AZlist.html. Accessed June 30, 2020.

Plakun EM: A view from Riggs: treatment resistance and patient authority-introduction to paper IX: integrative psychodynamic treatment of psychotic disorders. J Am Acad Psychoanal Dyn Psychiatry 36(4):737–738, 2008

President's Commission for the Study of Ethical Problems in Medicine and Biomedical and Behavioral Research: Making Health Care Decisions: A Report on the Ethical and Legal Implications of Informed Consent in the Patient–Practitioner Relationship. Washington, DC, U.S. Government Printing Office, 1982

Rudnick A: Recovery from schizophrenia: a philosophical framework. Am J Psychiatr Rehabil 11(3):267–278, 2008

Ryan RM, Deci EL: Self-determination theory and the facilitation of intrinsic motivation, social development, and well-being. Am Psychol 55(1):68–78, 2000

Shapiro ER: A view from Riggs: treatment resistance and patient authority—XII. Examined living: a psychodynamic treatment system. J Am Acad Psychoanal Dyn Psychiatry 37(4):683–698, 2009

Shay LA, Lafata JE: Where is the evidence? A systematic review of shared decision making and patient outcomes. Med Decis Making 35(1):114–131, 2015

Sheridan S, Harris R, Woolf S: Shared decision making about screening and chemoprevention. A suggested approach from the U.S. Preventive Services Task Force. Am J Prev Med 26(1):56–66, 2004

Solomon M, Wagner SL, Goes J: Effects of a Web-based intervention for adults with chronic conditions on patient activation: online randomized controlled trial. J Med Internet Res 14(1):e32, 2012

Szasz T: Coercion as Cure: A Critical History of Psychiatry. Piscataway, NJ, Transaction, 2007

Szasz TS, Hollender MH: A contribution to the philosophy of medicine; the basic models of the doctor-patient relationship. AMA Arch Intern Med 97(5):585–592, 1956

Towle A, Godolphin W: Framework for teaching and learning informed shared decision making. BMJ 319(7212):766–769, 1999

Townsend C: Review of the book "Challenges to the Human Rights of People With Intellectual Disabilities." Australian Social Work 63(1):135–136, 2010

Velligan DI, Weiden PJ, Sajatovic M, et al: Assessment of adherence problems in patients with serious and persistent mental illness: recommendations from the Expert Consensus Guidelines. J Psychiatr Pract 16(1):34–45, 2010

Vuckovich PK: Compliance versus adherence in serious and persistent mental illness. Nurs Ethics 17(1):77–85, 2010

Wennberg JE: Dealing with medical practice variations: a proposal for action. Health Aff (Millwood) 3(2):6–33, 1984

Williams GC, McGregor H, Zeldman A, et al: Promoting glycemic control through diabetes self-management: evaluating a patient activation intervention. Patient Educ Couns 56(1):28–34, 2005

CHAPTER 9

Healthy Living Skills

Erin L. Kelly, Ph.D.
John S. Brekke, Ph.D.

Individuals with serious mental illness (SMI), such as schizophrenia, major depression, bipolar disorder, and schizoaffective disorder, present clinicians with an array of issues beyond their mental illness symptoms. As part of the recovery process for those with SMI, it is key that they develop or regain basic skills needed to function adaptively within the world so that they not only manage their illness but also thrive (Drake and Whitley 2014; Lyman et al. 2014). Recovery from mental illness is therefore focused on improvement of not only clinical symptoms, which can wax and wane over the life course, but also overall health and well-being (Davidson and Roe 2007; Drake and Whitley 2014). In this chapter, we review healthy living skills that psychiatrists and other providers can assist their clients with for improving their health and well-being.

In recent decades, there has been increasing attention to the high rates of comorbid physical issues for those with SMI as there is significant evidence that individuals with SMI have high rates of morbidity and early mortality (Crump et al. 2013; De Hert et al. 2011b; Hjorthøj et al. 2017; Walker et al. 2015). There are numerous reasons for this health disparity, but across meta-analytic and systematic reviews, it is clear that the majority of deaths are attributable to acute and chronic illnesses (e.g., cardiovascular, metabolic, and pulmonary diseases) rather than other causes such as accidents or suicide

(Crump et al. 2013; Jayatilleke et al. 2017; Walker et al. 2015). The higher rates of health problems are often attributed to poor health habits (e.g., physical inactivity, poor diet, smoking, treatment nonadherence), and the side effects of psychiatric medications (De Hert et al. 2011b; Dombrovski and Rosenstock 2004; Stanley and Laugharne 2014); however, critical issues such as provider stigma, system bifurcation, and poor care coordination also contribute to the health disparities for individuals with SMI (De Hert et al. 2011a; Lawrence and Kisely 2010). It is critical for the care and functioning of this population to understand the processes that help them learn and maintain healthy attitudes and behaviors that support their physical well-being over time. In this chapter, we define healthy living skills and describe interventions developed for cultivating those skills to manage physical health and health care among those with SMI. Our goal is to provide practitioners with an overview of relevant interventions and the evidence supporting them so that they can make informed practice decisions.

Definition of Healthy Living Skills

Healthy living skills are broadly defined as any skills that allow individuals to complete their daily activities, facilitate their health and well-being, and prevent adverse outcomes (Dilk and Bond 1996; Lyman et al. 2014). Achieving these results requires cultivation of thoughts, attitudes, and behaviors that address physical health and health care use. Individuals with SMI often have a spectrum of skills that need to be developed or regained after the onset of their illness (Lyman et al. 2014). This need for skill development or recovery is due in part to the unfortunate timing of mental illness onset, which is typically within late adolescence or early adulthood, when living skills and habits are usually being developed and refined (Harrow et al. 2005; Levine 2012). In this chapter, we focus specifically on skills and interventions developed to address the physical health and health care issues of individuals with SMI. To develop this list, we examine barriers to better health and health care, survey examinations of theoretical models of health behaviors, and review the literature for domains that have been identified as intervention targets for physical health and health care among those with SMI.

Identifying Living Skills for Health and Health Care Among Individuals With SMI

To identify skills pertinent to the health and health care of those with SMI, it is useful to consider how health behaviors are created and maintained.

Numerous theoretical models attempt to explain health behaviors and deficits in health care use. The health belief model, one of the most widely used models since the 1950s (Champion and Skinner 2008), is predicated on the notion that people value their health and that they expect that their actions can prevent or ameliorate illness. The health belief model entails six main constructs to predict preventive behaviors: perceived susceptibility, perceived severity, perceived benefits, perceived barriers, self-efficacy, and cues to action. People need to think that it is possible for them to have a health issue, that it is serious enough to merit investigation, and that treatment can help them more than barriers can stop them. They also need to have strategies ready to address an issue (cues to action) and the confidence to address it. A limitation of this model is that it does not include emotional concerns, such as fear, which is associated with the avoidance of health care. However, some research suggests that individuals with SMI may have difficulty recognizing that their health needs attention (Hahm and Segal 2005), which means that they may need assistance in becoming attentive to their physical health needs. Further, individuals with SMI may have health beliefs that negatively affect their lifestyles, such as a diminished sense that they can control their behavior and doubts about the value of changing their behavior—for example, quitting smoking or consuming a high-fiber diet (Brunero and Lamont 2010).

Motivation is also a key factor in maintaining health. However, the negative symptoms common to several SMIs, such as anhedonia, blunted affect, apathy, reduced social drive and interest, and diminished sense of purpose and motivation, are all associated with adverse outcomes and, troublingly, are more persistent and difficult to treat than positive symptoms such as hallucinations and delusions. These clinical issues can make it more difficult to cultivate skills to alter the unhealthy habits, attitudes, and behaviors that contribute to chronic disease and mortality (Stanley and Laugharne 2014). In a qualitative study among individuals with mental illnesses generally, participants reported that thinking about lifestyle changes can be overwhelming and that negative symptoms and depression can make it difficult to be motivated to address physical health (Yarborough et al. 2019). This suggests that managing stress, depression, and anxiety around these issues is important as well. Other theoretical models, such as the theory of planned behavior (Ajzen 1985) and the self-determination theory (Deci and Ryan 2000), include motivation as the key factor for improving health behaviors. In a study comparing motivation for physical activity among individuals with SMI, individuals with bipolar disorder and major depressive disorder were found to be more motivated by pressures of guilt or self-criticism (introjected regulation) than individuals with schizophrenia (Vancampfort et al. 2015). The study also found across diagnoses that individuals with SMI who were early in their process of adopting change (precontemplation) had higher rates of amotivation than those in the more advanced stages of change (preparation, action, and maintenance), as outlined in the transtheoretical model. Finally, both intrinsic and extrinsic motivation for physical activity were higher among those who exercised more, which suggests that strategies that address both intrinsic and extrinsic motivation can play important roles in the long-term maintenance of health behavior.

Individuals with mental illnesses manage their health care within systems of care that, typically, are not tailored to their unique needs (Brekke et al. 2013). In addition, cognitive deficits, common to schizophrenia, can limit patients' abilities to communicate their symptoms and needs, which can lead to poor follow-up with care and poor comprehension of medical advice (Lambert et al. 2003). For example, individuals with schizophrenia may have reduced pain responses, which can cause them to not describe conditions as painful, and which in turn can cause diagnostic difficulties for doctors who are unaware of these irregularities. Other barriers to physical health and physical health care for those with SMI include issues of fear and trauma (Hahm et al. 2008). In a review of theoretical models that examined why those with mental illnesses did not receive health care, Hahm et al. (2008) identified individual-level factors such as a lack of transportation, financial resources, coping skills, verbal skills, and interpersonal relationship skills as potential barriers as well. In another systematic review of the impact of lifestyle factors (diet, exercise, smoking, and dental care) on the physical health of those with mental illnesses (Stanley and Laugharne 2014), deficits in social support, self-image, social skills, knowledge of risk factors for chronic health conditions, personal hygiene habits, ability to provide a medical history, transportation, and affordability were noted as issues. Stanley and Laugharne (2014) also noted how psychiatric medications can exacerbate health issues, have drug interactions with treatment for other issues, and enhance sedation (which can reduce motivation to address health issues). Provider stigma (which can lead providers to misattribute physical symptoms to mental causes) is a serious barrier to the treatment of this population, and individuals may avoid seeking help because of fear of coercion as a consequence of previous adverse experiences in hospitals after psychiatric emergencies (Hahm and Segal 2005).

As can be seen, health disparities among those with SMI are due to a host of individual and sociostructural factors. Poverty, homelessness, substance use, criminal justice involvement, race/ethnicity, gender, and other social determinants of health also create barriers to health and health care (Corrigan et al. 2014). When one reviews available interventions, it is important to consider how these elements have been accounted for in any intervention's development and how they may influence the effectiveness of the intervention.

Living Skills to Target for Intervention

Our literature review suggests that there are several skill sets that need to be cultivated and used adaptively to address multiple pertinent domains of health and health care use. Key outcomes include improvement of health through changing personal health habits (e.g., diet, exercise, reduced smoking and substance use), as well as improvement of skills to manage individuals' health care (e.g., awareness of illness, communication with practitioners). Although improving healthy living skills is a common goal for individuals with and without mental illness, remediation of deficits in these areas is particularly challenging for individuals with SMI. In the following subsections, we outline the skill sets that are useful for addressing physical health and health care among those with SMI (based on our literature review).

Self-Monitoring and Prioritizing Health

The ability to recognize the importance of health relative to other pressing concerns (e.g., housing, benefits, co-occurring substance use, clinical symptoms) and to notice physical symptoms is key to changing health beliefs, attitudes, and behaviors. Education about risk for common health conditions, particularly those exacerbated by psychiatric medications, and the preventive strategies or treatments available for these conditions may help individuals to recognize that maintaining their health is a priority. Enhancing individuals' abilities to self-monitor and to prioritize their health contributes to improving health and health care use.

Motivational Skills

Motivation is a multifaceted construct applied in a variety of contexts. Two overarching forms of motivation are intrinsic motivation and extrinsic motivation (Ryan and Deci 2000). *Intrinsic motivation* refers to an internal drive for behavior, wherein the behavior itself is rewarding. People may be motivated to pursue actions and achieve specific goals that are gratifying in and of themselves, enabling development of skills, a sense of competency, or a sense of meaning and purpose. Individuals who are intrinsically rewarded may enjoy the processes of exercise or feeling competent at negotiating the health care system. Conversely, *extrinsic motivation* involves behavior that is propelled by rewards that are external to the self, such as incentives or outcomes that are valued rather than the achievement of the goal itself. People may be motivated to improve their appearance in order to gain admiration and acceptance from others. Fear can also be a form of extrinsic motivation; individuals may fear the consequences of not achieving a goal or fear experiencing adverse outcomes. For example, individuals who fear developing cancer or want to prevent further health consequences of cardiovascular issues may be motivated to change their health habits.

Self-Efficacy and Self-Management Skills

Self-efficacy is the belief that one is capable of completing a task or goal, and this can be a key component of motivation and an antecedent to self-management behaviors. Self-management is both the enactment of healthy behaviors and the use of skills to successfully navigate health care services. Relatedly, individuals with SMI can have health beliefs that have adverse impacts on how they live, such as an inadequate sense that they can control their behavior (internal vs. external locus of control) (Brunero and Lamont 2010). Improving their senses of self-efficacy and internal locus of control is therefore critical to engagement in their own care. However, it is important to note that the health disparities experienced by this population are due to deficiencies not only in their lifestyle but also in their access, use, and coordination of health care services; development of their confidence and their abilities to negotiate the health care system is required.

Coping Skills

Development of coping skills to deal with anxieties around medical care is also important for the SMI population. Fear of learning adverse news about one's health, anticipation of frustrations (e.g., transportation challenges, long waits for appointments, long waits in the emergency room (ER) or doctors' waiting rooms, provider stigma), trauma symptoms related to prior psychiatric care, and being overwhelmed by required lifestyle changes all necessitate the development of coping strategies to manage these situations.

Medication and Treatment Adherence Skills

Development of habits that support medication and treatment adherence is key to successful treatment. As outlined in the section "Identifying Living Skills for Health and Health Care Among Individuals With SMI," negative symptoms, cognitive deficits, and depression can all make it more difficult to understand complex treatment regimens, such as those required to manage diabetes. Treatment nonadherence and medication nonadherence are common issues among individuals with SMI. Psychiatric medication can have unpleasant side effects, can interact with medications for other health conditions, and can cause somnolence. Medication adherence studies typically focus on whether individuals are taking their psychiatric medications rather than other physical health medications. Treatment adherence is also key to the health and well-being of those with SMI because they need to stay engaged in case management services and integrated health care interventions or follow nonpharmacological treatment regimens, such as changing dressings for wound care or monitoring blood pressure.

Communication and Interpersonal Relationship Skills

Communication and interpersonal relationship skills are both important to conveying health issues to doctors and building trusting relationships with them. Doctors are under a great deal of time pressure; they may not have the extra time that this population needs because of difficulties individuals with SMI face in conveying information to their clinicians. Individuals with SMI may need assistance in conveying their symptoms to clinicians, providing a medical history (including a list of all medications and conditions they are or have been treated for), and using online platforms to access their medical information. Instability in benefits or frequent housing changes may lead to particular difficulties for those with SMI in developing relationships with primary care providers who are knowledgeable about the health needs of patients with SMI.

Living Skills and Health in the General Population Compared With Individuals With SMI

Among the general population, poor lifestyle habits, such as smoking, poor diet, excessive alcohol use, and physical inactivity, often cluster together, meaning that people often have multiple poor habits rather than just one (Noble et al. 2015). Therefore, it is important to address these issues collectively rather than separately. In the intervention literature, interventions that focus on improving health do not typically focus on a single domain but try to redress multiple domains, although the combinations of those domains are highly variable across interventions. Physical health interventions typically target lifestyle factors, such as diet, exercise, and smoking, and less frequently target other outcomes, such as sleep, personal hygiene, or substance use. Some interventions focus on addressing the prevention, detection, or management of specific conditions and parameters (e.g., diabetes, obesity [body mass index; BMI], cardiovascular disease, blood pressure, cholesterol), while others focus on physical health conditions generally.

In a meta-review of the literature on lifestyle factors among the general population and individuals with SMI, improvements in diet and exercise emerged as important to enhancing health (Ward et al. 2015), and cognitive-behavioral approaches were critical to supporting those improvements. Among the general population, overall caloric restriction is more important than food content for weight loss, but different diets do have significant impacts on other health outcomes. Exercise needs to last at least 150 minutes per week to have an impact on weight. Physical activity is a critical issue for those with SMI. In a systematic review, Stubbs et al. (2016) found that individuals with psychosis self-report spending 11 hours a day in sedentary behavior, which is nearly 3 hours a day more than those without a mental illness. When objective measures are used, individuals with psychosis are sedentary for nearly 12.5 hours per day. Individualized rather than general diet and exercise advice are associated with improved adherence and outcomes (Ward et al. 2015). Lifestyle interventions need to be sustained for at least 4–6 months to be effective. Greater frequency of contact (regardless of the treatment length) is also associated with weight loss. Individuals in a variety of positions (both health care professionals and individuals who are in nonprofessional or peer positions) have delivered effective interventions when they have been sufficiently trained and experienced. In-person interactions are more effective than digital communication because relationship building is crucial to success. All these findings are applicable to the health of individuals with SMI. However, Ward et al. (2015) found that these principles are not always applied in interventions for individuals with SMI; consequently, support for lifestyle interventions among this population is weaker. For example, exercise regimens for those with SMI are often of lower intensity to allow for motivational deficits, and few interventions have been manualized. Ward et al. also found that many interventions were too short in duration, were group based rather than individually tailored, addressed a single issue rather than multiple issues, and often lacked specialized training for providers. Critical components of lifestyle interventions included activities that cultivated self-efficacy supported by a structured cognitive-behavioral curricula, including goal setting and self-monitoring of diet and exercise.

There are several systematic reviews that show that individuals with SMI can be responsive to interventions for physical health and/or physical health care (Cabassa et al. 2010, 2017; Faulkner et al. 2003; Firth et al. 2016; Kelly et al. 2014a; Mazoruk et al. 2019; Naslund et al. 2017; Siantz and Aranda 2014; Soundy et al. 2014; Teasdale et al. 2017; Vancampfort et al. 2017). However, not all articles or reviews describe the skills cultivated by the intervention, which limits evaluation of their specific components. We now turn to a description and an evidence assessment of specific interventions for improving the physical health and health care utilization of individuals with SMI.

Specific Programs for Physical Health and Health Care

For the purposes of this chapter, we reviewed interventions that focused on improving the skills used for addressing physical health and/or health care experiences of patients with SMI. This review included selected interventions found on PubMed and Google Scholar or in the library systems of the University of Southern California and University of California, Los Angeles. A search of the reference sections of articles, book chapters, and government reports was also used to help identify overlooked studies. Search terms included the following: "serious mental illness," "severe mental illness," "schizophrenia," "schizoaffective," "bipolar," "depression," "weight," "physical activity," "exercise," "lifestyle," "healthy living skills," "skills training," "intervention," "health," "health care," "integrated health care," and "collaborative care." We included interventions from the last 10 years, conducted in the United States, that identified which skills they help to cultivate with respect to physical health or health care. We excluded articles that only described interventions conceptually and those that did not provide quantitative results. The interventions included needed to target individuals with a primary diagnosis of SMI (e.g., schizophrenia, schizoaffective disorder, bipolar disorder, major depression). For the included interventions, we considered whether they were manualized, their intensity and duration, skills targeted, special populations targeted, format (individual or group), providers involved (e.g., psychiatrists, nurses, case managers, peers), training specific to the intervention, and outcomes addressed.

We note the sample size, sample characteristics, and the type of study design. When available, we also provide websites with information about the interventions.

We identified 16 studies (for 12 interventions) that primarily addressed skills for lifestyle (e.g., diet, exercise) and 19 studies (for 14 interventions) that addressed skills for health care and/or health experiences (e.g., health status, service access, satisfaction with health care practitioner, extent of service utilization). We include Cohen's *d*, when specified, as an estimate of effect size for outcomes (small=0.2–0.4, medium=0.5–0.7, large=≥0.8). Tables 9–1 and 9–2 provide an overview of our findings.

Interventions to Improve Lifestyle Skills

Study Design

Of the 16 studies on lifestyle interventions in Table 9–1, three studies were focused on the InSHAPE intervention from pilot to randomized controlled trial (RCT) (Bartels et al. 2013, 2015; Van Citters et al. 2010), two studies were on the STRIDE intervention (Green et al. 2015a, 2015b), two studies were on the MOVE! intervention (Goldberg et al. 2013b; Muralidharan et al. 2018), and the remainder focused on other unique approaches.

The majority of studies were pilots, although four were pre-post within-person studies (Aschbrenner et al. 2016; Daumit et al. 2011; McKibbin et al. 2010; Van Citters et al. 2010), and the six remaining were RCTs (Beebe et al. 2011; Erickson et al. 2017; Gillhoff et al. 2010; Goldberg et al. 2013b; Green et al. 2015a; Ratliff et al. 2012).

Skills Developed

All the studies described building of skills, including self-monitoring, motivation, and self-efficacy skills. However, only four included coping skills (Erickson et al. 2017; Gillhoff et al. 2010; Green et al. 2015a, 2015b). Most critically, only the InSHAPE (Bartels et al. 2013, 2015; Van Citters et al. 2010) and MOVE! (Goldberg et al. 2013b; Muralidharan et al. 2018) interventions included measures of skill development (although the Web-MOVE Intervention assessed these skills qualitatively only). This is a serious limitation to evaluating the effectiveness of these interventions, because it is unclear which skills or collection of skills was critical to lead to measurable changes in these outcomes.

Special Populations

The majority of studies specifically required that individuals be overweight or obese (Aschbrenner et al. 2016; Bartels et al. 2013, 2015; Daumit et al.

TABLE 9–1. Lifestyle interventions targeting skills for diet and/or physical activity

Intervention name, authors, and website (if applicable)	Study design and sample	Intervention, skills, and intervention training	Outcomes
Diabetes Prevention Program Group Lifestyle Balance intervention plus mobile health (mHealth) Aschbrenner et al. 2016	Pilot within-subjects, 6 months *N*=13 Age, mean (SD): 48.2 (11.2) 73% female, 91% white Diagnosis: 46% major depressive disorder, 27% bipolar disorder, 27% schizophrenia Special population: overweight individuals (BMI≥30)	Over 24 weeks, weekly (90-minute) group weight management sessions taught by two lifestyle coaches and one peer and biweekly exercise sessions with a fitness trainer (1 hour) and use of mHealth (Fitbit) and social media to increase motivation, self-monitoring, self-efficacy skills, and peer support. Attendance was 56% overall. Two mental health graduate students were trained in a 2-day workshop on healthy eating, nutrition, and skills training. Training for peer trainer was not specified.	Overall weight loss was not significant compared with control group of gym membership and health promotion education. Reduction in weight was reported for 45% of participants. Increased walking distance was reported for 45% of participants.

TABLE 9–1. Lifestyle interventions targeting skills for diet and/or physical activity (*continued*)

Intervention name, authors, and website (if applicable)	Study design and sample	Intervention, skills, and intervention training	Outcomes
InSHAPE Bartels et al. 2013 www.hprcd.org/inshape	RCT, 12 months *N*=133 (67 treatment group, 66 control group) Age, mean (SD): 43.8 (11.5) 62% female, 92% white Diagnosis: 18% schizophrenia, 13% schizoaffective disorder, 35% bipolar disorder, 34% major depression Special population: overweight individuals (BMI ≥25)	Health promotion intervention consisting of weekly individual sessions (45–60 minutes) for 12 months with a health promotion coach, fitness training and membership at a gym, and nutrition education (including classes, meeting with a dietitian, and grocery store tours). Skills included motivation, self-efficacy, and self-monitoring. Attendance of ≥50% weekly visits was 40% in treatment group vs. 7% in control group. Individual-based health mentoring from community mental health center staff certified as fitness trainers was provided. Mentors received three sets of trainings: 1) 3-day training in program with instruction in MI, goal setting, and tracking of diet and exercise; 2) 2-day training in healthy eating from nutrition educator; and 3) 3-day training in nutrition from doctoral candidate in nutrition services.	Significantly more days of physical activity, exercise minutes, vigorous activity, cardiorespiratory fitness, reduced dietary fat, and portion control.

TABLE 9–1. Lifestyle interventions targeting skills for diet and/or physical activity (*continued*)

Intervention name, authors, and website (if applicable)	Study design and sample	Intervention, skills, and intervention training	Outcomes
InSHAPE Bartels et al. 2015 www.hprcd.org/inshape	RCT, 18 months $N=210$ (104 treatment group, 106 control group) Age, mean: 43.9 51% female, 54% white, 34% Black Diagnosis: 23% schizophrenia, 32% schizoaffective disorder, 29% bipolar disorder, 16% major depression Special population: overweight individuals (BMI≥25)	Health promotion intervention consisting of weekly individual sessions (45–60 minutes) for 12 months with a health promotion coach/case manager, fitness training and membership at a gym, and nutrition education. Participants were monitored for an additional 6 months and could have some additional contact. Skills included motivation, self-efficacy, and self-monitoring. Attendance of InShape group: mean (SD)=21.3 (12.6) visits (of 50 possible health promotion coach visits) and mean (SD)=28.5 (36.9) gym visits vs. mean (SD)=10.7 (2.4) gym visits for control group. All coaches completed a 1-week training with instruction in MI, goal setting, nutrition, health behavior strategies, and tracking of eating and activity.	At 12 months, significant improvements in physical activity, fitness, walking performance; more readiness for change; greater weight loss (mean=−5.3 lb); lower BMI; and smaller waist circumference (mean=−1.7 inches).

TABLE 9–1. Lifestyle interventions targeting skills for diet and/or physical activity (*continued*)

Intervention name, authors, and website (if applicable)	Study design and sample	Intervention, skills, and intervention training	Outcomes
Walk, Address Sensations, Learn About Exercise, Cue Exercise Behavior for SSDs (WALC-S) Beebe et al. 2011	Pilot RCT, 5 months $N=97$ (48 treatment group, 49 control group) Age, mean (SD): 46.9 (2.0) 47% female, 55% white, 44% Black, 1% Asian Diagnosis: 71% schizo-affective disorder, 29% schizophrenia Special population: limited to individuals with schizoaffective and schizophrenia disorders	Intervention consisting of four weekly 1-hour groups (eight per group) including self-efficacy information, followed by 16 weeks of walking group three times per week with warm-up/cool-down exercises, assistance with setting exercise goals, exercise recovery, and calendars to monitor walking. Skills include self-monitoring, motivation, and self-efficacy. Attendance was 38.5% by treatment group. Groups were facilitated by graduate students. Training not specified.	Experimental group attended more groups, persisted for longer, and walked more minutes than control group.

TABLE 9–1. Lifestyle interventions targeting skills for diet and/or physical activity (*continued*)

Intervention name, authors, and website (if applicable)	Study design and sample	Intervention, skills, and intervention training	Outcomes
Recovering Energy Through Nutrition and Exercise for Weight Loss (RENEW) Brown et al. 2011 www.cmhsrp.uic.edu/health/weight-wellbeing.asp	RCT, 12 months *N*=136 enrolled, 89 completed study (47 treatment group, 42 control group) Demographics only provided on 89 completers Age, mean (SD): 44.6 (10.9) 61% female, 60% white, 34% Black, 6% other Diagnosis: not provided, but SMI	Group-based intervention delivered by nurse, occupational therapist, or dietitians in three phases: 1) intensive phase (3 months), with weekly 3-hour sessions on nutrition, exercise, goal setting, and meals; 2) maintenance phase (3 months), with monthly 3-hour meetings and phone support weekly, no meals; and 3) intermittent support (6 months). Skills included self-monitoring, motivation, and self-efficacy. Training manuals for a facilitator and participants and a series of exercise videos were designed collaboratively with occupational therapists and people in recovery. No detail on length of training provided.	Significant weight loss at 3 months (mean=−5.3 lb) and at 6 months (mean=−4.4 lb).

TABLE 9–1.   Lifestyle interventions targeting skills for diet and/or physical activity (*continued*)

Intervention name, authors, and website (if applicable)	Study design and sample	Intervention, skills, and intervention training	Outcomes
Based on PREMIER study Daumit et al. 2011	Pilot, within-subject, 6 months $N=63$ Age, mean (SD): 43.7 (10.8) 56% female, 49% white, 49% Black, 2% Asian Diagnosis: 34% schizophrenia, 20% schizoaffective disorder, 23% bipolar disorder, 20% depression, 4% other psychotic disorder Special population: overweight individuals (BMI ≥25)	Individual- and group-based intervention delivered by registered dietitian and health educator and consisting of three components: 1) weight management counseling (one 45-minute group session per week, one individual session every 6 weeks); 2) group physical activity of moderate intensity (45-minute sessions); and 3) education for kitchen staff about diet (met with staff two to four times over study). Skills included self-monitoring, motivation, and self-efficacy. Attendance was 70% of sessions. Training not specified.	Significant weight loss (mean=−4.5 lb at 6 months), decrease in waist circumference (mean=−3.1 cm), BMI reduction, and an increase in walking fitness from preintervention to postintervention.

TABLE 9–1. Lifestyle interventions targeting skills for diet and/or physical activity *(continued)*

Intervention name, authors, and website (if applicable)	Study design and sample	Intervention, skills, and intervention training	Outcomes
Achieving Healthy Lifestyles in Psychiatric Rehabilitation (ACHIEVE) Daumit et al. 2013	RCT, 18 months *N*=291 (144 treatment group, 147 control group) Age, mean (SD): 45.3 (11.3) 50% female, 56% white, 38% Black, 6% other Diagnosis: 58% schizophrenia/ schizoaffective disorder, 22% bipolar disorder, 12% major depression Special population: overweight individuals (BMI≥25)	Over 18 months, participants completed sessions that followed three phases of gradually reduced intensity. Participants completed three types of sessions: 1) group weight management, 2) individual weight management, and 3) group exercise sessions. Skills included self-monitoring, motivation, and self-efficacy. Median attendance was 2.5 per month for treatment group (median=46 contacts in first 6 months, 31 from months 7 to 18). Individual- and group-based with study staff leading exercise sessions for 6 months, then member of rehabilitation staff offered an exercise video. Training not specified.	Weight loss (net change) in treatment group compared with control group was 1.5 kg at 6 months and 3.2 kg at 18 months. Significantly greater mean reduction in BMI in the treatment group (−0.6) compared with the control group (−0.01).

TABLE 9–1. Lifestyle interventions targeting skills for diet and/or physical activity (*continued*)

Intervention name, authors, and website (if applicable)	Study design and sample	Intervention, skills, and intervention training	Outcomes
Lifestyle Balance Erickson et al. 2017	Pilot RCT, 12 months *N*=121 (62 treatment group, 59 control group) Sample characteristics provided on completers only Age, mean: 30 19% female, 31% Black, 44% white, 15% Latino Diagnosis: 30% schizophrenia, 31% schizoaffective, 13% bipolar disorder, 16% multiple, 10% other Special population: veterans	Individual- and group-based intervention with a dietitian. Participants met weekly (60 minutes per session on two topics) for 8 weeks in classes (one to four people) and for individual nutrition counseling (15–60 minutes) and then monthly until 12 months. Classes used handouts, written materials, and group discussions covering 16 topics. Sessions covered stage of change, motivational interviewing, and accountability tools. Skills included self-monitoring, motivation, self-efficacy, and coping. Attendance was 86% sessions in 8-week intervention. Training for the registered dietitian was provided by the PI; the registered dietitian and PI worked together for 6 months while training a second dietitian.	At 12 months, fewer empty calories consumed and decreased body fat (0.4) and waist circumference (mean=−1.04 cm). Weight loss significantly greater among female participants.

TABLE 9–1. Lifestyle interventions targeting skills for diet and/or physical activity (*continued*)

Intervention name, authors, and website (if applicable)	Study design and sample	Intervention, skills, and intervention training	Outcomes
Quality of Life for Persons With Bipolar Disorder Gillhoff et al. 2010	Pilot RCT, 11 months *N*=50 (26 treatment group, 24 control) Age, mean: 48 46% female Diagnosis: 100% bipolar disorder Special populations: individuals with bipolar disorder	Individual- and group-based intervention consisting of three modules (lifestyle, nutrition, and physical activity) delivered by a nutrition counselor, fitness trainer, psychotherapist, and psychiatrist. Over 5 months, 11 group sessions and weekly physical activity with a personal trainer. Sessions focused on weight control, cooking classes, education, and bipolar relapse prevention. Skills include self-monitoring, motivation, self-efficacy, and coping. Attendance was 77% of sessions. Training not specified.	Significantly lower BMI (in females only) at 5 months (mean=−0.9 kg) and 11 months postintervention (mean=−0.8 kg), but weight loss at trend level only.

TABLE 9–1.   Lifestyle interventions targeting skills for diet and/or physical activity (*continued*)

Intervention name, authors, and website (if applicable)	Study design and sample	Intervention, skills, and intervention training	Outcomes
MOVE! Goldberg et al. 2013b	Pilot, RCT, 6 months N=109 (53 treatment group, 56 control group) Age, mean (SD): 52.0 (9.1) 19% female, 60% Black Diagnosis: 37% schizophrenia, 25% bipolar, 14% depression, 25% PTSD Special population: veterans	Individual- and group-based intervention delivered by research staff in three phases: 1) weekly individual sessions in the first month, 2) weekly group sessions (60 minutes) for months 2–4, and 3) four biweekly sessions and two individual sessions in months 5 and 6. Training included psychoeducation focused on nutritional counseling, caloric expenditure, and portion control. Skills included self-monitoring, motivation, and self-efficacy. Mean attendance was 3.3 individual sessions in first month. Mean number of group sessions was 7.4. Training not specified.	Compared with control condition, no significant reduction in weight or metabolic or cardiovascular health indicators, increase in exercise, or improvement in diet. Confidence and importance of health activities also unchanged.

TABLE 9–1. Lifestyle interventions targeting skills for diet and/or physical activity (*continued*)

Intervention name, authors, and website (if applicable)	Study design and sample	Intervention, skills, and intervention training	Outcomes
STRIDE Green et al. 2015a www.kpchr.org/stridepublic	RCT pilot, 3 months *N*=36 (18 treatment group, 18 control group) Age mean (SD): 48.5 (10.6) 81% female, 94% white Diagnosis: 69% bipolar, 29% schizophrenia, 2% PTSD Special population: overweight individuals (BMI≥25)	Individual- and group-based intervention based on the PREMIER lifestyle intervention and the DASH diet and adapted for an SMI population. The intervention was delivered by a mental health counselor and a person with experience in nutritional interventions in two phases 1) weekly 2-hour group meetings for 6 months, followed by 2) 6 months of groups sessions focused on maintaining weight. Participants monitored diet, exercise, and coping with emotions, using a workbook and CalorieKing database, with individualized feedback. Skills included self-monitoring, motivation, self-efficacy, and coping. Attendance not specified. Attended 2-day training on intervention and 2-days on motivational interviewing. Refresher trainings were every 6 months.	Significant weight loss after 3 months (mean=−6.5 lb).

TABLE 9–1. Lifestyle interventions targeting skills for diet and/or physical activity (*continued*)

Intervention name, authors, and website (if applicable)	Study design and sample	Intervention, skills, and intervention training	Outcomes
STRIDE Goldberg et al. 2013b https://research.kpchr.org/Research/Research-Areas/Mental-Health/STRIDE	RCT, 12 months $N=200$ (194 treatment group, 96 control group) Age, mean (SD): 47.2 (10.6) 72% female, 88% white Diagnosis: 69% bipolar, 29% schizophrenia, 2% PTSD Special population: overweight individuals (BMI≥27)	Individual- and group-based intervention based on the PREMIER lifestyle intervention and the DASH diet and adapted for an SMI population and delivered by a mental health counselor and a person with experience in nutritional interventions in two phases: 1) 6 months of weekly 2-hour group meetings for 6 months, followed by 2) 6 months of monthly meetings focused on maintaining weight loss and lifestyle changes. Participants monitored diet, exercise, and sleep, using a workbook and CalorieKing book, in small groups and individual feedback. Skills included self-monitoring, motivation, self-efficacy, and coping. Mean (SD) attendance was 14.5 (7.2) for weekly sessions and 2.7 (2.17) for monthly maintenance phase. Attended 2-day training on intervention and 2-days on motivational interviewing. Refresher trainings were held every 6 months.	Significant weight loss (mean=−4.4 kg more than control group at 6 months; mean=−2.6 kg more than control group at 12 months) and reduction in BMI and fasting glucose from baseline to 12 months.

TABLE 9–1. Lifestyle interventions targeting skills for diet and/or physical activity (*continued*)

Intervention name, authors, and website (if applicable)	Study design and sample	Intervention, skills, and intervention training	Outcomes
Diabetes Awareness and Rehabilitation Training (DART) McKibbin et al. 2010	Within-subjects, 12 months N=64 Age, mean (SD)=55.6 (8.7) 39% female, 69% white, 31% other Diagnosis: 89% schizophrenia, 12% schizoaffective Special population: individuals with diabetes	24-week group-based intervention focused on diabetes education, nutrition, and lifestyle exercise. Four sessions each were devoted to these three topics (90 minutes per session). Groups (6–8 per group) were led by a mental health professional trained in diabetes management and incorporated self-monitoring, modeling, practice, goal setting, and reinforcement strategies. Skills included self-monitoring, motivation, and self-efficacy. Attendance and training not specified.	Significant reduction in BMI (mean=–1.0 vs. +0.5 control group) and waist circumference (mean=–0.9 vs. +0.9 control group) at 12 months and increased knowledge about diabetes.

TABLE 9–1.   Lifestyle interventions targeting skills for diet and/or physical activity (*continued*)

Intervention name, authors, and website (if applicable)	Study design and sample	Intervention, skills, and intervention training	Outcomes
WebMOVE Muralidharan et al. 2018	RCT, 6 months N=276 (93 WebMOVE, 95 MOVE! SMI, 88 control group) 6% female, 40% white, 50% Black Diagnosis: schizophrenia spectrum, affective spectrum, and PTSD Special population: veterans (BMI≥30)	Computerized version of MOVE! SMI delivered in 30 online interactive modules (15 diet, 15 physical activity) via text-, audio-, and video-based information, tracking activity, weight, and goal setting. Peers provided 25- to 30-minute coaching calls weekly. Sessions used positive reinforcement, motivational enhancement activity suggestions, and problem-solving. Skills included self-monitoring, motivation, and self-efficacy. Mean (SD) attendance for WebMove was 14.7 (12.2) out of 30 possible. Mean attendance for MOVE! SMI was 9.7 (6.2) out of 24 possible. Online training with peers and a psychologist. Peer coaches received 5 months of training with master's- and doctoral-level study staff. Manualized instructions provided for each coaching call. Training included didactic instruction (via manual) and experiential training in coaching. Experiential training was completed with master therapist or through live coaching sessions, with peer coach eventually leading sessions.	Compared with control group, significantly more physical activity at 3 months by MOVE! SMI group, more physical activity at 6 months by MOVE! SMI and WebMOVE groups, more walking at 6 months by MOVE! SMI group, and more moderate activity and vigorous activity after 6 months by MOVE! SMI group.

TABLE 9–1. Lifestyle interventions targeting skills for diet and/or physical activity (*continued*)

Intervention name, authors, and website (if applicable)	Study design and sample	Intervention, skills, and intervention training	Outcomes
Simplified Intervention to Modify Physical Activity, Lifestyle and Eating (SIMPLE) Ratliff et al. 2012 www.simpleprogram.org	Pilot RCT, 2 months $N=30$ (10 per group of paid for attendance, paid for weight loss, reimbursed for healthy food after wait period) 66% female, 50% white, 37% Black, 13% Latino Special population: individuals with BMI≥28	Tested different forms of contingency management with a lifestyle modification intervention delivered over 8 weeks in weekly, 1-hour sessions (8–10 individuals), rewarding individuals who succeed in losing weight, attending groups, or being reimbursed for health food purchases (only after serving as control group). Based on social cognitive theory; encouraged to use social support and change attitudes for diet and physical activity. Skills included self-monitoring, motivation, and self-efficacy. Group-based by unspecified leader. Attendance and training not specified.	More rewards given to participants in attendance group and reimbursement group than to those in the weight-loss group. Weight loss reported in all groups, but differences not significant across the three strategies. However, significant weight loss after reimbursement for health food purchases reported for the wait-list group.

TABLE 9–1.   Lifestyle interventions targeting skills for diet and/or physical activity (*continued*)

Intervention name, authors, and website (if applicable)	Study design and sample	Intervention, skills, and intervention training	Outcomes
InSHAPE Van Citters et al. 2010 www.hprcd.org/inshape	Pilot within–subjects, 9 months *N*=76 Age, mean (SD)=43.5 (11.4) 72% female, 91% white Diagnosis: 40% major depressive disorder, 25% bipolar disorder, 24% schizophrenia, 5% PTSD, 3% anxiety, 3% alcohol dependence Special population: overweight individuals (BMI≥25)	Individual- and group-based intervention with health mentor. Individualized intervention focused on diet and exercise delivered in community settings over 9 months. Participants met weekly with their health mentor (45–60 minutes per session) and were encouraged to attend group-based exercise and nutrition education classes (approximately 1 hour long with 6–8 participants). Skills included self-monitoring, motivation, and self-efficacy. Attendance not specified. Health mentors were trained in fitness training, CPR, goal setting, motivational interviewing, and healthy eating behaviors. Received instructions from dietitian on dietary goals and basic education about mental illnesses.	Increased exercise, vigorous activity, walking, satisfaction with fitness; improvement in mental health functioning; and decreased waist circumference and severity of negative symptoms.

Note.   BMI=body mass index; CPR=cardiopulmonary resuscitation; DASH=Dietary Approaches to Stop Hypertension; MI=motivational interviewing; PI=principal investigator; PREMIER=clinical trial of lifestyle interventions for blood pressure control; PTSD=posttraumatic stress disorder; RCT=randomized controlled trial; SD=standard deviation; SMI=serious mental illness.

2011, 2013; Green et al. 2015a, 2015b; Muralidharan et al. 2018; Ratliff et al. 2012; Van Citters et al. 2010). Three studies targeted veterans (Erickson et al. 2017; Goldberg et al. 2013b; Muralidharan et al. 2018), one focused on individuals with bipolar disorder only (Gillhoff et al. 2010), one focused on individuals with schizophrenia or schizoaffective disorder only (Beebe et al. 2011), two focused on diabetes or diabetes prevention (Aschbrenner et al. 2016; McKibbin et al. 2010), and one study did not identify a special population of interest (Brown et al. 2011).

Culturally specific interventions were not represented among the interventions that were only focused on lifestyle. Indeed, most of the study samples were primarily white or highly representative of whites. Few of the interventions included Latinos or Asians, and neither were a majority of the samples, which suggests a significant need for interventions specifically targeting these populations (Erickson et al. 2017; Ratliff et al. 2012). Only two interventions had a majority of individuals who were Black (Goldberg et al. 2013b; Muralidharan et al. 2018). The percentage of female participants ranged from 6% to 81%. The majority of studies included a range of diagnoses, although one included only participants with bipolar disorder (Gillhoff et al. 2010).

Form of the Intervention

There were wide variations in the forms of the interventions. All the interventions appeared to be manualized. Only two studies had Web-based components (Aschbrenner et al. 2016; Muralidharan et al. 2018). Five interventions were group based only (Aschbrenner et al. 2016; Beebe et al. 2011; Brown et al. 2011; McKibbin et al. 2010; Ratliff et al. 2012), although four of those interventions were pilots. The InSHAPE intervention was the only one that was delivered individually (Bartels et al. 2013, 2015). The rest of the studies were a combination of group-based and individual- and group-based interventions. The lengths of interventions ranged from 2 months to 18 months (Daumit et al. 2013). Only three interventions included a peer for delivery of services (Aschbrenner et al. 2016; McKibbin et al. 2010; Muralidharan et al. 2018).

Outcomes

Interventions that specifically targeted lifestyle mostly focused on weight loss as an outcome, but several also sought to alter physical activity as well. Eight studies found significant weight loss (Bartels et al. 2015; Brown et al. 2011; Daumit et al. 2011, 2013; Erickson et al. 2017; Green et al. 2015a,

2015b; Ratliff et al. 2012), six found reductions in BMI (Bartels et al. 2015; Daumit et al. 2011, 2013; Gillhoff et al. 2010; Green et al. 2015; McKibbin et al. 2010), and five found reduced waist circumferences (Bartels et al. 2015; Daumit et al. 2011; Erickson et al. 2017; McKibbin et al. 2010; Van Citters et al. 2010). Seven studies (three of which were the InSHAPE intervention) found increased physical activity (Aschbrenner et al. 2016; Bartels et al. 2013, 2015; Beebe et al. 2011; Daumit et al. 2011; Muralidharan et al. 2018; Van Citters et al. 2010). The InSHAPE program was the only program in which changes in weight loss intentions were reported.

Interventions to Develop Physical Health Care Skills

Study Design

There were 19 studies that focused on health care use and experiences, such as service access or communication with providers (Table 9–2). Multiple studies addressed the same intervention or were based on an adaptation of the Chronic Disease Self-Management Program (Health and Recovery Peer [HARP] Program, Living Well). Three of the studies addressed the Bridge model (Kelly et al. 2014b, 2017, 2018); three focused on the Life Goals Collaborative Care program, although in one the program was specifically adapted for cardiovascular issues (Kilbourne et al. 2012, 2013, 2017); two involved Targeted Training for Illness Management (Sajatovic et al. 2011, 2017); two focused on Helping Older People Experience Success (HOPES) (Bartels et al. 2014b; Pratt et al. 2017); two focused on the HARP Program (Druss et al. 2010b, 2018); and two were on the Living Well intervention (Goldberg et al. 2013a; Muralidharan et al. 2019).

Only four studies were pre-post, within-subject comparisons (Lorig et al. 2014; Pratt et al. 2017; Sajatovic et al. 2011; Teachout et al. 2011), five were pilot RCTs (Druss et al. 2010b; Goldberg et al. 2013a; Kelly et al. 2014b, 2018; Kilbourne et al. 2012), and 10 were fully powered RCTs (Bartels et al. 2014a, 2014b; Druss et al. 2010a, 2018; Katon et al. 2010; Kelly et al. 2017; Kilbourne et al. 2013, 2017; Muralidharan et al. 2019; Sajatovic et al. 2017).

Skills Developed

All the studies described skill-building activities targeting self-monitoring, motivation, and self-efficacy skills. Two studies included changes to knowledge

TABLE 9–2. Interventions targeting skills to address physical health care

Intervention name, authors, and website (if applicable)	Study design and sample	Intervention, skills, and intervention training	Outcomes
Integrated Illness Management and Recovery (I-IMR) Bartels et al. 2014a https://practicetransformation.umn.edu/clinicaltraining/imr	RCT, 14 months *N*=71 (36 treatment group, 35 control group) Age, mean (SD): 60.3 (6.5) 55% female, 97% white Diagnosis: 38% schizophrenia, 18% bipolar disorder, 44% depression Special population: older adults	8-month individual- and group-based program delivered by a social worker (master's) and a primary care nurse and consisting of 10 modules aimed at addressing SMI and chronic health conditions equally with self-management strategies. Program had four main components: 1) psychoeducation, 2) behavioral tailoring, 3) relapse prevention training, and 4) coping skills training. Nurse helped to coordinate care. Skills included self-monitoring, motivation, self-efficacy, coping, adherence, and access to care. Mean (SD) attendance was 15.8 (9.5) for I-IMR sessions and 8.2 (5.9) for nurse sessions. 1.5 days of training in I-IMR, using program tool kit and manual for social worker, was provided.	Significant improvements in self-management of psychiatric symptoms according to client (*d*=0.46) and clinician (*d*=0.29), diabetes self-management (*d*=0.15), knowledge seeking about health (*d*=0.88), and decreased hospitalizations.

TABLE 9–2. Interventions targeting skills to address physical health care *(continued)*

Intervention name, authors, and website (if applicable)	Study design and sample	Intervention, skills, and intervention training	Outcomes
Helping Older People Experience Success (HOPES) Bartels et al. 2014b	RCT, 36 months N=183 (90 treatment group, 93 control group) Age, mean (SD): 60.2 (7.9) 42% female, 86% white Diagnosis: 28% schizophrenia, 28% schizoaffective disorder, 20% bipolar disorder, 24% major depression Special population: older adults	Group-based intervention consisting of 1 year of weekly skills training classes (8–10 persons per group), two per day (one training on a specific skill and one role-play session—150 minutes total), followed by a 1-year maintenance phase with monthly booster sessions with a nurse. Skills included self-monitoring, motivation, self-efficacy, coping, communication, and access to care. Attendance was 75% in year 1 and 70% in year 2 for skills training, and 66% for nurse visits. Training was manualized, but details were not provided in article.	Significant improvements in community living skills (d=0.25), functioning (d=0.26), mental health symptoms (d=−0.17), performance skills (d=0.27), and self-efficacy (d=0.33). Increase in some physical health screenings (d=0.32–0.59), and fewer hospitalizations and ER visits.

TABLE 9–2. Interventions targeting skills to address physical health care (*continued*)

Intervention name, authors, and website (if applicable)	Study design and sample	Intervention, skills, and intervention training	Outcomes
Primary Care Access Referral, and Evaluation (PCARE) Druss et al. 2010a	RCT, 12 months N=407 (205 treatment group, 202 control group) Age, mean: 46 48% female, 78% Black Diagnosis: 43% schizo-phrenia/schizoaffective, 33% depression, 17% bipolar disorder, 7% PTSD	Individual-based intervention delivered by care manager and designed to address patient, provider, and system barriers to care. Care manager used MI, coached on communication with providers, monitored their readiness for change, and reinforced autonomy for medical care and lifestyle goals. Care manager also helped participants to obtain benefits and connect to transportation. Skills included self-monitoring, motivation, self-efficacy, adherence, communication, and access to care. Attendance and training not specified.	Compared with control group, increased physical exams (70.5% vs. 35.6%), screening (50.4% vs. 21.6%), health education (80.0% vs. 18.9%), vaccinations (24.7% vs. 3.8%), and access to care (21% vs. 4%). Improvements in mental health and social functioning, physical health functioning, and detection of undiagnosed conditions.

TABLE 9–2. Interventions targeting skills to address physical health care (*continued*)

Intervention name, authors, and website (if applicable)	Study design and sample	Intervention, skills, and intervention training	Outcomes
Health and Recovery Peer Program (HARP) Druss et al. 2010b	RCT pilot, 6 months $N=80$ (41 treatment group, 39 control group) Age, mean: 49 70% female, 83% Black, 17% white, 1% other Diagnosis: 29% schizophrenia, 33% bipolar disorder, 26% major depression, 11% PTSD	Intervention consisting of six sessions with mental health peers in a classroom-based format adapted from Chronic Disease Self-Management Program (CDSMP) training, including self-management skills, addressing lifestyle (diet, exercise), pain and fatigue management, money management, medication management, self-monitoring, motivation, coping, communication and health care access. Attendance was mean of 4.5 sessions. Interventionists received 1-week training in HARP intervention/study protocol. Training included didactic training, role-playing, and techniques for patient activation and health education. Peers completed 2-week certification course.	Significant increase in patient activation (8% improvement vs. 6% decline), medication adherence (14% improvement vs. 7% decline), health-related quality of life, and health care access (8% improvement vs. 17% decline) in treatment group, compared with control group, at 6 months.

TABLE 9–2. Interventions targeting skills to address physical health care (*continued*)

Intervention name, authors, and website (if applicable)	Study design and sample	Intervention, skills, and intervention training	Outcomes
Health and Recovery Peer Program (HARP) Druss et al. 2018	RCT, 6 months *N*=400 (198 treatment group, 202 control group) Age, mean: 49 67% female, 66% Black, 30% white, 4% other Diagnosis: 29% schizophrenia / schizoaffective, 39% bipolar disorder, 71% major depression, 22% PTSD	Intervention consisting of six sessions (2.5 hours per session) delivered by mental health peers in a classroom-based format adapted from CDSMP training, including self-management skills, addressing lifestyle (diet, exercise), general medical conditions, money management, medication management, health care access, and communication. Skills also included self-monitoring, motivation, self-efficacy, and coping. 70% attended at least four sessions. Peers received 1 week of training that included didactic training, role-playing, enhancement of patient activation (making an action plan, sharing and feedback, modeling, and persuasion), health education techniques (lecture with discussion, brainstorming, demonstration, feedback, problem-solving). A leader's manual was provided.	Significant improvement in physical health (*d*=0.11), mental health (*d*=0.17), quality of life (*d*=0.15), and recovery in treatment group, compared with control group, at 6 months, Increased patient activation present at 3-month, but not at 6-month, follow-up in the treatment group. No changes in diet, medication adherence, or usual source of medical care.

TABLE 9–2. Interventions targeting skills to address physical health care (*continued*)

Intervention name, authors, and website (if applicable)	Study design and sample	Intervention, skills, and intervention training	Outcomes
Living Well Goldberg et al. 2013a	RCT pilot, 6 months *N*=63 (32 treatment group, 31 control group) Age, mean (SD): 49.5 (9.1) 48% male, 29% white, 67% Black, 4% mixed Diagnosis: schizophrenia and bipolar disorder with psychotic features Special population: veterans	Group-based intervention delivered by two peer providers and a mental health professional. Intervention based on modified version of the CDSMP that converted 6 sessions into 13-session (60–75 minutes) peer-cofacilitated Living Well intervention. Focus was on action planning, peer feedback and support, modeling, problem-solving, disease-specific management techniques, lifestyle skills (sleep, medication, substance use), and integrated health care. Skills also included self-monitoring, motivation, self-efficacy, adherence, coping, and access to care. The PI, who had completed the 5-day CDSMP master training course, participated in modifying the intervention and trained all the leaders.	From baseline to end of intervention (13 weeks), significant improvement in self-management (generally *d*=0.57 and health care *d*=0.81), internal locus of control (*d*=0.66), general physical health, mental health, and general functioning. Less frequent ER use (20% less than use at baseline), but difference not significant compared with the control group. Two months postintervention, only locus of control and health care self-management still significant.

TABLE 9–2. Interventions targeting skills to address physical health care (*continued*)

Intervention name, authors, and website (if applicable)	Study design and sample	Intervention, skills, and intervention training	Outcomes
Collaborative care Katon et al. 2010 www.aims.uw.edu/teamcare	RCT, 12 months *N*=214 (106 treatment group, 108 control group) 49% female, 22% non-white Diagnosis: 100% depression (76% ≥2 years) Special population: individuals with depression	A clinic-based intervention delivered by a nurse over 12 months to provide collaborative care management, help with depression, and facilitate improvements in hemoglobin A1c, blood pressure, and lipid control. Nurses provided motivational coaching for problem-solving and health goals and offered support in a maintenance phase. Skills included self-monitoring, motivation, self-efficacy, adherence, communication, coping, and access to care. Individualized and delivered by a nurse. Mean attendance was 10 in-person contacts and 10.8 phone contacts over 12 months. A 2-day training course on depression management, behavioral strategies, and medical indicators (glycemic, blood pressure, and lipid control) was provided. The program was created by a psychiatrist, family physician, internist specializing in nephrology, endocrinologist, psychologist, and a nurse.	Significant changes to insulin and antihypertensive medications. Improvements in hemoglobin A1c, LDL cholesterol, and systolic blood pressure. No change in diet or exercise.

TABLE 9–2.   Interventions targeting skills to address physical health care (*continued*)

Intervention name, authors, and website (if applicable)	Study design and sample	Intervention, skills, and intervention training	Outcomes
Bridge Kelly et al. 2014b www.healthnavigation.org	RCT pilot, 12 months $N=23$ (12 treatment group, 11 control group) Age, mean (SD): 46.78 (8.45) 57% male, 26% white, 35% Black, 13% Latino, 26% mixed or other Diagnosis: not specified, but SMI	Three-phase individual-based intervention delivered by a mental health peer that begins intensively and then slowly tapers off to allow more self-management. The 6 months of health navigator sessions, provided in 1:1 coaching sessions, were field-based and addressed an array of issues, including prevention, detection, and management of chronic diseases. Skills include self-monitoring, motivation, self-efficacy, adherence, communication, coping, and access to care. Average of three contacts per month. Peers completed a peer specialist training course and 3-day intervention training, and coaching continued for 10 weeks.	Significant reductions in pain ($d=0.91$), decreased preference for ER use (0% treated group vs. 56% of control group), and a trend for fewer health problems.

TABLE 9–2. Interventions targeting skills to address physical health care (*continued*)

Intervention name, authors, and website (if applicable)	Study design and sample	Intervention, skills, and intervention training	Outcomes
Bridge Kelly et al. 2017 www.healthnavigation.org	RCT, 12 months *N*=151 (76 treatment group, 75 control group) Age, mean (SD): 45.63 (10.95) 54% female, 25% white, 8% Black, 60% Latino, 8% other Diagnosis: 37% schizophrenia/schizoaffective disorder, 19% bipolar disorder, 39% depression, 5% other	Three-phase individual-based intervention delivered by a mental health peer that begins intensively and then slowly tapers off. The 6 months of health navigator sessions, provided in 1:1 coaching sessions, were field-based and addressed an array of issues, including prevention, detection, and management of chronic diseases. Skills included self-monitoring, motivation, self-efficacy, adherence, communication, coping, and access to care. Mean (SD) attendance was 4.91 (5.02) for in-person and 6.27 (6.70) for phone contacts. Peers completed a peer specialist training course and 3-day intervention training, and coaching continued for 10 weeks. Training and implementation manuals provided. Supervisors completed 1-day training on intervention and supervision.	Significantly more visits to routine care provider (d=0.46), improved relationship quality with PCP (*d*=−0.51), increased preference for non-ER services, increased detection of chronic diseases (*d*=0.38), reduced bodily pain severity (*d*=−0.36), and increased self-efficacy for health care after 6 months (*d*=0.36).

TABLE 9–2.   Interventions targeting skills to address physical health care (*continued*)

Intervention name, authors, and website (if applicable)	Study design and sample	Intervention, skills, and intervention training	Outcomes
Bridge Kelly et al. 2018 www.healthnavigation.org	RCT pilot, 12 months $N=20$ (11 treatment group, 9 wait-list group) Age, mean (SD): 50.60 (9.89) 50% female, 20% Black, 35% white, 15% Latino, 30% mixed race Special population: individuals who are homeless or history of homelessness	Three-phase individual-based intervention delivered by a mental health peer that begins intensively and then slowly tapers off. The 6 months of health navigator sessions, provided in 1:1 coaching sessions, were field-based and addressed an array of issues (prevention, detection, and management of chronic diseases). Participants were also trained to access electronic health records. Skills included self-monitoring, motivation, self-efficacy, adherence, communication, coping, and access to care. Peers completed a peer specialist training course and 4-day intervention training, received coaching for 10 weeks, and met with PI for individual training on use of iPad and EHR system. Training and implementation were manualized. Supervisors completed 1-day training.	Significant increase in visits to routine care providers ($d=0.66$) and health screenings ($d=0.41$), and significantly improved relationship with PCP ($d=-0.51$). Self-management of communication with providers also significantly improved. Homeless individuals had reduced pain ($P=0.04$) and a trend for increased self-management of following doctors' instructions ($P=0.07$).

TABLE 9–2. Interventions targeting skills to address physical health care *(continued)*

Intervention name, authors, and website (if applicable)	Study design and sample	Intervention, skills, and intervention training	Outcomes
Life Goals Collaborative Care (LGCC) Kilbourne et al. 2012	RCT pilot, 12 months $N=65$ (32 treatment group, 33 control group) Age, mean (SD): 45.3 (12.8) 61% female, 78% white, 19% Black Diagnosis: 100% bipolar disorder Special population: veterans and individuals with bipolar disorder	Intervention delivered by master's-level social worker consisting of four 2-hour weekly group self-management sessions to LGCC patients, then brief care management contacts for up to 6 months. Each group session included 8–10 participants and featured guided discussions and exercises designed to help patients set personal self-management goals. Skills included self-monitoring, motivation, self-efficacy, adherence, communication, coping, and access to care. Mean (SD) attendance was 4.5 (1.5). Care manager received 3 days of training.	No reductions in cardio-metabolic risk factors or health well-being; reduced functional disability ($d=-0.20$) and de-pressive symptoms ($d=-0.23$).

TABLE 9–2. Interventions targeting skills to address physical health care (*continued*)

Intervention name, authors, and website (if applicable)	Study design and sample	Intervention, skills, and intervention training	Outcomes
Self-Management Addressing Health Risk Trial (SMAHRT) Kilbourne et al. 2013	RCT, 24 months $N=116$ (57 treatment group, 59 control group) Age, mean (SD): 52.8 (9.9) 17% female, 95% white Diagnosis: 100% bipolar disorder	12-month clinic- and classroom-based group intervention adapted from the LGCC program designed to address cardiometabolic risk. Intervention was delivered by master's-level trained health specialists. Adaptation used four of six components of the chronic care model but also used social cognitive theory to address health behavior change. Skills included self-monitoring, motivation, self-efficacy, adherence, communication, coping, and access to care. Mean (SD) attendance was 4.6 (3.6) during 12 months of treatment; 1.2 (1.0) with mental health specialist, 0.3 (0.6) with PCP. Health specialists received 2 days of training led by study investigators using established protocol.	Reduced systolic ($d=-0.22$) and diastolic ($d=-0.23$) blood pressure and symptoms of mania after 24 months.

TABLE 9–2. Interventions targeting skills to address physical health care *(continued)*

Intervention name, authors, and website (if applicable)	Study design and sample	Intervention, skills, and intervention training	Outcomes
Life Goals Collaborative Care (LGCC) Kilbourne et al. 2017 www.lifegoalscc.com	RCT, 12 months N=293 (146 treatment group, 147 control group) Age, mean (SD): 55.5 (10.8) 15% female, 82% white, 18% Black Diagnosis: 58% depression, 24% bipolar disorder, 7% schizophrenia, 11% other SMI Special population: overweight individuals (BMI≥28 or chronic health condition)	Group-based intervention delivered by trained master's-level social workers to promote healthy behavior changes. Over first 2 months, five weekly sessions of guidance on physical and mental health symptoms were provided. Over 12 months, care coordination services were incorporated, including 6 months of contacts about self-management, ongoing assistance with communication with doctors, and mental health clinic support services to providers. Skills included self-monitoring, motivation, self-efficacy, adherence, communication, coping, and access to care. Attendance was not specified. Social workers received 2 days of training led by study investigators using established protocol.	After 12 months, significantly reduced BMI (d=−0.27) and improvements in physical health (d=0.39) and LDL levels (d=−0.30) in the treatment group compared with the control group. No significant change in physical activity or Framingham risk score.

TABLE 9–2. Interventions targeting skills to address physical health care *(continued)*

Intervention name, authors, and website (if applicable)	Study design and sample	Intervention, skills, and intervention training	Outcomes
Chronic Disease Self-Management Program (CDSMP) Lorig et al. 2014 www.selfmanagementresource.com/programs/smallgroup/programs/smallgroup/chronicdisease-selfmanagement	Within-subjects, 6 months $N=137$ Age, mean (SD): 48.2 (11.0) 73% female, 24% Black Diagnosis rates not provided	Modified version of CDSMP consisting of six classroom-based sessions conducted by peer support specialists over 6 months. Sessions covered self-management education, chronic disease management, action planning, and feedback on progress. Skills included self-monitoring, motivation, self-efficacy, adherence, communication, coping, and access to care. Mean (SD) attendance was 4.2 (1.6). Peer support specialists completed a 60-hour program through the official training center. CDSMP leaders also completed 18 hours of additional training in how to facilitate the program.	After 6 months, significant improvement in fatigue ($d=0.22$), quality of life ($d=0.29$), health distress ($d=0.42$), communication with providers ($d=0.25$), and adherence to medical care ($d=0.30$), and significantly fewer bad physical health days ($d=0.25$) and bad mental health days ($d=0.39$).

TABLE 9–2. Interventions targeting skills to address physical health care *(continued)*

Intervention name, authors, and website (if applicable)	Study design and sample	Intervention, skills, and intervention training	Outcomes
Living Well Muralidharan et al. 2019	RCT, 6 months $N=242$ (124 in Living Well, 118 in control group) Age, mean (SD): 57.8 (7.7) 13% female, 29% white, 62% Black, 9% other Diagnosis: 12% schizophrenia, 16% schizoaffective, 35% bipolar disorder, 5% major depressive disorder with psychotic features, 5% psychosis NOS, 29% PTSD Special populations: veterans	Modified version of the CDSMP delivered in a group format with a master's-level clinician over 12 sessions (75 minutes each). Sessions were co-led by a peer and a non-peer facilitator. Content included goal setting, action planning, and problem-solving, with positive reinforcements. Skills included self-monitoring, motivation, self-efficacy, adherence, communication, coping, and access to care. Attendance mean (SD) was 6.4 (4.2). Trainings were completed by PI.	After 3 months, improvement in mental health quality of life ($d=0.24$), physical health quality of life ($d=-0.21$), self-efficacy ($d=0.43$), internal locus of control ($d=0.23$), patient activation ($d=0.21$), symptom management ($d=0.29$), and overall BASIS ($d=-0.23$). At 3 months postintervention, significant improvement in self-management ($d=0.32$) remained, and there was significant improvement in physical activity ($d=0.29$) and BASIS relationships ($d=-0.32$).

TABLE 9–2. Interventions targeting skills to address physical health care (*continued*)

Intervention name, authors, and website (if applicable)	Study design and sample	Intervention, skills, and intervention training	Outcomes
Helping Older People Experience Success—Individually Tailored (HOPES-I) Pratt et al. 2017	Pilot, within-subjects, 6 months N=47 Age, mean (SD): 62 (6.5) 76% female, 100% white Diagnosis: 36% schizophrenia, 26% schizoaffective disorder, 23% bipolar disorder, 15% depression Special population: older adults	Individual- and group-based intervention based on HOPES model and a skills training model that was modified to be individually delivered. Intervention was delivered by interns, case managers, and master's-level therapists and consisted of weekly sessions for 9–12 months. Five modules, on leisure, relationships, living independently, communication about health, and self-management of health, were offered. Skills included self-monitoring, motivation, self-efficacy, adherence, communication, and coping. Mean (SD) attendance was 29.6 (9.4) sessions; mean number of modules completed was 3.32. Coaches completed 2-day training in skills training techniques, instruction on curriculum, and weekly supervision.	Increased engagement in leisure activities, more effective communication about health, and increased confidence in social relationships, community living skills, and self-management of health.

TABLE 9–2. Interventions targeting skills to address physical health care (*continued*)

Intervention name, authors, and website (if applicable)	Study design and sample	Intervention, skills, and intervention training	Outcomes
Targeted Training for Illness Management Sajatovic et al. 2011	Pilot within-subjects, 4 months *N*=12 Age, mean: 49.5 Diagnosis: SMI	Group-based intervention based on LGP and DART program and delivered by peer and nurse. Over 12 weeks, participants completed weekly group sessions (60–90 minutes each) and four weekly telephone follow-up sessions. Sessions focused on psychoeducation, problem identification, goal setting, and behavioral modeling and reinforcement. Skills included self-monitoring, motivation, self-efficacy, adherence, communication, coping, and access to care. Attendance was not specified. Training was led by nurse educators and took place in groups. Training manual covered lifestyle, nutrition, communication skills, group leading, assistance in help seeking, and crisis management.	Significant improvement in hemoglobin A1c for eight participants and improvement in dietary behaviors. Weight loss not significant, but improvement in diet.

TABLE 9–2. Interventions targeting skills to address physical health care (*continued*)

Intervention name, authors, and website (if applicable)	Study design and sample	Intervention, skills, and intervention training	Outcomes
Targeted Training for Illness Management Sajatovic et al. 2017	RCT, 15 months $N=200$ (100 treatment group, 100 control group) Age, mean (SD): 52.7 (9.5) 64% female, 37% white, 54% Black, 9% other Diagnosis: 48% depression, 25% schizophrenia, 28% bipolar disorder Special population: individuals with diabetes	Group-based intervention based on LGP and DART program and delivered by peer and nurse over two phases: Phase 1: a group-based, peer-led illness self-management program for diabetes and SMI with 12 weekly sessions (6–10 participants) covered medication management, nutrition, exercise, substance use, problem-solving, goal setting, and social support. Phase 2: for 48 weeks, participants had bimonthly phone calls with interventionists for 3 months, then monthly calls for 9 months. Skills also included self-monitoring, motivation, self-efficacy, communication, coping, and access to care. Mean (SD) attendance was 7.2 (4.6). 2-day training groups were led by nurse educators. Training manual covered lifestyle, nutrition, communication skills, group leading, assistance in help seeking, and crisis management.	Significant improvement in psychiatric symptoms, general functioning, and knowledge about diabetes.

TABLE 9–2. Interventions targeting skills to address physical health care *(continued)*

Intervention name, authors, and website (if applicable)	Study design and sample	Intervention, skills, and intervention training	Outcomes
Diabetes Management Program Teachout et al. 2011	Pilot within-subjects, 6 months $N=13$ Age, mean (SD): 45 (6.9) 23% female, 69% Black, 31% white Diagnosis: 46% schizophrenia, 31% schizoaffective, 15% depression, 8% psychotic disorder NOS Special population: individuals with diabetes in supportive housing	Diabetes education classes led by teaching residents (advance practice nurses) about self-care, healthy lifestyle, and food shopping (in addition to other supports routinely provided). Skills included self-monitoring, motivation, self-efficacy, adherence, coping, and access to care. Attendance and training not specified.	Weight loss in 100% of the sample; improved glucose levels in 27% of participants after 6 months.

Note. BASIS=Behavior and Symptom Identification Scale; BMI=body mass index; CDSMP=Chronic Disease Self-Management Program; d=Cohen's d: estimate of effect size; DART=Diabetes Awareness and Rehabilitation Training; EHR=electronic health record; ER=emergency room; LDL=low-density lipoprotein; LGP=Life Goals Program; MI=motivational interviewing; NOS=not otherwise specified; PCP=primary care provider; PHR=personal health record; PI=principal investigator; PTSD=posttraumatic stress disorder; RCT=randomized controlled trial; SD=standard deviation; SMI=serious mental illness.

about health (Bartels et al. 2014a; Druss et al. 2010a), and two included changes to diabetes knowledge (Bartels et al. 2014a; Sajatovic et al. 2017), both of which could be considered proxies for some aspects of self-monitoring, although no studies included this as an outcome. The Living Well intervention included changes to locus of control (Goldberg et al. 2013a; Muralidharan et al. 2019). Seven studies (for the HOPES, Integrated Illness Management and Recovery, Bridge, and Living Well interventions) found significant improvements in self-efficacy or self-management (Bartels et al. 2014a, 2014b; Goldberg et al. 2013a; Kelly et al. 2017, 2018; Muralidharan et al. 2019; Pratt et al. 2017), and the HARP intervention was associated with improvement in patient activation (Druss et al. 2010b, 2018).

Treatment adherence skills were not described in the curriculum for only one intervention (Bartels et al. 2014b), and only one study specifically included medication adherence as an improved outcome (Druss et al. 2010b). Communication skills with providers were not included in three studies (Bartels et al. 2014a; Goldberg et al. 2013a; Teachout et al. 2011), and only four studies (across three interventions) found improved communication with providers (Kelly et al. 2017, 2018; Lorig et al. 2014; Pratt et al. 2017). Coping skills were addressed by all but the Primary Care Access, Referral, and Evaluation (PCARE) study (Druss et al. 2010a), although only one study detected improvements in health distress (Lorig et al. 2014). Access-to-care skills were not included in the individually tailored HOPES intervention (Pratt et al. 2017) but were included in the other studies. There were two studies (one intervention) that found changed attitudes about accessing nonemergency care (Kelly et al. 2014b, 2017), although other studies also found improvements in health care access (Bartels et al. 2014a, 2014b; Druss et al. 2010a, 2010b).

Special Populations

Three studies described interventions tailored for older adults (Bartels et al. 2014a, 2014b; Pratt et al. 2017). Three studies were focused on treatment of individuals with diabetes (Sajatovic et al. 2011, 2017; Teachout et al. 2011). One was developed for individuals who were homeless or had a history of homelessness (Kelly et al. 2018). Veterans were targeted in four studies, two of which also targeted individuals with bipolar disorder (Goldberg et al. 2013a; Kilbourne et al. 2012, 2013; Muralidharan et al. 2019). One intervention was developed for individuals with depression only (Katon et al. 2010).

None of the studies were designed to target individuals of a specific culture, although there were seven studies that had a majority of participants who were Black (Druss et al. 2010a, 2010b, 2018; Goldberg et al. 2013a; Muralidharan et al. 2019; Sajatovic et al. 2017; Teachout et al. 2011) and one other that had a majority of Latinos (Kelly et al. 2017). Female participants ranged from 13% to 76%.

Form of the Intervention

All but two interventions were manualized (Katon et al. 2010; Teachout et al. 2011). Interventions to address physical health and health care are more effective when they are intensive and individualized. Individualized approaches were more common for physical health care interventions than they were for the lifestyle-only interventions (Druss et al. 2010a; Katon et al. 2010; Kelly et al. 2014b, 2017, 2018). Twelve studies were group based only (Bartels et al. 2014b; Druss et al. 2010b, 2018; Goldberg et al. 2013a; Kilbourne et al. 2012, 2013, 2017; Lorig et al. 2014; Muralidharan et al. 2019; Sajatovic et al. 2011, 2017; Teachout et al. 2011). Mental health peers delivered independently or in conjunction with another leader for 10 studies (across a subset of studies with pilot trials and fully powered RCTs) (Druss et al. 2010b, 2018; Goldberg et al. 2013a; Kelly et al. 2014b, 2017, 2018; Lorig et al. 2014; Muralidharan et al. 2019; Sajatovic et al. 2011, 2017), and six studies were delivered by nurses—three alone, two with peers, and one with a master's-level social worker (Bartels et al. 2014a, 2014b; Katon et al. 2010; Sajatovic et al. 2011, 2017; Teachout et al. 2011). The remainder involved a master's-level-trained person alone or with others.

Outcomes

The targets for physical health care interventions ranged considerably, including self-management/self-efficacy, patient activation, locus of control, improvements in physical and mental health, detection of illnesses, psychoeducation, access to primary or specialty care, physical activity, diet, sleep, leisure, independent living skills, and functional status, as well as decreased use of ER services/hospitalizations and weight loss. Effect sizes were typically small or moderate. There were significant improvements in self-efficacy, locus of control, or empowerment in nine studies (Bartels et al. 2014a, 2014b; Druss et al. 2010b, 2018; Goldberg et al. 2013a; Kelly et al. 2017, 2018; Muralidharan et al. 2019; Pratt et al. 2017) and a trend in another (Bartels et al. 2014b).

Improvements in physical health were found by 12 studies (Druss et al. 2010a, 2010b, 2018; Goldberg et al. 2013a; Katon et al. 2010; Kelly et al. 2014b, 2017; Kilbourne et al. 2013, 2017; Lorig et al. 2014; Sajatovic et al.

2011; Teachout et al. 2011). Lifestyle outcomes of diet or exercise were improved in three studies (Muralidharan et al. 2019; Sajatovic et al. 2011; Teachout et al. 2011). Physical health care access or use was improved in five studies (Bartels et al. 2014b; Druss et al. 2010a, 2010b; Kelly et al. 2017, 2018), and improved communication with providers was found in four studies (Kelly et al. 2017, 2018; Lorig et al. 2014; Pratt et al. 2017). There were detectable decreases in use of ERs or hospitalizations in two studies (Bartels et al. 2014a, 2014b).

This review highlights several promising interventions for improving the healthy living skills of individuals with SMI. However, successful implementation of any skill-building program requires coordination and partnership with the existing mental health team and physical health care providers. To illustrate this, we describe a prototypical participant in the Bridge peer health navigator intervention in the following case vignette.

Case Vignette

Jorge is a 38-year-old Latino man. His situation with regard to health care is quite typical for someone with an SMI who is engaged in mental health services. He has Medicaid coverage for his health and mental health services; yet, he has not established an ongoing relationship with a primary care provider and often goes to the ER when he feels ill. Other than infrequent trips to the ER, he does not seek medical care. He believes that the ER is his primary care provider.

Once he is engaged by a Bridge peer health navigator and connected to an outpatient primary care physician whom he likes, he begins receiving routine care there. As part of his health navigation, he works with his navigator to develop wellness goals for himself. Typical wellness goals include exercise, weight loss, diet, recreational activities, building social networks, and educational activities. He chooses to begin with exercise. He develops a step-by-step plan with his navigator for how he will achieve his goal and then discusses it with his primary care physician. The doctor is very supportive of the plan as it sets incremental goals for walking that include things like days, times, and locations for the walks and even a discussion of neighborhood safety. After a month, Jorge is walking 5 times a week for 30 minutes. He then decides to focus on his eating habits, including food choices.

For each issue addressed through the Bridge, the health navigator seeks input from agency social workers about how to implement the intervention protocols and has joint sessions with them. The protocols are highly individualized and use physician support for motivation. Jorge is also asked to share his plans with one or two of his fellow consumers. On-site nurses also reinforce the intervention plans. After years of neglecting his routine health care needs and his wellness needs, Jorge begins to see routine health care as part of his life. He also begins to take control of two issues that have an impact on his health and wellness: exercise and diet. In addition, he talks about how he sees very clearly how improving his health and wellness routines positively impacts his mental health. Jorge begins attending wellness groups at the agency as a support for his ongoing wellness efforts. For Jorge, the critical issues for change are having a peer navigator, experiencing success with health care access and use, individualizing his wellness goals, having agency support for the navigator implementing the wellness protocols, physician support for his goals, and peer involvement in his change.

Considerations for the Future

Preparing the partners in care to anticipate the changes in their patients during a healthy living skills intervention can help to facilitate positive response and support for their nascent skills. Medical providers who understand the role and function of the health navigator are more likely to accept the assistance of this additional person in medical appointments and to encourage his or her development. These newly acquired skills may have benefits in other domains, and coordinating the response of the mental health team can ensure that there is consistent messaging across the treatment team, which can further reinforce their development. Regardless of the intervention that an agency may select as appropriate for its population and context, training supervisors about how to manage the new role or intervention, as well as advertising this new role to the treatment team and local community, can help to ensure its successful adoption.

There has been a proliferation of evidence-based practices for improving the physical health and health care of individuals with SMI in the last decade. The majority of these interventions are designed to build multiple skills, although the degree to which these skills are developed could be better evaluated in future assessments of these interventions. Practitioners have a set of manualized interventions that they can select that target improvements in healthy living skills and habits or improvements in the access, use, and experience of health care services. The decision about which intervention to employ depends on the outcomes desired. Overall, the level of evidence for the interventions ranges from modest (within-subject pre-post designs) to robust (fully powered RCTs). We suggest that practitioners consider the level of evidence for any intervention they select. We have included interventions with a range of evidence, as practitioners might want to select a promising intervention because of its specific features. It is also likely that promising interventions will be investigated with more rigorous designs, so practice decisions should be based on recent literature searches for particular interventions of interest.

Dissemination and implementation of these programs are important next steps to ensure that improvements in the health and well-being of this high-need population are realized. Mental health services to support and assist the population with SMI must devote attention to the development of healthy living skills to foster patient management of all aspects of living activities. This can be challenging because the development of healthy living skills requires attention to a broad array of issues, and addressing these deficits requires an understanding of how healthy living skills are developed and maintained for this population. Given the heterogeneity of the critical ingredients in various programs, more work is needed to compare the relative value of addressing skills in each of the targeted domains.

Knowledge and interventions are evolving rapidly in this area. In future studies, it will be critical to explore how these interventions affect the range of subpopulations that exist within the SMI population (e.g., housed vs. unhoused, male vs. female, multicultural) and to conduct comparative effectiveness trials to understand which programs have the most real-world utility for these subgroups. It is also important to consider the context in which individuals with SMI may live. Individuals with SMI often have low socioeconomic status and may reside in high-poverty neighborhoods. In addition to their stigmatized identity based on mental illness, they may also have other devalued identities, such as being a member of a racial/ethnic minority, being homeless, being involved with the criminal justice system, or being LGBTQ. Few of the interventions in this chapter focus on the spectrum of multiple social determinants or health disparities that may affect individuals with SMI, although several did note making adaptations for culture or poverty. Nonetheless, there are a growing number of interventions that practitioners can use to improve the physical health and health care utilization of individuals diagnosed with an SMI.

Key Points

- There are a variety of high-quality, evidence-based interventions that providers can select to help their patients develop a common set of healthy living skills.

- Interventions involving skill building are most likely to be effective when they are intensive and individualized.

- Attention to health disparities and to the social determinants of care can be important when determining the utility and fit of an intervention.

- Increasing attention to subpopulations and the diversity of individuals with serious mental illness will increase the applicability of interventions for healthy living skills

- Peer coaches have been shown to be effective facilitators or co-facilitators in several interventions.

- Physical health care interventions were much more likely to assess and find healthy skills development than lifestyle-only interventions—but few meaningfully affected both lifestyle and physical health care, both of which must be taken into account to truly address the health needs of this population.

References

Ajzen I: From intentions to actions: a theory of planned behavior, in Action Control (SSSP Springer Series in Social Psychology). Edited by Kuhl J, Beckmann J. New York, Springer, 1985, pp 11–39

Aschbrenner KA, Naslund JA, Shevenell M, et al: Feasibility of behavioral weight loss treatment enhanced with peer support and mobile health technology for individuals with serious mental illness. Psychiatr Q 87(3):401–415, 2016

Bartels SJ, Pratt SI, Aschbrenner KA, et al: Clinically significant improved fitness and weight loss among overweight persons with serious mental illness. Psychiatr Serv 64(8):729–736, 2013

Bartels SJ, Pratt SI, Mueser KT, et al: Integrated IMR for psychiatric and general medical illness for adults aged 50 or older with serious mental illness. Psychiatr Serv 65(3):330–337, 2014a

Bartels SJ, Pratt SI, Mueser KT, et al: Long-term outcomes of a randomized trial of integrated skills training and preventive healthcare for older adults with serious mental illness. Am J Geriatr Psychiatry 22(11):1251–1261, 2014b

Bartels SJ, Pratt SI, Aschbrenner KA, et al: Pragmatic replication trial of health promotion coaching for obesity in serious mental illness and maintenance of outcomes. Am J Psychiatry 172(4):344–352, 2015

Beebe LH, Smith K, Burk R, et al: Effect of a motivational intervention on exercise behavior in persons with schizophrenia spectrum disorders. Community Ment Health J 47(6):628–636, 2011

Brekke JS, Siantz E, Pahwa R, et al: Reducing health disparities for people with serious mental illness. Best Pract Ment Health 9(1):62–82, 2013

Brown C, Goetz J, Hamera E, et al: Weight loss intervention for people with serious mental illness: a randomized controlled trial of the RENEW program. Psychiatr Serv 62(7):800–802, 2011

Brunero S, Lamont S: Health behaviour beliefs and physical health risk factors for cardiovascular disease in an outpatient sample of consumers with a severe mental illness: a cross-sectional survey. Int J Nurs Stud 47(6):753–760, 2010

Cabassa LJ, Ezell JM, Lewis-Fernandez R: Lifestyle interventions for adults with serious mental illness: a systematic literature review. Psychiatr Serv 61(8):774–782, 2010

Cabassa LJ, Camacho D, Velez-Grau CM, et al: Peer-based health interventions for people with serious mental illness: a systematic literature review. J Psychiatr Res 84:80–89, 2017

Champion VL, Skinner CS: The health belief model, in Health Behavior and Health Education: Theory, Research, and Practice. Edited by Glanz K, Rimer B, Viswanath K. San Francisco, CA, Jossey-Bass, 2008, pp 45–65

Corrigan PW, Pickett S, Batia K, et al: Peer navigators and integrated care to address ethnic health disparities of people with serious mental illness. Soc Work Public Health 29(6):581–593, 2014

Crump C, Sundquist K, Winkleby MA, et al: Comorbidities and mortality in bipolar disorder: a Swedish national cohort study. JAMA Psychiatry 70(9):931–939, 2013

Daumit GL, Dalcin A, Jerome G, et al: A behavioral weight-loss intervention for persons with serious mental illness in psychiatric rehabilitation centers. Int J Obes (Lond) 35(8):1114–1123, 2011

Daumit GL, Dickerson FB, Wang N-Y, et al: A behavioral weight-loss intervention in persons with serious mental illness. N Engl J Med 368(17):1594–1602, 2013

Davidson L, Roe D: Recovery from versus recovery in serious mental illness: one strategy for lessening confusion plaguing recovery. J Ment Health 16(4):459–470, 2007

Deci EL, Ryan RM: The "what" and "why" of goal pursuits: human needs and the self-determination of behavior. Psychol Inq 11(4):227–268, 2000

De Hert M, Cohen D, Bobes J, et al: Physical illness in patients with severe mental disorders, II: barriers to care, monitoring and treatment guidelines, plus recommendations at the system and individual level. World Psychiatry 10(2):138–151, 2011a

De Hert M, Correll CU, Bobes J, et al: Physical illness in patients with severe mental disorders, I: prevalence, impact of medications and disparities in health care. World Psychiatry 10(1):52–77, 2011b

Dilk MN, Bond GRJ: Meta-analytic evaluation of skills training research for individuals with severe mental illness. J Consult Clin Psychol 64(6):1337–1346, 1996

Dombrovski A, Rosenstock J: Bridging general medicine and psychiatry: providing general medical and preventive care for the severely mentally ill. Curr Opin Psychiatry 17(6):523–529, 2004

Drake RE, Whitley R: Recovery and severe mental illness: description and analysis. Can J Psychiatry 59(5):236–242, 2014

Druss B, von Esenwein S, Compton M, et al: A randomized trial of medical care management for community mental health settings: the Primary Care Access, Referral, and Evaluation (PCARE) study. Am J Psychiatry 167(2):151–159, 2010a

Druss B, Zhao L, von Esenwein S, et al: The Health and Recovery Peer (HARP) Program: a peer-led intervention to improve medical self-management for persons with serious mental illness. Schizophr Res 118(13):264–270, 2010b

Druss B, Singh M, von Esenwein SA, et al: Peer-led self-management of general medical conditions for patients with serious mental illnesses: a randomized trial. Psychiatr Serv 69(5):529–535, 2018

Erickson ZD, Kwan CL, Gelberg HA, et al: A randomized, controlled multisite study of behavioral interventions for veterans with mental illness and antipsychotic medication-associated obesity. J Gen Intern Med 32(1):32–39, 2017

Faulkner G, Soundy A, Lloyd K: Schizophrenia and weight management: a systematic review of interventions to control weight. Acta Psychiatr Scand 108(5):324–332, 2003

Firth J, Rosenbaum S, Stubbs B, et al: Motivating factors and barriers towards exercise in severe mental illness: a systematic review and meta-analysis. Psychol Med 46(14):2869–2881, 2016

Gillhoff K, Gaab J, Emini L, et al: Effects of a multimodal lifestyle intervention on body mass index in patients with bipolar disorder: a randomized controlled trial. Prim Care Companion J Clin Psychiatry 12(5):PCC.09m00906, 2010

Goldberg R, Dickerson F, Lucksted A, et al: Living well: an intervention to improve self-management of medical illness for individuals with serious mental illness. Psychiatr Serv 64(1):51–57, 2013a

Goldberg R, Reeves G, Tapscott S, et al: "MOVE!": outcomes of a weight loss program modified for veterans with serious mental illness. Psychiatr Serv 64(8):737–744, 2013b

Green CA, Yarborough BJH, Leo MC, et al: The STRIDE weight loss and lifestyle intervention for individuals taking antipsychotic medications: a randomized trial. Am J Psychiatry 172(1):71–81, 2015

Green CA, Yarborough BJH, Leo MC, et al: Weight maintenance following the STRIDE lifestyle intervention for individuals taking antipsychotic medications. Obesity 23(10):1995–2001, 2015b

Hahm HC, Segal SP: Failure to seek health care among the mentally ill. Am J Orthopsychiatry 75(1):54–62, 2005

Hahm HC, Speliotis AE, Bachman SS: Failure to receive health care among people with mental illness: theory and implications. J Soc Work Disabil Rehabil 7(2):94–114, 2008

Harrow M, Grossman LS, Jobe TH, et al: Do patients with schizophrenia ever show periods of recovery? A 15-year multi-follow-up study. Schizophr Bull 31(3):723–734, 2005

Hjorthøj C, Stürup AE, McGrath JJ, et al: Years of potential life lost and life expectancy in schizophrenia: a systematic review and meta-analysis. Lancet Psychiatry 4(4):295–301, 2017

Jayatilleke N, Hayes R, Dutta R, et al: Contributions of specific causes of death to lost life expectancy in severe mental illness. Eur Psychiatry 43:109–115, 2017

Katon WJ, Lin E, Von Korff M, et al: Collaborative care for patients with depression and chronic illnesses. N Engl J Med 363(27):2611–2620, 2010

Kelly EL, Fenwick KM, Barr N, et al: A systematic review of self-management health care models for individuals with serious mental illnesses. Psychiatr Serv 65(11):1300–1310, 2014a

Kelly EL, Fulginiti A, Pahwa R, et al: A pilot test of a peer navigator intervention for improving the health of individuals with serious mental illness. Community Ment Health J 50(4):435–446, 2014b

Kelly EL, Duan L, Cohen H, et al: Integrating behavioral healthcare for individuals with serious mental illness: a randomized controlled trial of a peer health navigator intervention. Schizophr Res 182:135–141, 2017

Kelly EL, Braslow JT, Brekke JS: Using electronic health records to enhance a peer health navigator intervention: a randomized pilot test for individuals with serious mental illness and housing instability. Community Ment Health J 54(8):1172–1179, 2018

Kilbourne AM, Goodrich DE, Lai Z, et al: Life Goals Collaborative Care for patients with bipolar disorder and cardiovascular disease risk. Psychiatr Serv 63(12):1234–1238, 2012

Kilbourne AM, Goodrich D, Lai Z, et al: Randomized controlled trial to assess reduction of cardiovascular disease risk in patients with bipolar disorder: the Self-Management Addressing Heart Risk Trial (SMAHRT). J Clin Psychiatry 74(7):e655–e662, 2013

Kilbourne AM, Barbaresso MM, Lai Z, et al: Improving physical health in patients with chronic mental disorders: 12-month results from a randomized controlled collaborative care trial. J Clin Psychiatry 78(1):129, 2017

Lambert TJ, Velakoulis D, Pantelis C: Medical comorbidity in schizophrenia. Med J Aust 178(S9):S67–S70, 2003

Lawrence D, Kisely S: Inequalities in healthcare provision for people with severe mental illness. J Psychopharmacol 24(4 suppl):61–68, 2010

Levine ES: Facilitating recovery for people with serious mental illness employing a psychobiosocial model of care. Prof Psychol Res Pract 43(1):58–64, 2012

Lorig K, Ritter P, Pifer C, et al: Effectiveness of the Chronic Disease Self-management Program for persons with a serious mental illness: a translation study. Community Ment Health J 50(1):96–103, 2014

Lyman D, Kurtz M, Farkas M, et al: Skill building: assessing the evidence. Psychiatr Serv 65(6):727–738, 2014

Mazoruk S, Meyrick J, Taousi Z, et al: The effectiveness of health behavior change interventions in managing physical health in people with a psychotic illness: a systematic review. Perspect Psychiatr Care 56(1):121–140, 2019

McKibbin CL, Golshan S, Griver K, et al: A healthy lifestyle intervention for middle-aged and older schizophrenia patients with diabetes mellitus: a 6-month follow-up analysis. Schizophr Res 121(1–3):203–206, 2010

Muralidharan A, Niv N, Brown CH, et al: Impact of online weight management with peer coaching on physical activity levels of adults with serious mental illness. Psychiatr Serv 69(10):1062–1068, 2018

Muralidharan A, Brown C, Peer J, et al: Living well: an intervention to improve medical illness self-management among individuals with serious mental illness. Psychiatr Serv 70(1):19–25, 2019

Naslund JA, Whiteman KL, McHugo GJ, et al: Lifestyle interventions for weight loss among overweight and obese adults with serious mental illness: a systematic review and meta-analysis. Gen Hosp Psychiatry 47:83–102, 2017

Noble N, Paul C, Turon H, et al: Which modifiable health risk behaviours are related? A systematic review of the clustering of Smoking, Nutrition, Alcohol and Physical activity ('SNAP') health risk factors. Prev Med 81:16–41, 2015

Pratt SI, Mueser K, Wolfe R, et al: One size doesn't fit all: a trial of individually tailored skills training. Psychiatr Rehabil J 40(4):380–386, 2017

Ratliff JC, Palmese LB, Tonizzo KM, et al: Contingency management for the treatment of antipsychotic-induced weight gain: a randomized controlled pilot study. Obes Facts 5(6):919–927, 2012

Ryan RM, Deci EL: Intrinsic and extrinsic motivations: classic definitions and new directions. Contemp Educ Psychol 25(1):54–67, 2000

Sajatovic M, Dawson N, Perzynski A, et al: Best practices: optimizing care for people with serious mental illness and comorbid diabetes. Psychiatr Serv 62(9):1001–1003, 2011

Sajatovic M, Gunzler DD, Kanuch SW, et al: A 60-week prospective RCT of a self-management intervention for individuals with serious mental illness and diabetes mellitus. Psychiatr Serv 68(9):883–890, 2017

Siantz E, Aranda MP: Chronic disease self-management interventions for adults with serious mental illness: a systematic review of the literature. Gen Hosp Psychiatry 36(3):233–244, 2014

Soundy A, Freeman P, Stubbs B, et al: The transcending benefits of physical activity for individuals with schizophrenia: a systematic review and meta-ethnography. Psychiatry Res 220(12):11–19, 2014

Stanley S, Laugharne J: The impact of lifestyle factors on the physical health of people with a mental illness: a brief review. Int J Behav Med 21(2):275–281, 2014

Stubbs B, Williams J, Gaughran F, et al: How sedentary are people with psychosis? A systematic review and meta-analysis. Schizophr Res 171(1–3):103–109, 2016

Teachout A, Kaiser SM, Wilkniss SM, et al: Paxton House: integrating mental health and diabetes care for people with serious mental illnesses in a residential setting. Psychiatr Rehabil J 34(4):324–327, 2011

Teasdale SB, Ward PB, Rosenbaum S, et al: Solving a weighty problem: systematic review and meta-analysis of nutrition interventions in severe mental illness. Br J Psychiatry 210(2):110–118, 2017

Vancampfort D, Stubbs B, Venigalla SK, et al: Adopting and maintaining physical activity behaviours in people with severe mental illness: the importance of autonomous motivation. Prev Med 81:216–220, 2015

Vancampfort D, Rosenbaum S, Schuch F, et al: Cardiorespiratory fitness in severe mental illness: a systematic review and meta-analysis. Sports Med 47(2):343–352, 2017

Van Citters AD, Pratt SI, Jue K, et al: A pilot evaluation of the In SHAPE individualized health promotion intervention for adults with mental illness. Community Ment Health J 46(6):540–552, 2010

Walker ER, McGee RE, Druss BG: Mortality in mental disorders and global disease burden implications: a systematic review and meta-analysis. JAMA Psychiatry 72(4):334–341, 2015

Ward MC, White DT, Druss BG: A meta-review of lifestyle interventions for cardiovascular risk factors in the general medical population: lessons for individuals with serious mental illness. J Clin Psychiatry 76(4):e477–e486, 2015

Yarborough BJH, Stumbo SP, Cavese JA, et al: Patient perspectives on how living with a mental illness affects making and maintaining healthy lifestyle changes. Patient Educ Couns 102(2):346–351, 2019

CHAPTER 10

Health Navigators to Address Wellness

Lindsay Sheehan, Ph.D.
Carla Kundert, M.S.
Jonathon E. Larson, Ed.D.

Case Vignette

Charlie lives on the West Side of Chicago and is being treated for several chronic health conditions, including bipolar disorder. Although his psychiatrist is nearby, he sees a physician for his chronic respiratory problem at John H. Stroger, Jr. Hospital of Cook County in the Illinois Medical District, then has to travel more than an hour on public transportation to his podiatrist located on the North Side. Charlie fills his prescriptions at a pharmacy downtown. He also has a referral for lab testing at Loyola University Medical Center, which is in the suburbs and even more difficult to get to on public transportation, and he sometimes resorts to paying for a cab. His respiratory therapist, whom he sees weekly, is located at Mercy Hospital on the South Side. Charlie struggles to manage all these appointments given their scattered locations; he is often at the mercy of providers' availability (and the travel time required to get between them). He has struggled to find providers in his area, or even just in close proximity to one another, but he is restricted by his insurance. He is also hesitant to change physicians because he knows of the headache of trying to coordinate records and billing with a new provider, not to mention the potential for lapses in continuity of care. As a result of this fractured system, Charlie often misses appointments with his providers. He is unsure how he will get to his next respiratory therapy appointment, because he used all his bus fare this week getting back and forth to other appointments. Charlie also has some challenges with his memory, so implementing doctors' recommendations in his daily life, including about his diet, exercise, sleep hygiene, and over-the-counter medication usage, is difficult. Charlie's psychiatrist has been trying to get him enrolled in a case management program to help him manage these challenges, but although Charlie went for a first appointment, he did not really connect with the caseworker. In addition, he does not have regular access to the internet, so accessing his electronic records and viewing test results from doctors is quite challenging. He often receives paperwork from providers but has lost track of some of it. Consequently, Charlie's chronic conditions have continued to worsen, and he fears that his health will impact his ability to live independently as he ages.

Unfortunately, Charlie's story is not unusual given the fragmented nature of the health care service system. Chapter 7 focused on addressing the failure of physical and mental health services to adequately coordinate with one another to address the needs of people with psychiatric disability through the implementation of patient care medical homes. This failure, known as *system bifurcation*, is a structural issue that complicates health care (Brekke et al. 2013). For example, mental health providers are not well versed in chronic physical illness and struggle to assist individuals with psychiatric disabilities with complications of diabetes or manage chronic pain. Likewise, medical providers often lack a comprehensive understanding of a patient's psychiatric symptoms and have insufficient capacity to provide the level of support needed for managing diabetes. This results in individuals with psychiatric disability floundering between mental health and medical services, which are often located in disparate areas, do not share information about common patients, maintain different funding mechanisms, and have different philosophical approaches to care (Druss and Newcomer 2007). This chapter will address another reality of services: that various services are often scattered and rarely are a variety of services available in one geographical location.

As alluded to in the vignette about Charlie, individuals with psychiatric disabilities may struggle to engage in a wide range of health- and health care–related activities. As summarized in Table 10–1, challenges to health care utilization and wellness are categorized into difficulties with 1) health coordination, 2) wellness self-management, and 3) communication. In terms of health coordination, people with psychiatric disabilities have to manage the complexities of maintaining insurance coverage and determine which health care services are accessible for them, often while living in unstable

TABLE 10–1. Challenges to health care utilization and wellness activities for individuals with psychiatric disabilities

Health coordination	Selecting, enrolling in, and maintaining health insurance coverage
	Finding and selecting health providers that accept insurance
	Scheduling and keeping medical appointments
	Interacting with technology (e.g., accessing online medical records and health-related information)
	Transportation to medical appointments
	Finding and enrolling in substance use treatment
	Procuring and affording medications and medical devices
	Transitioning health care between community settings and institutions (hospital, nursing home, jail, or prison)
Wellness self-management	Understanding and implementing medical recommendations
	Monitoring and managing chronic conditions (e.g., diabetes, hypertension)
	Filling prescriptions and administering prescription drugs
	Maintaining healthy diet and exercise regimen
	Problem-solving health challenges
	Maintaining personal safety
	Managing daily structure activities
	Having access to food
	Budgeting for health-related costs
	Obtaining and maintaining safe and affordable housing
	Engaging in self-care, including emotional, social, spiritual, and sexual activities
Communication	Understanding and responding to medical bills and correspondence
	Communicating with health care providers about physical and mental health symptoms and treatment adherence
	Determining the appropriate urgency of care (emergency room versus urgent care or primary care appointment)
	Expressing frustration, apathy, and mistrust with health care providers

TABLE 10–1. Challenges to health care utilization and wellness activities for individuals with psychiatric disabilities *(continued)*

Communication *(continued)*	Following up with specialist care
	Utilizing social and emotional support
	Cultural misunderstandings, lack of culturally competent and/ or bilingual providers

Source. Adapted from Burt et al. 1995; Green 1996; Green et al. 2004; Kêdoté et al. 2008; Ness et al. 2014.

or unsafe housing situations and experiencing severe financial hardship. Physical or mental health limitations present barriers to using public transportation or owning a car. Transportation systems designed for people with disabilities are inconvenient and unreliable, such that traveling to frequent health care appointments can become the equivalent of a full- or part-time job. Wellness self-management activities such as following up on health care provider recommendations, eating a healthy diet, and exercising may be undermined by poverty, cognitive functioning, and mental health symptoms (e.g., anxiety, depression). Finally, communication can pose barriers to health care when people with psychiatric disabilities struggle to adequately describe symptoms to their array of health care providers or are hesitant to communicate about their level of adherence to treatment.

Health Navigators

Health navigators are one solution to help patients through the complexities of chronic illness. Health navigation originated in cancer care; called *patient navigators*, these individuals were typically social workers or nurses who guided patients with cancer among various services within a single system (Robinson-White et al. 2010). Navigators for cancer typically provide emotional support, accompany patients to appointments, and help patients understand doctor recommendations and attain affordable care (Parker et al. 2010; Wells et al. 2008; Yosha et al. 2011). Research shows that patient navigation in cancer treatment, as an adjunct to standard care, has improved screening, diagnostic testing, and treatment engagement (Robinson-White et al. 2010). Improvements in patient care are specifically seen earlier in the health care continuum of services, specifically with screening rates and follow-up with diagnostic care after an abnormality has been detected (Wells et al. 2008).

While patient navigators from heterogeneous backgrounds can be effective in improving patient outcomes, there is evidence that patient navigators who are also peers may be additionally impactful. Navigators of similar ethnic backgrounds are often viewed as more emotionally present and better listeners, leading to their being more trusted (Han et al. 2009; Nguyen et al. 2011). Additionally, further research is warranted about how navigators who are of similar backgrounds can assist with addressing other barriers unique to ethnic minority backgrounds, such as limited English proficiency and limited health literacy. Possible interventions include assisting with translation or medical terminology, education about health behaviors, skill building, and decision making (Han et al. 2009). Peers—patients with past experiences with cancer—have also joined the ranks of navigators. Navigators who had themselves experienced breast cancer led to better engagement in cancer care (Giese-Davis et al. 2006; Nguyen et al. 2011). Furthermore, peer navigators with breast cancer experience have demonstrated increases in patient outcomes outside of health engagement, such as trauma responses and emotional well-being (Giese-Davis et al. 2006).

The health navigator model has subsequently been applied to address other chronic illnesses, including diabetes, heart disease, kidney disease (leading to transplant), obesity, and asthma (Kelly et al. 2014; Shommu et al. 2016). A systematic review on navigators found that programs are usually implemented to promote cultural understanding and engagement of vulnerable populations (Shommu et al. 2016). Evidence for the effectiveness of peer support models for chronic physical illnesses such as diabetes is mounting, especially for difficult-to-engage ethnic communities, and the provision of emotional support appears to be an important component of navigation (Fisher et al. 2012). For example, the Peers for Progress model specifies four functions of peer support for chronic illness, including 1) help with illness self-management, 2) social and emotional support, 3) linkage to health care and community resources, and 4) ongoing support to address the chronicity of needs (Fisher et al. 2012).

Health navigators also have roles and responsibilities strictly defined by federal policy. With the advent of the Patient Protection and Affordable Care Act (ACA), health navigators were funded to assist uninsured individuals in enrolling in health coverage (Vargas 2016). ACA health navigators are laypeople with specific training in health insurance enrollment who are stationed in the community. They provide information about insurance enrollment, help patients compare insurance plans, and complete the online enrollment process.

Community Health Workers

Another group of health care providers deserves mention here. Community health workers (CHWs) are employed in a similar space as are health navigators but have some distinct roles and responsibilities within health care engagement. CHWs are paraprofessionals (often from ethnic minority communities) who address chronic illness through management and prevention (Centers for Disease Control and Prevention 2015; Perry et al. 2014). CHWs can reach difficult-to-engage populations through shared culture and language, benefiting from trust and unique knowledge of the community (Kim et al. 2016). While CHWs and health navigators both have a goal of engaging people in care, CHWs are more often employed in the initial stages of this process on the screening and prevention side. Thus, their efforts are generally targeted at the broader community, with the goal of educating patients about health conditions and encouraging them in regular doctor visits and health screenings. In contrast, health navigators more often work with individuals already diagnosed with a health condition, with the goal of managing illness and producing more favorable outcomes. Table 10–2 outlines distinctions between CHWs and health navigators. Typically, CHWs are laypeople with no licensure who provide most of their services in the community; they connect individuals earlier in the health care continuum and do outreach, engagement, linkage to services, and transportation assistance. Health navigators, on the other hand, may be peers, may be laypeople, or may have a clinical license (such as a nurse or social worker), and often engage with individuals later in the continuum of care to provide care coordination, health education, illness management, and ongoing support. Health navigators may work in the community like CHWs but may also serve individuals in specific hospitals or clinics.

Research on CHWs indicates efficacy in promoting immunizations, reducing respiratory infections, and improving diabetes self-care (Lewin et al. 2005; Norris et al. 2006). A systematic review by Jack and colleagues (2017) of CHW randomized controlled trials (RCTs) and pre-post studies found significant reductions in emergency room visits, urgent care use, and hospitalization for patients assigned to CHWs. Additionally, the review indicated that CHWs can reduce preventable health care use for individuals with chronic conditions, as well as increase appropriate health care use among those whose conditions are not yet severe and chronic (Jack et al. 2017).

Health Navigation for Psychiatric Disability

Health navigation has been applied to address navigation of the mental health system as well. Compton and colleagues (2014) implemented navigation teams for people with psychiatric disabilities, with the goals of reducing psychiatric hospitalization. Their team approach combined peers,

TABLE 10–2. Distinctions between community health workers (CHWs) and health navigators

Community health workers	Health navigators
Also called *promotores de salud*, community health advisors, lay health educators, community health representatives	Also called patient navigators, peer navigators, patient advocates, service navigators
Usually do not have professional license	May be peers, may be laypeople, or have clinical license (nurse or social worker)
Provide general services in community (health fairs, door-to-door, community events)	Work one-on-one with specific individuals
CHW usually considered an occupation	Navigator usually defined by function or role
Are usually employed earlier in the health care continuum for linkage to care, screenings, outreach, education, and transportation	Are usually employed later in health care process (care coordination, health education, ongoing support, illness management)
Work in community settings	May work in community settings or at hospitals and clinics

Source. Adapted from Centers for Disease Control and Prevention 2015; Patient Navigator Training Collaborative 2011; Roland et al. 2017.

social workers, and family members to help patients engage in 1) developing day structure, 2) promoting healthcare access, 3) obtaining housing, and 4) technology access (Compton et al. 2014). Navigators completed a five-day training, which included components such as recovery orientation, listening skills, person-centered goal setting, and stress management. A pre-post study found decreased number of hospitalizations, decreased in days hospitalized, and greater self-reported recovery with use of navigation team (Compton et al. 2014).

Two research groups have developed and evaluated models for engaging individuals with psychiatric disability in health navigation, specifically targeting both physical and mental health (Corrigan et al. 2017a; Kelly et al. 2017). Central to both of these interventions seems to be the role of peers. In fact, services for people with psychiatric disability have a rich history of including peer-provided interventions (Davidson et al. 2006). These include treatments delivered by peer providers to address the health needs of participants with psychiatric disability. Four RCTs showed that people who received versions of psychiatric case management services from peers demonstrated the same level of functional and symptom stability as those who received services provided by professional or paraprofessional staff (Clarke et al. 2000; Davidson et al. 2004). Additionally, people with serious mental illness in hospitals who received peer mentoring had significantly fewer hospitalizations and inpatient days during the 9 months of the study than those who did not work with a mentor (Sledge et al. 2011). However, health navigation is a different approach from other peer-led services that have been developed and tested for people with mental illness (e.g., psychoeducational programs meant to teach participants medical self-management living skills; Druss et al. 2010). As outlined further below, navigation allows peers to work alongside the consumer as they manage their multiple health needs, rather than instructing or teaching. Additionally, *peer* is a multilayered idea here: people from a similar community background but also (more importantly) individuals in recovery from mental illness who may have similar life experiences (e.g., poverty, homelessness, or involvement in the criminal justice system) (Corrigan et al. 2017a).

Components of Health Navigation Programs

Practice guidelines and consensus reports have identified services that positively impact health goals of people with psychiatric disability (Salzer and Evans 2006). Below we review two components of health navigation that may be especially relevant for supporting people with serious mental illness.

Shared Decision Making

Shared decision making (SDM), as delineated further in Chapter 8, combines several principles and procedures that help people with psychiatric disability make self-determined health decisions (Joosten et al. 2008). SDM has been shown to help people make more personally relevant decisions related to 1) diet and exercise (Liberatore and Nydick 2008); 2) substance use programs (Joosten et al. 2009); 3) homelessness, victimization, and criminal court involvement (Tarzian et al. 2005); and 4) resources that address health needs (Stiggelbout et al. 2012). Health navigators may be essential agents in efforts like SDM that are meant to promote self-determination in health care decisions.

Navigators as In Vivo Supports

Supports are an essential part of services for people with psychiatric disability and are useful for finding and availing health resources (Corrigan et al.

2017a, 2017b). *In vivo* refers to services that are provided in a person's home or community setting and that are practical in nature. For example, navigators travel via public transportation to patient appointments, help patients fill out an insurance application, or call the doctor's office to discuss a medical bill. Navigators who are "in the field" providing these supports have been shown to have significant effects on engagement in services (Corrigan et al. 2017b) and subsequent self-report of health, recovery, and quality of life (Corrigan et al. 2017a).

Models of Peer-Led Health Navigation for Psychiatric Disability

Here we describe two models that provide evidence for health navigation in psychiatric disability.

Bridge Program

The Bridge program is a manualized health navigation program focused on building skills and experiences for self-management of both physical and mental illnesses (Brekke et al. 2013). Navigators are paraprofessionals with either personal lived experience of mental illness or experience with a family member's mental illness. Navigators are trained through shadowing and manualized training. The Bridge program has four primary components: 1) assessment and planning, 2) coordinated linkage, 3) consumer education, and 4) cognitive-behavioral strategies. In assessment and planning, navigators engage and motivate patients to be involved in their health by helping patients develop a health navigation plan and wellness goals. In the linkage component, navigators help patients make appointments, develop treatment plans, communicate with the pharmacy, follow up on treatment recommendations, and speak with doctors. These activities are performed during real-life interactions rather than through didactic instruction. For the educational component, navigators provide information on health-related topics, including adherence to treatment, self-advocacy, diet, exercise, health insurance, and communication. Finally, patients are coached in cognitive-behavioral exercises, in which the navigator uses techniques such as modeling, role-playing, and fading to reinforce lessons in health care navigation (e.g., making a doctor appointment by phone).

The intervention is split into an initial 4-month phase during which there is frequent contact between navigator and patient, followed by a 2-month phase in which meetings are less frequent and the patient is encouraged to develop more independent self-management skills. Researchers conducted a 6-month RCT of the Bridge program; patients in the navigator group saw their physicians more, reported less severe pain, better understood health problems, and were more confident in managing future health problems (Kelly et al. 2017).

Peer Navigator Program

A manualized peer navigator program for African Americans with psychiatric disability and homelessness was developed by a community-based participatory research (CBPR) team (Corrigan et al. 2017b). CBPR, which is discussed in Chapter 2, includes community members with lived experience of the health condition, in the development and evaluation of services. Thus, this program was developed in collaboration with individuals with psychiatric disabilities. The goal of this program is to facilitate engagement in health care to improve personal health, wellness, and quality of life. Peer navigators are defined as people in recovery from serious mental illness and are hired and supervised by an integrated care health provider. Peer navigators complete a 2-week manualized training prior to providing services and adhere to accompanying fidelity standards. The training includes didactic instruction, role-play activities, worksheets, and activity templates for peer navigators to use with program participants. In the training, peer navigators practice basic helping skills (e.g., active listening) and discuss problem-solving strategies, illness management, cultural competency, and time management, among others. Corrigan and colleagues tested the program in a yearlong RCT with 67 participants assigned to treatment as usual (TAU) or TAU plus the navigator program. Compared with the control group, patients who worked with navigators had improved service engagement as assessed by scheduled and achieved appointments (Corrigan et al. 2017b). Findings also showed those assigned to the navigator program demonstrated significantly greater improvement in perceived health, quality of life, and recovery over the control group (Corrigan et al. 2017a).

The same peer navigation model was adapted by another CBPR team to address the health and wellness needs of Latinos with psychiatric disability. Latinos ($N=110$) with serious mental illness were randomly assigned to TAU (integrated care) or TAU plus a peer navigator (Corrigan et al. 2018). Significant improvements were found in service engagement for the navigator group compared with the control group, which corresponded with significant improvement in recovery, empowerment, and quality of life. For Latinos with psychiatric disability, program participants reported receiving emotional support, informational support, and in-the-field navigation services (Sheehan et al. 2018). Individualization of services, rapport, accessibility, and peer connection were highlighted by program participants as among the most important components (Sheehan et al. 2018).

Challenges of Peer Health Navigation

Given the relative recency of health navigation services to address physical health for individuals with psychiatric disability, many implementation challenges remain and research questions remain unanswered. Here we describe challenges with peer health navigation programs and suggest ways these challenges might be ameliorated. These challenges are summarized in Table 10–3.

Time-Limited and Dependent on Funding

Health navigation services are largely grant funded, which complicates program sustainability (Balcazar et al. 2011). Given the complex and chronic needs of individuals with psychiatric disabilities, it is especially crucial to provide ongoing services that result in continuity of care (Sheehan et al. 2018) as is the best practice for provision of other psychiatric services (Corrigan et al. 2016). Organizations that pilot navigation programs can collect evaluative data to justify cost-effectiveness and can consult with other organizations on sustainable implementation strategies. Certification programs for peers may create opportunities for peer health navigators to bill for services. Additionally, many payers are moving toward performance-based funding (pay-for-performance, or P4P, services) in place of standard fee-for-service programs (Stewart et al. 2017). In response, behavioral health providers may consider incorporating more health navigation services to improve patient outcomes and increase consistent revenue streams. Organizations that wish to implement health navigation may benefit from a champion who is invested in surmounting these challenges.

Navigator Integration With Other Health Services

Sometimes navigators do not feel that they are a valued part of the organization or that their role within the health care system is distinct (Brekke et al. 2013; Sheehan et al. 2018). An organizational champion can highlight the importance of the program to other health care workers and help with role differentiation (Davidson et al. 2012). Especially when no existing peer-led services are available in the organization, policies and procedures may be needed to introduce the concept of peer services. For full integration, health navigators should go through orientations, trainings, and team meetings with other agency staff.

TABLE 10–3. Challenges in peer health navigation and strategies for addressing them

Challenge	Potential solutions
Health navigation programs are often time-limited and dependent on grant funding.	Advocate routes for health navigators to obtain certification and qualifications for billing insurance. Conduct research to justify cost-effectiveness.
Health navigator services may not be fully integrated with other health services within an organization.	Develop a health navigator champion within the organization, especially if there are no existing peer services. Have navigators complete onboarding process along with other employees.
Health navigator programs have unique recruitment, selection, supervision, training, and program fidelity needs.	Give health navigators regular access to supervisors who endorse the goals of the program and can provide ongoing training and support. Ensure that health navigator roles are differentiated from other roles within the organization so navigators can develop an identity as navigators. Provide peer health navigators additional support, especially in regard to self-care, self-disclosure, and role boundaries. Provide ongoing and frequent staff training, supervision, and program fidelity.
Stigma and lack of high-level support impact health care systems and services.	Identify and challenge stigmatizing attitudes and systems. Arrange for organization leadership to publicly endorse and support navigation programming. Engage in program evaluation efforts that highlight program outcomes.
There is a lack of clarity in essential components of health navigation programs.	Conduct research to compare components (e.g., educational versus in vivo) of navigator services and role of peerness in program efficacy.
Health navigators may be unable to address systemic barriers to care.	Encourage health navigators to engage in advocacy for disenfranchised populations. Partner with other community services to maximize resources. Collect data that will highlight need for systemic change.

Recruitment, Selection, Supervision, Training, and Fidelity Needs

Health navigation programs need well-defined job descriptions, but a flexible hiring process that will recognize barriers that people in recovery may have (e.g., criminal justice history, lack of access to a car) and that can discern individuals who can connect with others. Given that health navigators are paraprofessionals who have little formal training, they should have regular access to supervisors who endorse the goals of the program and can provide ongoing training and support. Health navigator roles can be differentiated from other roles within the organization so navigators can develop a shared identity within the navigator program. Peer health navigators may need additional support, especially to learn about self-care, stress management, self-disclosure, and role boundaries (Brekke et al. 2013; Sheehan et al. 2018). An effective program supervisor will be able to advocate for the program and be able to provide frequent support and mentorship to health navigators (Sheehan et al. 2018). Agency leadership should be prepared to conduct program evaluation, including determining fidelity to the program goals.

Stigma and Lack of High-Level Support

Another potential barrier to recruiting and filling peer navigator positions in some communities is stigma. An investigation into new integrated health care systems in Los Angeles County indicated that providers endorsed beliefs that consumers—specifically in ethnic minority communities—would be unlikely to engage with peers who identified as having lived mental health experience, so providers were thus unlikely to incorporate peer engagement services in their health care systems (Siantz et al. 2016). This is problematic as certain cultural communities may be excluded in engaging with peer navigators from the start.

Lack of Clarity in Essential Components

Whereas some health navigator programs (e.g., Brekke et al. 2013) include a didactic component, other models of navigation (e.g., Corrigan et al. 2017a) are focused on in vivo supports. The essential components of health navigation have not been elucidated in the research literature. For peer health navigation, peerness can be viewed in terms of race/ethnicity, language, shared diagnosis, gender, country of origin, religion, or a variety of other factors (Sheehan et al. 2018). It is unclear what aspects of peerness are most important or even if health navigation services provided by peers are more effective than those provided by nonpeers. Is it more important that my health navigator is from my home country or shares my gender? Is my personal rapport with my health navigator more important than health care knowledge or navigational savvy in terms of health care engagement outcomes? Methodologically sound research is needed to answer these questions.

Failure to Address Systemic Issues

Health navigation services cannot fully ameliorate concerns experienced by the most disenfranchised populations, such as undocumented immigrants who lack funding and insurance (Sheehan et al. 2018) and those who are discriminated against in health care settings (e.g., transgender). Services that lack cultural competency, are not in locations accessible to people with psychiatric disabilities, require specific types of insurance to enroll, or have complicated enrollment processes may be difficult challenges for even health navigators to address. However, health navigators could be trained and encouraged to engage in more advocacy efforts and collect data that will highlight the need for systemic change in the health care system.

Key Points

- Fragmented health care systems compromise health outcomes for people with psychiatric disabilities.

- Health navigation, which originally emerged to help breast cancer patients, is one solution to help individuals with chronic illness manage their health.

- Health navigators are typically employed to bridge cultural or language barriers and engage vulnerable individuals in health care.

- Health navigation for people with psychiatric disabilities is usually provided by peers, focusing on shared decision making and in vivo supports.

- Research on health navigation to address physical health needs of individuals with psychiatric disability suggests health navigation improves engagement in health, perceived health, knowledge, and confidence in managing health challenges.

- Challenges of health navigation include lack of funding, integration of health navigation with existing services, training and supervision needs, stigma, and limited research on essential components of navigation.

References

Balcazar H, Rosenthal EL, Brownstein JN, et al: Community health workers can be a public health force for change in the United States: three actions for a new paradigm. Am J Public Health 101(12):2199–2203, 2011

Brekke JS, Siantz E, Pahwa R, et al: Reducing health disparities for people with serious mental illness. Best Pract Ment Health 9(1):62–82, 2013

Burt DB, Zembar MJ, Niederehe G: Depression and memory impairment: a meta-analysis of the association, its pattern, and specificity. Psychol Bull 117(2):285–305, 1995

Centers for Disease Control and Prevention: Addressing Chronic Disease Through Community Health Workers: A Policy and Systems-Level Approach, 2nd Edition. Atlanta, GA, National Center for Chronic Disease Prevention and Health Promotion, April 2015. Available at: www.cdc.gov/dhdsp/docs/chw_brief.pdf. Accessed August 14, 2019.

Clarke GN, Herinckx HA, Kinney RF, et al: Psychiatric hospitalizations, arrests, emergency room visits, and homelessness of clients with serious and persistent mental illness: findings from a randomized trial of two ACT programs vs. usual care. Ment Health Serv Res 2(3):155–164, 2000

Compton MT, Reed T, Broussard B, et al: Development, implementation, and preliminary evaluation of a recovery-based curriculum for community navigation specialists working with individuals with serious mental illnesses and repeated hospitalizations. Community Ment Health J 50(4):383–387, 2014

Corrigan PW, Mueser KT, Bond GR, et al: Principles and Practice of Psychiatric Rehabilitation: An Empirical Approach, 2nd Edition. New York, Guilford, 2016

Corrigan PW, Kraus D, Pickett S, et al: Peer navigators that address the integrated healthcare needs of African Americans with serious mental illness who are homeless. Psychiatr Serv 68(3):264–270, 2017a

Corrigan PW, Pickett S, Schmidt A, et al: Peer navigators to promote engagement of homeless African Americans with serious mental illness in primary care. Psychiatry Res 255:101–103, 2017b

Corrigan PW, Sheehan L, Morris S, et al: The impact of a peer navigator program in addressing the health needs of Latinos with serious mental illness. Psychiatr Serv 69(4):456–461, 2018

Davidson L, Shahar G, Stayner DA, et al: Supported socialization for people with psychiatric disabilities: lessons from a randomized controlled trial. J Community Psychol 32:453–477, 2004

Davidson L, Chinman M, Sells D, Rowe M: Peer support among adults with serious mental illness: a report from the field. Schizophr Bull 32:443–450, 2006

Davidson L, Bellamy C, Guy K, Miller R: Peer support among persons with severe mental illnesses: a review of evidence and experience. World Psychiatry 11(2):123–128, 2012

Druss BG, Newcomer JW: Challenges and solutions to integrating mental and physical health care. J Clin Psychiatry 68(4):e09, 2007

Druss BG, Zhao L, von Esenwein SA, et al: The Health and Recovery Peer (HARP) Program: a peer-led intervention to improve medical self-management for persons with serious mental illness. Schizophr Res 118:264–270, 2010

Fisher EB, Boothroyd RI, Coufal MM, et al: Peer support for self-management of diabetes improved outcomes in international settings. Health Aff (Millwood) 31(1):130–139, 2012

Giese-Davis J, Bliss-Isberg C, Carson K, et al: The effect of peer counseling on quality of life following diagnosis of breast cancer: an observational study. Psychooncology 15:1014–1022, 2006

Green MF: What are the functional consequences of neurocognitive deficits in schizophrenia? Am J Psychiatry 153(3):321–330, 1996

Green MF, Kern RS, Heaton RK: Longitudinal studies of cognition and functional outcome in schizophrenia: implications for MATRICS. Schizophr Res 72(1):41–51, 2004

Han H, Lee HH, Kim MT, et al: Tailored lay health worker intervention improves breast cancer screening outcomes in nonadherent Korean-American women. Health Educ Res 24:318–329, 2009

Jack HE, Arabadjis SD, Sun L, et al: Impact of community health workers on use of healthcare services in the United States: a systematic review. J Gen Intern Med 32(3):325–344, 2017

Joosten EA, DeFuentes-Merillas L, De Weert GH, et al: Systematic review of the effects of shared decision-making on patient satisfaction, treatment adherence and health status. Psychother Psychosom 77(4):219–226, 2008

Joosten EA, De Jong CAJ, De Weert-van Oene GH, et al: Shared decision-making reduces drug use and psychiatric severity in substance-dependent patients. Psychother Psychosom 78(4):245–253, 2009

Kêdoté MN, Brousselle A, Champagne F: Use of health care services by patients with co-occurring severe mental illness and substance use disorders. Ment Health Subst Use 1(3):216–227, 2008

Kelly E, Fulginiti A, Pahwa R, et al: A pilot test of a peer navigator intervention for improving the health of individuals with serious mental illness. Community Ment Health J 50(4):435–446, 2014

Kelly E, Duan L, Cohen H, et al: Integrating behavioral healthcare for individuals with serious mental illness: a randomized controlled trial of a peer health navigator intervention. Schizophr Res 182:135–141, 2017

Kim KB, Kim MT, Lee HB, et al: Community health workers versus nurses as counselors or case managers in a self-help diabetes management program. Am J Public Health 106(6):1052–1058, 2016

Lewin SA, Dick J, Pond P, et al: Lay health workers in primary and community health care. Cochrane Database Syst Rev (1):CD004015, 2005

Liberatore MJ, Nydick RL: The analytic hierarchy process in medical and health care decision making: a literature review. Eur J Oper Res 189(1):194–207, 2008

Ness O, Borg M, Davidson L: Facilitators and barriers in dual recovery: a literature review of first-person perspectives. Adv Dual Diagn 7(3):107–117, 2014

Nguyen TN, Tran JH, Kagawa-Singer M, et al: A qualitative assessment of community-based breast health navigation services for Southeast Asian women in Southern California: recommendations for developing a navigator training curriculum. Am J Public Health 101:87–93, 2011

Norris SL, Chowdhury FM, Van Le K, et al: Effectiveness of community health workers in the care of persons with diabetes. Diabet Med 23(5):544–556, 2006

Parker VA, Clark JA, Leyson J, et al: Patient navigation: development of a protocol for describing what navigators do. Health Serv Res 45(2):514–531, 2010

Patient Navigator Training Collaborative: Community Health Workers and Patient Navigators. Module 3: Healthcare Team. 2011. Available at: http://patientnavigatortraining.org/healthcare_system/module3/1_index.htm. Accessed August 15, 2019.

Perry HB, Zulliger R, Rogers MM: Community health workers in low-, middle-, and high-income countries: an overview of their history, recent evolution, and current effectiveness. Annu Rev Public Health 35:399–421, 2014

Robinson-White S, Conroy B, Slavish KH, Rosenzweig M: Patient navigation in breast cancer: a systematic review. Cancer Nurs 33(2):127–140, 2010

Roland KB, Milliken EL, Rohan EA, et al: Use of community health workers and patient navigators to improve cancer outcomes among patients served by federally qualified health centers: a systematic literature review. Health Equity 1(1):61–76, 2017

Salzer MS, Evans AC: CATIE and the value of atypical antipsychotics in the context of creating a recovery-oriented behavioral health system. Adm Policy Ment Health 33(5):536–540, 2006

Sheehan L, Torres A, Lara JL, et al: Qualitative evaluation of a peer navigator program for Latinos with serious mental illness. Adm Policy Ment Health 45(3):495–504, 2018

Shommu NS, Ahmed S, Rumana N, et al: What is the scope of improving immigrant and ethnic minority healthcare using community navigators: a systematic scoping review. Int J Equity Health 15:6, 2016

Siantz E, Henwood B, Gilmer T: Implementation of peer providers in integrated mental health and primary care settings. J Soc Social Work Res 7(2):231–246, 2016

Sledge WH, Lawless M, Sells D, et al: Effectiveness of peer support in reducing readmissions of persons with multiple psychiatric hospitalizations. Psychiatr Serv 62(5):541–544, 2011

Stewart RE, Lareef I, Hadley TR, Mandell DS: Can we pay for performance in behavioral health care? Psychiatr Serv 68(2):109–111, 2017

Stiggelbout AM, Van der Weijden T, De Wit MP, et al: Shared decision making: really putting patients at the centre of healthcare. BMJ 344:e256, 2012

Tarzian AJ, Neal MT, O'Neil JA: Attitudes, experiences, and beliefs affecting end-of-life decision-making among homeless individuals. J Palliat Med 8(1):36–48, 2005

Vargas R: How health navigators legitimize the Affordable Care Act to the uninsured poor. Soc Sci Med 165:263–270, 2016

Wells KJ, Battaglia TA, Dudley DJ, et al: Patient navigation: state of the art or is it science? Cancer 113(8):1999–2010, 2008

Yosha AM, Carroll JK, Hendren S, et al: Patient navigation from the paired perspectives of cancer patients and navigators: a qualitative analysis. Patient Educ Couns 82(3):396–401, 2011

CHAPTER 11

Smoking

Janis Sayer, Ph.D.
Marisa D. Serchuk, M.S.

Rates of smoking among the general population
have decreased substantially since the Surgeon General first warned of the
devastating health effects of smoking (U.S. Public Health Service 1964);
however, persons with serious mental illness (SMI) have not enjoyed similar declines (Lê Cook et al. 2014). Compared with persons in the general
population, individuals with SMI smoke at higher rates and smoke more
heavily (Drope et al. 2018; Lipari and Van Horn 2017). In turn, tobacco-
related conditions are the leading cause of mortality among persons with
mental illness (Callaghan et al. 2014).

We begin this chapter with a focus on the prevalence of smoking among
persons with SMI, factors contributing to smoking disparities, and morbidity and mortality caused by smoking. This is followed by a discussion of
smoking cessation strategies among persons with SMI and cessation interventions. Topics covered include the benefits of quitting smoking, quit rates,
and factors influencing smoking cessation among persons with SMI. We
then discuss what can be done to help individuals stop smoking and strategies
to help lower rates of smoking among persons with SMI. We close the chapter by detailing assessment and treatment strategies, as well as structural barriers to smoking cessation, especially in terms of how psychiatrists might
adopt these strategies in their practices.

Smoking Prevalence

Persons with SMI are two to three times more likely to smoke than persons without SMI (Lawrence et al. 2009). A recent analysis of nationally representative survey data between the years 2009 and 2014 found that the prevalence of cigarette smoking was 27.9% among people with SMI in the past year, compared with only 12.9% for those without a past-year mental illness (Drope et al. 2018).

In contrast to persons with no mental illness, prevalence of smoking among persons with mental illness appears to be remaining fairly stable over time. Trends in smoking behavior demonstrate markedly different rates of decline in smoking between the two groups. Between 2004 and 2011, Lê Cook et al. (2014) revealed that after adjustment for covariates, smoking rates among persons without mental illness decreased from 19.2% to 16.2%, while rates of smoking among persons with mental illness declined less than 1%, from 25.3% to 24.9%.

Prevalence of smoking varies by mental health diagnosis. The prevalence is highest among persons with schizophrenia, at three to seven times higher than persons in the general population (de Leon and Diaz 2005). For persons with bipolar disorder, smoking prevalence is three to four times higher (Jackson et al. 2015). Individuals with depression are two times as likely to smoke as others (Lasser et al. 2000). Among persons with posttraumatic stress disorder, smoking prevalence is about five times as high as persons without mental illness (Fu et al. 2007). In a recent analysis of data collected prior to enrollment in a research study, Dickerson et al. (2017) concluded that 62% of persons with schizophrenia and 37% of persons with bipolar disorder were current smokers, compared with 17% of persons without a psychiatric disorder. In addition, smoking prevalence is higher with increasing numbers of mental disorders (Lasser et al. 2000). Eriksen and colleagues (2015) showed that the prevalence of smoking among persons with more than two mental disorders was 61%.

Among persons with mental illness, certain groups are more likely to smoke. These differences are similar to those among persons without mental illness (Gfroerer et al. 2013). Income affects the likelihood of smoking; 48% of persons with mental illness with incomes below poverty level smoke compared with 33% of persons living above the poverty line (Gfroerer et al. 2013). Smoking also varies by age, level of education, and race/ethnicity. Data from the 2009–2011 National Survey on Drug Use and Health showed that smoking was more common among younger adults with mental illness. Forty-two percent of adults with mental illness ages 18–24 and 41% of adults ages 25–44 were smokers, followed by 34% of persons ages 45–64 and 13% of those age 65 or older. Persons with less education are more likely to smoke, with the largest percentage of smokers among individuals with a less than high school level of education (47%), compared with 19% among college graduates. By racial and ethnic group, 55% of American Indian/Alaska Native, non-Hispanic individuals with mental illness smoked, followed by 40% of those identifying as an "other" race; 38% of white, non-Hispanic individuals; and 34% of Black, non-Hispanic persons with mental illness (Gfroerer et al. 2013).

Persons with SMI who smoke are typically heavier smokers than persons in the general population. Lipari and Van Horn (2017) examined the National Survey on Drug Use and Health data from 2012 to 2014 to determine the quantity of cigarettes smoked by adults with a mental illness compared with persons without a mental illness. Persons with a mental illness smoked approximately two packs more cigarettes each month than did those without mental illness (Lipari and Van Horn 2017). By diagnosis, individuals with schizophrenia are almost four times as likely, and persons with bipolar disorder are almost three times as likely, to smoke a greater number of cigarettes than individuals with no psychiatric disorder (Dickerson et al. 2017).

Nicotine dependence and nicotine withdrawal syndrome are more likely among persons with mental illness (Smith et al. 2014). Among respondents to a two-wave cohort telephone survey of a national sample of 751 adult smokers, persons with psychological distress had reduced odds of quitting smoking compared with smokers without psychological distress, and the relationship between psychological distress and quit success was found to be completely mediated by nicotine dependence and withdrawal (Smith et al. 2014).

Causes of Smoking Disparities

Multiple and complex factors play a role in the increased smoking rates of persons with SMI. Individuals with SMI may face a number of challenges that increase the odds of smoking, as well as a number of barriers that make smoking cessation difficult. The tobacco industry, health systems, health care professionals, and social and biochemical factors contribute to smoking disparities. Psychiatry needs to account for these factors in addressing smoking concerns.

The tobacco industry has a disturbing history of promoting smoking among vulnerable persons, including persons with SMI (Prochaska et al. 2008). The industry fostered relationships with mental health care providers and advocacy groups, directed advertisements to persons with mental illness, donated money and cigarettes to organizations that serve persons with SMI, and tried to prevent legislation that would ban smoking in psychiatric hospitals (Prochaska et al. 2008). Further, the tobacco industry influenced research questions related to smoking among persons with schizophrenia (Prochaska et al. 2008). Industry-supported research aimed to provide evidence that smoking is less harmful and even helpful in some respects for persons with schizophrenia. For example, some studies aimed to show that persons with schizophrenia were less likely to get cancer from smoking. Other studies demonstrated that persons with schizophrenia were self-medicating by smoking, helping to improve their symptoms (Prochaska et al. 2008). This myth still prevents persons with SMI from getting the help needed to quit smoking today (Prochaska et al. 2008), even though there is good evidence that quitting smoking improves psychiatric symptoms (Taylor et al. 2014).

Unfortunately, psychiatric hospitals have historically supported smoking among patients. It was once commonplace for health care providers to incentivize and reward patients for attending programs, taking medications, or following rules with cigarettes (Prochaska et al. 2008). Even as recently as the year 2000, there is documentation of health care providers requesting cigarettes for patients (Prochaska et al. 2008). Although smoking in general hospitals was banned in 1993, mental health advocacy groups that considered smoking a right of patients with SMI fought to allow designated smoking areas in psychiatric hospitals (Prochaska et al. 2008). Over time, smoking bans in psychiatric hospitals have increased, but a substantial proportion of mental health treatment facilities still do not have smoke-free campuses (Marynak et al. 2018).

Health professionals, sometimes including psychiatrists, unknowingly contribute to smoking disparities by not providing smoking cessation referral and intervention as often as needed. Health professionals report that they lack the training, time, or ability to provide interventions (Sheals et al. 2016). This holds true across different types of health professionals, including psychiatric nurses (Sharp et al. 2009), mental health counselors (Sidani et al. 2011), and psychiatrists (Price et al. 2007).

In addition, social and environmental factors drive up smoking rates among persons with SMI. Persons with SMI are more likely to be in a low-income category, and persons with low income have an increased likelihood of smoking (Drope et al. 2018). Because persons with mental illness have reduced access to quality medical care, this decreases the chances of receiving smoking cessation interventions from a health care provider. Persons with SMI are also more likely to live in areas with a higher density of tobacco retailers, a factor that increases the likelihood of smoking (Young-Wolff et al. 2014).

Finally, biochemical and neurobiological factors likely contribute to increased smoking rates among persons with SMI. Once smoking has been initiated, tobacco use can temporarily ameliorate symptoms of mental illness. Nicotine, a stimulant, can make persons feel increased energy (Herman et al. 2014). Nicotine also increases the ability to concentrate and can enhance mood (Herman et al. 2014). Neurobiological features among persons with schizophrenia are believed to help drive increased tobacco use and make it harder for individuals to stop smoking. More intense cravings, alleviation of symptoms, and genetic vulnerability may contribute to high smoking rates (Wing et al. 2012). In addition, smoking increases the rate at which some antipsychotic medications are metabolized, and therefore can reduce medication side effects, a benefit that may act as a facilitator of smoking (Forchuk et al. 2000).

Morbidity and Mortality

Smoking increases the risk of many diseases, including cancer, stroke, respiratory disease, cardiovascular disease, and diabetes (U.S. Department of Health and Human Services 2014). Mortality rates among smokers in the general population are three times higher than those among nonsmokers (U.S. Department of Health and Human Services 2014). In fact, tobacco-related illnesses are the most common cause of death among persons with SMI (Callaghan et al. 2014). Callaghan and colleagues (2014) found that among persons with SMI, one-half of deaths were attributable to tobacco-related diseases. The researchers examined records for persons hospitalized in California with a primary psychiatric diagnosis between 1990 and 1995 to estimate age-, race-, and race-adjusted mortality rates for tobacco-related conditions. Tobacco-related cancers, respiratory diseases, and cardiovascular diseases were the cause of about 53% of deaths for persons with schizophrenia, 48% of deaths for persons with bipolar disorder, and 50% of deaths for persons with depression (Callaghan et al. 2014). Kelly et al. (2009) examined mortality risk among persons hospitalized for schizophrenia and similar psychotic disorders between 1994 and 2000. They reported a substantial increase in cardiac conditions as a cause of death among smokers, with 43% of the deaths of smokers due to a cardiac condition, compared with 19% for nonsmokers (Kelly et al. 2009).

Smoking Cessation

Quitting smoking can dramatically improve health and increase length of life. After smoking stops, the risk of coronary heart disease is reduced; risks due to smoking 15 years after quitting are the same as those for persons who have never smoked. Within 5 years, the odds of stroke are the same as the odds for those who have never smoked, and lung cancer risk is reduced by one-half within 10 years (U.S. Department of Health and Human Services 1990). Quitting smoking between the ages of 25 and 34 improves longevity by 10 years; quitting between the ages of 35 and 44 adds 8 years of life; and quitting between the ages of 45 and 54 adds 8 years of life (Jha et al. 2013).

Smoking cessation has additional important benefits for persons with SMI. Persons with SMI who have quit smoking have experienced an improvement in symptomatology, including depression, anxiety, and stress, along with improved quality of life and positive mood (Taylor et al. 2014). Quitting can reduce barriers to finding and maintaining housing, already difficult for many with SMI. In addition, because smoking is expensive, cessation can dramatically improve the finances of persons with SMI who have limited income (Williams et al. 2014).

Motivation to Quit

Contrary to what many health professionals believe, persons with SMI and persons without mental illness have similar levels of motivation to quit smoking (Siru et al. 2009). More specifically, results of nine combined studies demonstrate that over one-half of smokers with mental illness are thinking about quitting during the upcoming 6 months or are planning to quit within 30 days. However, there appear to be differences in motivation depending on the type of mental illness; persons with psychotic disorders seem to be less ready to quit than persons with depressive disorders (Siru et al. 2009).

Quit Rates

Although many persons with SMI are as motivated to quit as others in the general population, quit rates are lower among persons with SMI than among the general population. A recent study analyzing cigarette quit rates revealed that past-month quit rates were lower among individuals with serious psychological distress, every year from 2008 to 2016—about one-half of the rate of persons without serious psychological distress (Streck et al. 2020). Whereas quit rates among persons without psychological distress increased over time, quit rates among persons with serious psychological distress remained the same (Streck et al. 2020). Among persons with mental illness, individuals with schizophrenia or schizoaffective disorder have the lowest quit rate (Grand et al. 2007). Despite a similar number of quit attempts being taken (Etter et al. 2004), quit rates for persons with schizophrenia are estimated to be between 10% and 30% (Baker et al. 2006), compared with 38% for individuals with major depression (Lasser et al. 2000).

Barriers to and Facilitators of Quitting

A number of factors may challenge smoking cessation among persons with SMI. As discussed earlier in the section "Smoking Prevalence," persons with SMI may have more trouble quitting because of increased tobacco use, dependence, and withdrawal (Smith et al. 2014). Among some with SMI, cognitive impairment presents a barrier to planning and follow-through on goals, a necessity for smoking cessation. Persons with SMI may lack the self-efficacy needed to improve their health (Schmutte et al. 2008). Smoking may temporarily improve symptoms (Herman et al. 2014) and alleviate side effects of medications as it decreases levels of psychotropic medication in the body (Desai et al. 2001), and this can present additional barriers to quitting. In addition, social factors play a role in cessation. For example, among persons with SMI, approval from others is an important factor predicting the use of pharmacological cessation treatment (Aschbrenner et al. 2015).

Another hurdle standing in the way of smoking cessation among persons with SMI is the myth that they are improving their symptoms through smoking. This attitude, common among some health care professionals, including psychiatrists, contributes to smoking disparities because of reduced efforts to help patients quit (Manzella et al. 2015). The self-medication hypothesis as a cause of smoking among persons with schizophrenia became popular in the 1980s; although some studies offer limited support for this theory, many other studies provide evidence to the contrary (Manzella et al. 2015). In fact, research shows that quitting is linked to a decrease in symptoms and better quality of life (Taylor et al. 2014).

Other factors may facilitate successful quit attempts among smokers with SMI. Persons with SMI who have engaged in mental health treatment in the previous year are more likely to quit smoking than those who are not involved in mental health treatment (Lê Cook et al. 2014). Persons who successfully quit smoking frequently cite health concerns, cost, advice from a doctor, and advice from others as reasons for quitting smoking. Social support, guidance from a doctor, nicotine replacement therapy (NRT), and guidance from friends were described as the ways in which individuals with SMI were able to quit (Dickerson et al. 2011).

Psychiatrists' Role in Smoking Cessation

The American Psychiatric Association (APA Workgroup on Tobacco Use Disorder, Council on Addiction Psychiatry 2015) has adopted policy statements regarding tobacco use that urge professionals to provide smoking cessation interventions to their patients. Indeed, psychiatrists and other behavioral health professionals are well positioned to provide cessation interventions. Psychiatrists and behavioral health professionals often have training in intervention for addiction, promoting behavior change, and understanding psychological factors. Further, behavioral health providers often consult with persons with SMI more frequently and for longer periods of time than do other types of health care providers, providing opportunities for intervention (Williams et al. 2014). Just a doctor's recommendation to quit has been found to significantly increase cessation rates in patients (Fiore et al. 2008).

Nicotine dependence is a recognized medical condition in the International Classification of Diseases (ICD-10) (World Health Organization 1992), and tobacco-related disorders, including tobacco use disorder and tobacco withdrawal, are recognized medical conditions in the *Diagnostic and Statistical Manual of Mental Disorders* (DSM-5; American Psychiatric Association 2013). Documentation of nicotine dependence/tobacco use disorder as a comorbid diagnosis for patients with SMI provides an opportunity for treatment as well as the possibility for reimbursement.

Interventions for Individuals

Although the American Psychiatric Association (Kleber et al. 2010) and the U.S. Department of Health and Human Services (Fiore et al. 2008) identify behavioral/psychosocial and pharmacological interventions as effective stand-alone treatments for cessation, they recognize that these treatments are complementary such that the combination of treatments is more successful than either alone. Research has found that individuals with SMI can yield quit rates comparable with the general population when provided the opportunity to engage in multifaceted treatments involving both behavioral/psychosocial and pharmacological interventions (Schwindt et al. 2017). Taking an individualized approach to smoking cessation treatment (e.g., tailoring aspects of the proposed treatment plan to the patient's specific needs and motivations) can increase the patient's willingness as well as ability to adhere to the treatment (Fiore et al. 2008; Kleber et al. 2010; Steinberg et al. 2016). Treatments used for the general public can be successfully implemented with patients with SMI. However, when treatment is adjusted to the specific needs of this population, its efficacy can increase (Steinberg et al. 2016). Further, a significant dose effect of treatment intensity (e.g., multiple sessions, longer duration per session, combination of treatments) has been found to increase cessation rates (Baker et al. 2006; Centers for Disease Control and Prevention 2013; Fiore et al. 2008). Individuals typically make multiple quit attempts before they can maintain abstinence.

Assessment and Stages of Change

Practice guidelines recommend engaging in frequent assessment of patients' tobacco use (Fiore et al. 2008; Kleber et al. 2010). Accurate identification of tobacco use status and willingness to quit can aid psychiatrists in identifying, recommending, and engaging in appropriate interventions for their patients. The stages of change model, derived from Prochaska's transtheoretical model, is frequently used by health care providers and researchers as a foundation for conceptualizing motivation to quit in patients who smoke tobacco products (DiClemente et al. 2004; Fiore et al. 2008).

The model characterizes intentional behavior change as a cyclical, multidimensional five-stage process of attitudes, intentions, and behaviors (DiClemente et al. 2004). The five stages of this model are 1) precontemplation, in which individuals have little or no interest in considering smoking cessation within the next 6 months; 2) contemplation, characterized by awareness of the problem and serious consideration of quitting during the next 6 months but without commitment to taking action within the next 30 days; 3) preparation, in which individuals make a commitment to action within the next 30 days and make a plan to quit; 4) action, when individuals begin to actively modify their behavior (e.g., discarding smoking cues at home, engaging in therapy, beginning psychopharmacological treatment, abstinence); and 5) maintenance, during which the individual demonstrates sustained change (e.g., abstinence) for at least 6 months (DiClemente et al. 2004).

Recognizing the stage of change is effective for identification and implementation of appropriate assessment as well as treatment. For instance, individuals in the precontemplation stage have been found to benefit from evaluating their options (e.g., identifying costs and benefits to smoking), a different approach than for those in the preparation stage, who benefit from setting goals and priorities (DiClemente et al. 2004; Fiore et al. 2008). The cognitive impairments of some individuals with SMI can be a barrier to accurate assessment of motivation to change (DiClemente et al. 2008). Although research is limited, simple assessments with few questions have been used successfully to assess motivation among persons with schizophrenia, major depression, and bipolar disorder (Etter et al. 2004).

Effective smoking cessation requires a systematic approach to treatment and repeated interventions. Patients often move back and forth or cycle through stages rather than progress linearly (DiClemente et al. 2004, 2011).

As difficulties in life in any area—interpersonal problems, job stress, financial problems, housing issues, legal trouble—impact motivation, persons with SMI having difficulties may experience decreased motivation, making smoking cessation more difficult. Psychiatrists should anticipate the waxing and waning of motivation and provide additional resources, problem solving, or case management as needed (DiClemente et al. 2004).

Relapse is common among individuals who quit smoking and is sometimes considered a stage in the stages of change model. Relapse rates are particularly high among persons with SMI. Among persons with a psychotic disorder, 60%–100% relapse after they quit (Horst et al. 2005). Research has also shown that persons with major depressive disorder or even a history of major depressive disorder are more likely to relapse than those who have not had major depression (Zvolensky et al. 2015). Maintenance pharmacotherapy may be helpful in assisting individuals with SMI in sustaining abstinence (Evins et al. 2017).

The 5 A's

The U.S. Public Health Service Clinical Practice Guideline "Treating Tobacco Use and Dependence" (Clinical Practice Guideline Treating Tobacco Use and Dependence 2008 Update Panel, Liaisons, and Staff 2008) recommends use of the 5 A's as an assessment during every patient visit, regardless of the current stage of change (DiClemente et al. 2011; Fiore et al. 2008). Originally developed by the National Cancer Institute and adapted by the Canadian Task Force on Preventive Health Care, the 5 A's model is also considered an effective form of brief intervention for smoking cessation (DiClemente et al. 2011; Dixon et al. 2009; Fiore et al. 2008). The 5 A's model, shown in Figure 11–1, which can be administered in as little as 10 minutes, is described as follows:

1. Ask—Identify and document tobacco use status for every patient at every visit.
2. Advise—Urge every tobacco user to quit in a clear, strong, and personal manner.
3. Assess—Determine whether the patient is willing and ready to make a quit attempt. (When? At this time? Within the next 30 days?)
4. Assist—For patients willing to make a quit attempt, use behavioral/psychosocial interventions and pharmacotherapy to aid in smoking cessation. For patients unwilling to make a quit attempt, employ motivational interviewing and the 5 R's (discussed later in this section).
5. Arrange—Schedule follow-up contact (either in person or via telephone). Provide appropriate encouragement.

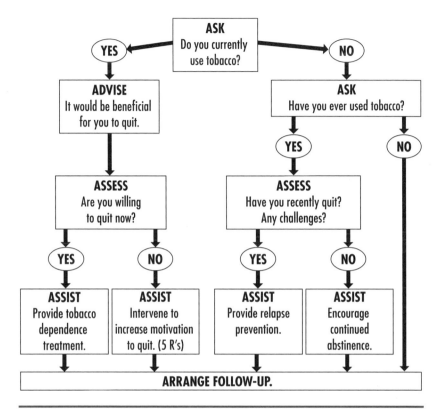

FIGURE 11–1. The 5 A's model.

Source. Adapted from Fiore et al. 2008.

Use of the 5 A's by psychiatrists is supported by research. Dixon et al. (2009) investigated the effectiveness of psychiatrists in a community mental health setting implementing the 5 A's of smoking cessation with patients with SMI, including 6- and 12-month follow-up. Using chart and patient report, the study authors found that psychiatrists were able to offer at least the first 3 of the 5 A's to a majority of the patients on an ongoing basis. Although abstinence rates were unchanged, there was a significant decrease in number of cigarettes typically smoked in a week at both 6- and 12-month follow-up. Further analyses of this study examining stages of change performed by DiClemente and colleagues (2011) found that almost 60% of individuals reported movement in terms of their stages at follow-up appointments.

A brief version, which can be completed in roughly 3 minutes, is "2 A's+R" or Ask, Advise, and Refer (Fiore et al. 2008). Psychiatrists faced with time constraints and/or limited resources to provide intervention can offer referrals to tobacco dependence treatment services (Fiore et al. 2008). However, a survey of 5,726 physicians by Steinberg et al. (2006) found that psychiatrists were among the least likely to be familiar with existing smoking cessation programs compared with their peers (e.g., general/family practitioners, cardiologists, obstetricians and gynecologists). Later, doctors were provided information on treatment resources. After familiarization with smoking cessation services, referral rates increased and were similar to those of their colleagues (Steinberg et al. 2006).

Psychosocial and Behavioral Interventions

The American Psychiatric Association (Kleber et al. 2010) and the U.S. Public Health Service Clinical Practice Guideline (Fiore et al. 2008) recommend that all smokers use behavioral interventions in combination with pharmacological interventions to quit smoking. A range of behavioral and psychosocial intervention strategies are employed for smoking cessation treatment, including education (e.g., risks of smoking), motivational interviewing, social support, and elements of cognitive-behavioral therapies (e.g., skills training and relapse prevention planning) (Fiore et al. 2008; Kleber et al. 2010).

Effective tobacco cessation counseling interventions can be delivered individually, in a group setting, and/or by telephone (Fiore et al. 2008; Kleber et al. 2010). Counseling for smoking cessation involves teaching behavioral strategies while incorporating support aimed at addressing the complex variables involved in the habit of smoking (Prochaska et al. 2017). Although available research among persons with SMI suggests that psychosocial interventions are beneficial when combined with psychopharmacological treatments, little evidence is available to definitively denote the ideal length or frequency or key intervention components (Evins et al. 2017).

Motivational Interviewing

A key element for successful smoking cessation is the patient's motivation to quit smoking (DiClemente et al. 2004, 2011; Fiore et al. 2008). Motivation to quit includes desire to stop smoking, goals and aims focused on quitting, commitment to stop smoking, and persistence or incentive toward sustaining cessation (DiClemente et al. 2004).

Motivational interviewing is a brief, empirically supported intervention designed to facilitate behavior change; it has been found to be effective for increasing motivation for smoking cessation (Fiore et al. 2008; Kleber et al. 2010; Miller and Rollnick 2002; Steinberg et al. 2016; Williams et al.

2006). Engagement in motivational interviewing permits greater flexibility in treatment, thus providing the ability to tailor interventions to the patient's movement through the stages of change (Williams et al. 2006). Overall, motivational interviewing is based on the premise that ambivalence is normal, and by working collaboratively and empathetically with patients, this motivational hurdle can be overcome (DiClemente et al. 2004; Steinberg et al. 2016).

Motivational interviewing is guided by five general principles: 1) expressing empathy through reflective listening (e.g., expressing understanding and acceptance of the patient's perspective); 2) drawing attention to the discrepancy between the patient's goals/values and his or her current behavior (e.g., highlighting the difference between the goal of good health and smoking behavior); 3) avoiding argument and direct confrontation, which can lead to defensiveness; 4) rolling with resistance (e.g., adjusting rather than directly opposing); and 5) supporting self-efficacy (Miller and Rollnick 2002).

Adapted versions of motivational interviewing have also shown success. Steinberg and colleagues (2016) conducted a study of adults with schizophrenia, schizoaffective disorder, or bipolar I disorder to test a motivational interviewing adaptation. A single 45-minute session involving motivational interviewing with personalized feedback delivered individually was compared with interactive education delivered in a group setting. Persons in the motivational interviewing group were significantly more likely to make a serious quit attempt by the 1-month follow-up assessment (Steinberg et al. 2016).

The 5 R's

The U.S. Public Health Service Clinical Practice Guideline "Treating Tobacco Use and Dependence" (Clinical Practice Guideline Treating Tobacco Use and Dependence 2008 Update Panel, Liaisons, and Staff 2008) identifies the 5 R's as a brief intervention for smoking cessation for patients who are unwilling to quit. The 5 R's can be an effective intervention for addressing patient ambivalence during any stage of change and can provide a structured approach for psychiatrists engaging in motivational interviewing (Fiore et al. 2008). This technique may be the main intervention used for patients identified as in the precontemplative or contemplative stage of change (DiClemente et al. 2004). Use of the guiding principles of motivational interviewing is recommended when implementing this 5 R's framework (Miller and Rollnick 2002):

1. Relevance—Ask the patient to indicate why quitting is personally relevant to him or her.

2. Risks—Ask the patient to identify potential risks of tobacco use (e.g., acute, long-term, environmental).
3. Rewards—Encourage the patient to identify benefits of stopping tobacco use.
4. Roadblocks—Ask the patient to discuss barriers to quitting. It may be helpful to note specific elements of treatment that can address barriers (e.g., medication, problem-solving skills, exercise).
5. Repetition—Repeat this motivational intervention during every visit with patients identified as unmotivated to quit. Remind patients that most people make repeated quit attempts before they are successful.

Quitlines

State tobacco quitlines are designed to provide accessible, evidence-based cessation services for smokers seeking assistance and health care providers seeking referral. Quitlines provide callers with telephone access to free practical counseling, self-help materials, referrals, and, in some cases, free or discounted pharmacological interventions (Fiore et al. 2008; Schwindt et al. 2017). It has been estimated that as many as 50% of quitline callers have a mental illness (Lukowski et al. 2015). Quitlines are an especially important cessation resource for persons with mental illness, who may experience financial barriers to treatment and difficulty accessing health care (Prochaska et al. 2017).

Quitline services for the general population are effective for smoking cessation. Schwindt and colleagues (2017) performed a systematic review to evaluate the utility of quitlines for assisting individuals with mental illness with smoking cessation. Only four studies were found to meet inclusion criteria (English language, peer-reviewed studies published between 2005 and 2016 evaluating quitline efficacy or effectiveness; study using an experimental or quasi-experimental design; sample of adult participants with a DSM-IV or DSM-5 diagnosis of mental illness). Still, overall study findings were positive, with the best outcomes reported for interventions combining a quitline with an additional intervention. Schwindt et al. (2017) recommend the continued use of quitlines among persons with mental illness, although more research is needed.

Technological Interventions

Technological interventions to address smoking cessation, including smartphone apps, websites, and social media, have become popular. There is evidence that these are more and more accessible to persons with SMI; the majority of persons with SMI have mobile phones, although owning a smartphone is less common (Naslund et al. 2016). Internet and social media use is growing among persons with SMI and these media are often a favored means to get support and manage health (Gay et al. 2016).

Some research shows that Web-based smoking cessation interventions can be effective tools for smoking cessation among people in the general population, including interactive Web-based interventions and smartphone cessation apps (Whittaker et al. 2016). Other researchers point out that evidence-based content in smoking cessation smartphone apps is lacking (Haskins et al. 2017). A small number of studies have reported positive outcomes, including increased rates of abstinence, reduced odds of relapse, and greater numbers of quit attempts, among persons utilizing social media interventions to quit smoking (Naslund et al. 2017). However, more research is needed to evaluate the effectiveness of technological interventions for persons with SMI (Prochaska et al. 2017).

Importantly, Web-based interventions may not be appropriately designed for persons with SMI (Ferron et al. 2017). Indeed, persons with cognitive impairment and/or little experience using the internet or smartphones may find technological interventions difficult to use (Rotondi et al. 2013). Brunette et al. (2011) assessed the content and usability of four commonly used smoking cessation websites and found that one website had acceptable content, but the majority of the 16 participants with SMI could not navigate the site. Similarly, in a study of a random selection of top-rated apps, Ferron et al. (2017) found that among 21 smokers with psychotic disorders, the apps tended to be difficult for participants to navigate. Participants also reported difficulty comprehending the content. In addition, the research revealed that app adherence to practice guidelines for treating tobacco use and dependence was low (Ferron et al. 2017).

Pharmacological Interventions

Pharmacological interventions for smoking cessation include both over-the-counter and prescription medications. First-line treatments are NRTs, varenicline (e.g., Chantix), and bupropion (e.g., Wellbutrin, Zyban). Each has been shown to be safe and effective and is approved by the U.S. Food and Drug Administration (except in the event of contraindications or for populations in which there is insufficient evidence) (Fiore et al. 2008). Each treatment is discussed here with a focus on its use among persons with SMI.

NRTs include over-the-counter skin patches, chewing gum, and lozenges as well as prescription inhalers and nasal sprays. NRT improves cessation rates and helps reduce symptoms of withdrawal (Stead et al. 2012). NRT provides a safer form of nicotine at a lower dose so that dependence and withdrawal are addressed while the user adjusts to not smoking (Stead et al. 2012). Using a single NRT product has been found to increase long-term cessation rates by 50%–70% compared with placebo among the general population (Stead et al. 2012). However, a meta-analysis conducted by Roberts et al. (2016) determined that no randomized controlled trials have assessed efficacy (abstinence at 6 months or longer) and tolerability of NRT for persons with SMI.

Varenicline and bupropion sustained release (SR) are prescription medications that promote abstinence from tobacco (Ebbert et al. 2010). Varenicline is a partial agonist for the neuronal nicotinic acetylcholine receptor subtype $\alpha_4\beta_2$ and has been shown to weaken the response to nicotine and reduces cravings, smoking satisfaction, smoking reinforcement, and withdrawal (Ebbert et al. 2010). Bupropion SR is an atypical antidepressant prescription medication that inhibits dopamine and norepinephrine and is a nicotine receptor antagonist (Kleber et al. 2010).

Both varenicline and bupropion SR have been shown to be safe and effective for persons with SMI in clinical trials (Roberts et al. 2016). The Evaluating Adverse Events in a Global Smoking Cessation Study (EAGLES), an international project with over 4,000 psychiatric patients and over 4,000 persons who were not psychiatric patients, was conducted to evaluate the safety of varenicline and bupropion. Use of varenicline and bupropion, compared with NRT or placebo, did not have a significantly different risk of adverse events (Anthenelli et al. 2016). Although some studies suggest that varenicline is more effective than bupropion (Evins et al. 2019), a meta-analysis of 14 randomized controlled trials among persons with SMI found no significant difference in the effectiveness of the two medications (Roberts et al. 2016). Because of the severity of nicotine dependence and high relapse rates among persons with SMI compared with the general population, once pharmacological interventions are discontinued for patients with SMI, maintenance pharmacological treatments may be needed to achieve sustained abstinence (Evins et al. 2017).

At the outset, psychiatrists should be aware of potential drug interactions that may influence treatment. Chemicals in cigarette smoke interact with enzymes that play a role in medication absorption, distribution, metabolism, and elimination. In particular, polycyclic aromatic hydrocarbons in smoke are linked to induction of cytochrome P450 enzymes (Maideen 2019). For some medications, including antipsychotics and antidepressants, quitting or reducing cigarette smoking results in higher drug concentrations in the blood; smokers may need a higher medication dose (Maideen 2019). In addition, nicotine interacts with benzodiazepines and opioids. Psychiatrists should carefully monitor drug levels and may need to adjust medication dosage when individuals change patterns of cigarette and nicotine use (Maideen 2019).

Harm Reduction

For persons with SMI who have been unsuccessful at quit attempts or who are unmotivated to quit, harm reduction is an alternative strategy. Harm reduction is used to lower the risks associated with a risky behavior such as substance use. Common alternatives to cigarettes that may be used for tobacco harm reduction are the long-term use of NRT, smokeless tobacco products, and e-cigarettes (electronic cigarettes) (Gartner and Hall 2015).

E-cigarettes have become commonly used as an alternative to smoking cigarettes and as a smoking cessation aid (National Institute on Drug Use 2018). The battery-operated devices emit an aerosol composed of chemicals, flavoring, and often nicotine (National Institute on Drug Use 2018). A systematic review and meta-analysis of six studies among smokers in the general population examined the use of e-cigarettes for smoking cessation and reduction. The authors found that nicotine-filled e-cigarettes were more effective for smoking cessation than e-cigarettes without nicotine, but both types of e-cigarettes were effective at reducing the number of cigarettes participants smoked (Rahman et al. 2015). However, to date, there have been few high-quality studies on the use of e-cigarettes for smoking cessation or reduction among persons with SMI (Gentry et al. 2018). Evidence of effectiveness of other tobacco harm reduction methods for persons with SMI is also limited (Gartner and Hall 2015).

Structural Interventions

The policy, systems, and environmental context for smoking cessation is fundamental to reducing smoking disparities among persons with SMI. Interventions that impact policy, systems, or the environment can be very effective ways to improve health. Individual cessation intervention is most effective when it is coordinated and rooted in a system in which health care administrators, insurers, and health care providers are working toward the same goal. Tobacco cessation treatment must be accessible and affordable for patients, and health care providers must be trained and supported in identifying patients and providing cessation treatment (Fiore et al. 2008). Psychiatrists should be aware of the structural barriers to smoking cessation that their patients encounter and advocate for changes that will best support patient health.

Many behavioral health service organizations do not provide tobacco cessation treatment. The Substance Abuse and Mental Health Services Administration's annual survey of all known, nonprivate, mental health and substance use treatment providers finds that only 37.6% of mental health facilities and 47.4% of substance abuse treatment facilities offer tobacco cessation counseling, with 25.2% of mental health and 26.2% of substance use treatment facilities offering NRT (Marynak et al. 2018). In addition, a review by Krauth and Apollonio (2015) conducted between May 2013 and October 2014 found that only 13 of the 50 states require tobacco cessation interventions to be provided routinely in alcohol, drug rehabilitation, and/ or mental health centers. Christiansen et al. (2016) conducted a review of the integration of policies to support tobacco cessation in Wisconsin's behavioral health care system. About 40% of the programs surveyed had integrated policies addressing the use of tobacco, treatment, and ability to support employees in quitting. Surveyed providers reported a need for training and technical assistance in the treatment of tobacco dependence (Christiansen et al. 2016).

Indeed, the need for tobacco treatment training for psychiatry residents was revealed in a 2006 national survey of residency program training directors. Only one-half of the programs provided training, which lasted a median of 1 hour (Prochaska et al. 2006b). Those programs without such training cited a lack of faculty with the education needed to provide training on tobacco treatment as the reason (Prochaska et al. 2006b).

A lack of insurance coverage presents additional barriers to smoking cessation. Almost all states have limitations on coverage for tobacco cessation treatment under Medicaid (DiGiulio et al. 2018), the insurer of 22% of nonelderly adults with mental illness and 26% of nonelderly adults with SMI (Kaiser Family Foundation 2017). For example, 33 states provide coverage for individual smoking cessation treatment counseling for all Medicaid beneficiaries; however, only 10 states cover group smoking cessation treatment. Twenty-four states impose annual limits on covered quit attempts, and 16 states require copays for tobacco cessation treatment. The nicotine patch, bupropion, and varenicline are covered by the vast majority of states, but coverage for other forms of NRT is less common (DiGiulio et al. 2018). Complete coverage would be expected to increase access to treatment and improve health of beneficiaries.

The American Psychiatric Association supports and advocates for smoke-free policies in health care facilities (APA Workgroup on Tobacco Use Disorder, Council on Addiction Psychiatry 2015). Psychiatric hospital smoking bans have not led to significant long-term posthospitalization changes in smoking behavior (el-Guebaly et al. 2002; Prochaska et al. 2006a). However, in tandem with coordinated individualized pharmacological and behavioral cessation interventions and posthospitalization treatment, they could play an important role in smoking cessation (Campion et al. 2008). Complete smoke-free policies in psychiatric settings provide patients with a model setting in which health professionals provide cessation support and monitor the impact of cessation on medication. If not immediately successful, short-term quit attempts in smoke-free settings can promote self-efficacy among patients for subsequent quit attempts (Campion et al. 2008). In contrast, partial smoking bans at psychiatric hospitals—generally those that allow patients to smoke outside—create conditions in which patients have ongoing withdrawal symptoms; intermittent reinforcement through cigarettes strengthens addiction (Lawn and Campion 2013).

Case Vignette

Dr. Brooks is a newly hired psychiatrist at Anderson Clinic. She meets with Paul Thompson today for the first time. Mr. Thompson is a 36-year-old African American man who lives on the South Side of Chicago. He has a history of bipolar disorder and was hospitalized because of self-harm and suicidal ideation approximately 10 years ago. Mr. Thompson participated in psychotherapy for several years in the past, but he hasn't seen a psychotherapist regularly for 3 years. He consistently attends his psychiatry appointments each month for medication management. He worked with a job coach during the last 6 months and successfully obtained full-time employment at a shipping warehouse. Mr. Thompson reports that he enjoys work and has been getting along with his coworkers. When asked about tobacco use, he reports that he is a smoker. Mr. Thompson has smoked since he was 16 and currently smokes a pack a day. He has made a few quit attempts in the past.

Dr. Brooks implements the 5 A's. She urges Mr. Thompson to stop smoking in a strong and clear manner. Next, Dr. Brooks assesses Mr. Thompson's willingness and readiness to quit. He endorses a desire to quit within the next 6 months but says he doesn't feel capable of quitting within the next 30 days. He has no specific plan to quit. Mr. Thompson also notes that smoking seems to help with his mood and energy level.

On the basis of this information, Dr. Brooks determines that Mr. Thompson is currently in the contemplation stage of change. She utilizes motivational interviewing and the 5 R's to guide further discussion with him. Mr. Thompson is able to identify personally relevant reasons for quitting smoking, including the desire to save more money. He also understands that lung cancer is a risk of continuing to smoke. Mr. Thompson identifies improving health and saving money as some rewards for quitting. He also identifies symptoms of withdrawal, increased psychiatric symptoms, and weight gain as potential roadblocks to a successful quit attempt. Dr. Brooks helps to clarify Mr. Thompson's misconceptions regarding smoking during this part of the discussion, specifically highlighting that smoking tobacco products does not help alleviate psychiatric symptoms. She also provides education regarding experiencing symptoms of withdrawal. Dr. Brooks validates his concerns and discusses the importance of having adequate support from friends and professionals. Dr. Brooks then provides Mr. Thompson with a handout that includes a quitline number, information regarding smoking cessation treatment, and Anderson Clinic cessation resources.

During his next appointment, Mr. Thompson reports that he called the quitline. He feels more motivated to quit. He has been engaging in small "quit challenges" each week, which make him feel like he could be successful in quitting this time. He reports a desire to join the smoking cessation group held at Anderson Clinic and would like to quit within the next 30 days. Dr. Brooks determines that Mr. Thompson is now in the action stage of change. Dr. Brooks enthusiastically validates his decision to quit smoking and works with Mr. Thompson to create a quit plan. Together, they identify various supports and barriers to a successful quit attempt and select a quit date. Mr. Thompson and Dr. Brooks decide that, in addition to engaging in group therapy, adding a pharmacological intervention would be a helpful tool to aid in Mr. Thompson's quit attempt.

During the next 2 months, Mr. Thompson actively engages in various cessation supports, including group therapy and pharmacotherapy, as well as reaching out to his friends as social supports throughout the process. Each month, Dr. Brooks checks in regarding Mr. Thompson's tobacco use status and progress on his quit plan. He initially struggles with resisting his urges to smoke and opts to reengage in individual psychotherapy for a short period of time to help him with his coping skills. As his progress continues, he reports feeling more confident.

Key Points

- Smoking contributes substantially to the heavy burden of disease and lost life among persons with serious mental illness (SMI).

- Many factors play a role in the smoking disparities between persons with mental illness and the general population. Historically, the tobacco industry marketed tobacco products to persons with SMI and spread misconceptions about smoking that helped to maintain smoking among this group. In addition, in the recent past, smoking was acceptable in psychiatric facilities, and cigarettes were used to reward patients.

- Additional social, environmental, biochemical, and neurochemical factors play a role in unacceptably high rates of smoking and smoking-related deaths among persons with SMI. Among them, misconceptions that smoking improves psychiatric symptoms and that persons with SMI are not motivated to quit have decreased efforts among health professionals to provide cessation opportunities.

- Research shows that persons with SMI want to quit smoking and are generally motivated to quit. However, quitting smoking is not easy, and persons with SMI may experience challenges, such as increased dependence and withdrawal, that make quitting harder.

- Persons with SMI should be given every opportunity to quit. Advocacy for optimal conditions and resources to improve quit rates for persons with SMI are needed. The best environment for quitting requires policies and systems that fully support smoking cessation. This includes psychiatrists who are well trained and supported in providing smoking cessation, behavioral health organizations that provide cessation treatment, insurance that covers the range of evidence-based treatment for unlimited quit attempts, and smoke-free health care facilities.

- In clinical practice, psychiatrists should engage in frequent assessment of patients' willingness and motivation to quit. Brief interventions to increase the motivation of patients who are unwilling to quit should be provided, such as motivational interviewing and the 5 R's.

- For patients who are willing to quit, a combination of psychosocial and pharmacological interventions is associated with the best chance of quit success. Nicotine replacement therapy, varenicline, and bupropion are first-line treatments shown to be safe and effective for persons with SMI in clinical trials.

- Psychiatrists can anticipate that quitting will require multiple attempts and should work with patients to problem-solve and address barriers to cessation as they come up. Harm reduction interventions should be considered for patients who are not willing to quit.

- Although smoking cessation is not easy, there are safe and effective ways to help individuals with SMI quit. Psychiatrists are uniquely trained and positioned to address their needs. Persistent efforts to provide cessation interventions to individuals, educate health professionals, and promote systems and policy change can help close the smoking disparities gap.

References

American Psychiatric Association: Diagnostic and Statistical Manual of Mental Disorders, 5th Edition. Arlington, VA, American Psychiatric Association, 2013

Anthenelli RM, Benowitz NL, West R, et al: Neuropsychiatric safety and efficacy of varenicline, bupropion, and nicotine patch in smokers with and without psychiatric disorders (EAGLES): a double-blind, randomised, placebo-controlled clinical trial. Lancet 387(10037):2507–2520, 2016

APA Workgroup on Tobacco Use Disorder, Council on Addiction Psychiatry: Position statement on tobacco use disorder. 2015. Available at: www.psychiatry.org/File%20Library/About-APA/Organization-Documents-Policies/Policies/Position-2015-Tobacco-Use-Disorder.pdf. Accessed July 14, 2020.

Aschbrenner KA, Ferron JC, Mueser KT, et al: Social predictors of cessation treatment use among smokers with serious mental illness. Addict Behav 41:169–174, 2015

Baker A, Richmond R, Haile M, et al: A randomized controlled trial of a smoking cessation intervention among people with a psychotic disorder. Am J Psychiatry 163(11):1934–1942, 2006

Brunette MF, Ferron JC, Devitt T, et al: Do smoking cessation websites meet the needs of smokers with severe mental illnesses? Health Educ Res 27(2):183–90, 2011

Callaghan RC, Veldhuizen S, Jeysingh T, et al: Patterns of tobacco-related mortality among individuals diagnosed with schizophrenia, bipolar disorder, or depression. J Psychiatr Res 48(1):102–110, 2014

Campion J, Checinski K, Nurse J, et al: Smoking by people with mental illness and benefits of smoke-free mental health services. Advances in Psychiatric Treatment 14(3):217–228, 2008

Centers for Disease Control and Prevention: Tobacco use cessation. 2013. Available at: www.cdc.gov/workplacehealthpromotion/implementation/topics/tobacco-use.html. Accessed July 14, 2020.

Christiansen BA, Macmaster DR, Heiligenstein EL, et al: Measuring the integration of tobacco policy and treatment into the behavioral health care delivery system: how are we doing? J Health Care Poor Underserved 27(2):510–526, 2016

Clinical Practice Guideline Treating Tobacco Use and Dependence 2008 Update Panel, Liaisons, and Staff: A clinical practice guideline for treating tobacco use and dependence: 2008 update. A U.S. Public Health Service Report. Am J Prev Med 35(2):158–176, 2008

de Leon J, Diaz FJ: A meta-analysis of worldwide studies demonstrates an association between schizophrenia and tobacco smoking behaviors. Schizophr Res 76(2–3):135–157, 2005

Desai HD, Seabolt J, Jann MW: Smoking in patients receiving psychotropic medications: a pharmacokinetic perspective. CNS Drugs 15:469–494, 2001

Dickerson F, Bennett M, Dixon L, et al: Smoking cessation in persons with serious mental illnesses: the experience of successful quitters. Psychiatr Rehabil J 34(4):311–316, 2011

Dickerson F, Schroeder J, Katsafanas E, et al: Cigarette smoking by patients with serious mental illness, 1999–2016: an increasing disparity. Psychiatr Serv 69(2):147–153, 2017

DiClemente CC, Schlundt D, Gemmell L: Readiness and stages of change in addiction treatment. Am J Addict 13(2):103–119, 2004

DiClemente CC, Nidecker M, Bellack AS: Motivation and the stages of change among individuals with severe mental illness and substance abuse disorders. J Subst Abuse Treat 34(1):25–35, 2008

DiClemente CC, Delahanty JC, Kofeldt MG: Stage movement following a 5A's intervention in tobacco dependent individuals with serious mental illness (SMI). Addict Behav 36(3):261–264, 2011

DiGiulio A, Jump Z, Yu A, et al: State Medicaid coverage for tobacco cessation treatments and barriers to accessing treatments—United States, 2015–2017. MMWR Morb Mortal Wkly Rep 67(13):390–395, 2018

Dixon LB, Medoff D, Goldberg R, et al: Is implementation of the 5 A's of smoking cessation at community mental health centers effective for reduction of smoking by patients with serious mental illness? Am J Addict 18(5):386–392, 2009

Drope J, Liber AC, Cahn Z, et al: Who's still smoking? Disparities in adult cigarette smoking prevalence in the United States. CA Cancer J Clin 68(2):106–115, 2018

Ebbert JO, Wyatt KD, Hays JT, et al: Varenicline for smoking cessation: efficacy, safety, and treatment recommendations. Patient Prefer Adherence 4:355–362, 2010

el-Guebaly N, Cathcart J, Currie S, et al: Public health and therapeutic aspects of smoking bans in mental health and addiction settings. Psychiatr Serv 53(12):1617–1622, 2002

Eriksen M, Mackay J, Schluger N, Drope J: The Tobacco Atlas, 5th Edition. Atlanta, GA, American Cancer Society, 2015

Etter M, Mohr S, Garin C, et al: Stages of change in smokers with schizophrenia or schizoaffective disorder and in the general population. Schizophr Bull 30(2):459–468, 2004

Evins AE, Hoeppner SS, Schoenfeld DA, et al: Maintenance pharmacotherapy normalizes the relapse curve in recently abstinent tobacco smokers with schizophrenia and bipolar disorder. Schizophr Res 183:124–129, 2017

Evins AE, Benowitz NL, West R, et al: Neuropsychiatric safety and efficacy of varenicline, bupropion, and nicotine patch in smokers with psychotic, anxiety, and mood disorders in the EAGLES trial. J Clin Psychopharmacol 39(2):108–116, 2019

Ferron JC, Brunette MF, Geiger P, et al: Mobile phone apps for smoking cessation: quality and usability among smokers with psychosis. JMIR Hum Factors 4(1):e7, 2017

Fiore MC, Jaen CR, Baker TB, et al: Treating Tobacco Use and Dependence: 2008 Update. Rockville, MD, U.S. Department of Health and Human Services, 2008

Forchuk C, Norman R, Malla A, et al: Schizophrenia and the motivation for smoking. Perspect Psychiatr Care 38(2):41–49, 2000

Fu SS, McFall M, Saxon AJ, et al: Post-traumatic stress disorder and smoking: a systematic review. Nicotine Tob Res 9(11):1071–1084, 2007

Gartner C, Hall W: Tobacco harm reduction in people with serious mental illnesses. Lancet Psychiatry 2(6):485–487, 2015

Gay K, Torous J, Joseph A, et al: Digital technology use among individuals with schizophrenia: results of an online survey. JMIR Ment Health 3(2):e15, 2016

Gentry S, Forouhi NG, Notley C: Are electronic cigarettes an effective aid to smoking cessation or reduction among vulnerable groups? A systematic review of quantitative and qualitative evidence. Nicotine Tob Res 21(5):602–616, 2018

Grand RBG, Hwang S, Han J, et al: Short-term naturalistic treatment outcomes in cigarette smokers with substance abuse and/or mental illness. J Clin Psychiatry 68(6):892–898, 2007

Gfroerer J, Dube SR, King BA, et al: Vital signs: current cigarette smoking among adults aged ≥18 years with mental illness—United States, 2009–2011. MMWR Morb Mortal Wkly Rep 62(5):81–87, 2013

Haskins BL, Lesperance D, Gibbons P, et al: A systematic review of smartphone applications for smoking cessation. Transl Behav Med 7(2):292–299, 2017

Horst WD, Klein MW, Williams D, et al: Extended use of nicotine replacement therapy to maintain smoking cessation in persons with schizophrenia. Neuropsychiatr Dis Treat 1(4):349–355, 2005

Herman AI, DeVito EE, Jensen KP, et al: Pharmacogenetics of nicotine addiction: role of dopamine. Pharmacogenomics 15(2):221–234, 2014

Jackson JG, Diaz FJ, Lopez L, et al: A combined analysis of worldwide studies demonstrates an association between bipolar disorder and tobacco smoking behaviors in adults. Bipolar Disord 17(6):575–597, 2015

Jha P, Ramasundarahettige C, Landsman V: 21st-century hazards of smoking and benefits of cessation in the United States. N Engl J Med 368(4):341–350, 2013

Kaiser Family Foundation: Facilitating access to mental health services: a look at Medicaid, private insurance, and the uninsured. 2017. Available at: http://files.kff.org/attachment/Fact-Sheet-Facilitating-Access-to-Mental-Health-Services-A-Look-at-Medicaid-Private-Insurance-and-the-Uninsured. Accessed April 28, 2019.

Kelly DL, McMahon RP, Wehring HJ: Cigarette smoking and mortality risk in people with schizophrenia. Schizophr Bull 37(4):832–838, 2009

Kleber HD, Weiss RD, Anton RF: Practice Guideline for the Treatment of Patients With Substance Use Disorders, 2nd Edition. Arlington, VA, American Psychiatric Association, 2010, pp 71–88. Available at: https://psychiatryonline.org/pb/assets/raw/sitewide/practice_guidelines/guidelines/substanceuse.pdf. Accessed July 14, 2020.

Krauth D, Apollonio DE: Overview of state policies requiring smoking cessation therapy in psychiatric hospitals and drug abuse treatment centers. Tob Induc Dis 13:33, 2015

Lasser K, Boyd JW, Woolhandler S, et al: Smoking and mental illness: a population-based prevalence study. JAMA 284(20):2606–2610, 2000

Lawn S, Campion J: Achieving smoke-free mental health services: lessons from the past decade of implementation research. Int J Environ Res Public Health 10(9):4224–4244, 2013

Lawrence D, Mitrou F, Zubrick SR: Smoking and mental illness: results from population surveys in Australia and the United States. BMC Public Health 9:285, 2009

Lê Cook B, Wayne GF, Kafali EN, et al: Trends in smoking among adults with mental illness and association between mental health treatment and smoking cessation. JAMA 311(2):172–182, 2014

Lipari R, Van Horn S: Smoking and Mental Illness Among Adults in the United States. Rockville, MD, Substance Abuse and Mental Health Services Administration, 2017

Lukowski AV, Morris CD, Young SE, Tinkelman D: Quitline outcomes for smokers in 6 states: rates of successful quitting vary by mental health status. Nicotine Tob Res 17(8):924–930, 2015

Maideen NMP: Tobacco smoking and its drug interactions with comedications involving CYP and UGT enzymes and nicotine. World Journal of Pharmacology 8(2):14–25, 2019

Manzella F, Maloney SE, Taylor GT: Smoking in schizophrenic patients: a critique of the self-medication hypothesis. World J Psychiatry 5(1):35–46, 2015

Marynak K, VanFrank B, Tetlow S: Tobacco cessation interventions and smoke-free policies in mental health and substance abuse treatment facilities—United States, 2016. MMWR Morb Mortal Wkly Rep 67(18):519–523, 2018

Miller WR, Rollnick S: Motivational Interviewing, 2nd Edition: Preparing People for Change. New York, Guilford, 2002

Naslund JA, Aschbrenner KA, Bartels SJ: How people with serious mental illness use smartphones, mobile apps, and social media. Psychiatr Rehabil J 39(4):364–367, 2016

Naslund JA, Kim SJ, Aschbrenner KA, et al: Systematic review of social media interventions for smoking cessation. Addict Behav 73:81–93, 2017

National Institute on Drug Use: Vaping devices (electronic cigarettes) DrugFacts: What are vaping devices? 2018. Available at: www.drugabuse.gov/publications/drugfacts/electronic-cigarettes-e-cigarettes. Accessed July 14, 2020.

Price JH, Ambrosetti LM, Sidani JE, et al: Psychiatrists' smoking cessation activities with Ohio community mental health center patients. Community Ment Health J 43(3):251–266, 2007

Prochaska JJ, Fletcher L, Hall SE, et al: Return to smoking following a smoke-free psychiatric hospitalization. Am J Addict 15(1):15–22, 2006a

Prochaska JJ, Fromont SC, Louie AK, et al: Training in tobacco treatments in psychiatry: a national survey of psychiatry residency training directors. Acad Psychiatry 30(5):372–378, 2006b

Prochaska JJ, Hall SM, Bero LA: Tobacco use among individuals with schizophrenia: what role has the tobacco industry played? Schizophr Bull 34(3):555–567, 2008

Prochaska JJ, Das S, Young-Wolff KC: Smoking, mental illness, and public health. Annu Rev Public Health 38:165–185, 2017

Rahman MA, Hann N, Wilson A, et al: E-cigarettes and smoking cessation: evidence from a systematic review and meta-analysis. PLoS One 10(3):e0122544, 2015

Roberts E, Evins EA, McNeill A, Robson D: Efficacy and tolerability of pharmacotherapy for smoking cessation in adults with serious mental illness: a systematic review and network meta-analysis. Addiction 111(4):599–612, 2016

Rotondi AJ, Eack SM, Hanusa BH, et al: Critical design elements of e-health applications for users with severe mental illness: singular focus, simple architecture, prominent contents, explicit navigation, and inclusive hyperlinks. Schizophr Bull 41(2):440–448, 2013

Schmutte T, Flanagan E, Bedregal L, et al: Self-efficacy and self-care: missing ingredients in health and healthcare among adults with serious mental illnesses. Psychiatr Q 80(1):1–8, 2008

Schwindt R, Hudmon KS, Knisely M, et al: Impact of tobacco quitlines on smoking cessation in persons with mental illness: a systematic review. J Drug Educ 47(1–2):68–81, 2017

Sheals K, Tombor I, McNeill A, et al: A mixed-method systematic review and meta-analysis of mental health professionals' attitudes toward smoking and smoking cessation among people with mental illnesses. Addiction 111(9):1536–1553, 2016

Sharp DL, Blaakman SW, Cole RE, et al: Report from a national tobacco dependence survey of psychiatric nurses. J Am Psychiatr Nurses Assoc 15(3):172–181, 2009

Sidani J, Price J, Dake J, et al: Practices and perceptions of mental health counselors in addressing smoking cessation. Journal of Mental Health Counseling 33(3):264–282, 2011

Siru R, Hulse GK, Tait RJ: Assessing motivation to quit smoking in people with mental illness: a review. Addiction 104(5):719–733, 2009

Smith PH, Homish GG, Giovino GA, et al: Cigarette smoking and mental illness: a study of nicotine withdrawal. Am J Public Health 104(2):e127–e133, 2014

Stead LF, Perera R, Bullen C: Nicotine replacement therapy for smoking cessation. Cochrane Database Syst Rev 11:CD000146, 2012

Steinberg MB, Alvarez MS, Delnevo CD, et al: Disparity of physicians' utilization of tobacco treatment services. Am J Health Behav 30(4):375–386, 2006

Steinberg ML, Williams JM, Stahl NF, et al: An adaptation of motivational interviewing increases quit attempts in smokers with serious mental illness. Nicotine Tob Res 18(3):243–250, 2016

Streck JM, Weinberger AH, Pacek LR, et al: Cigarette smoking quit rates among persons with serious psychological distress in the United States from 2008 to 2016: are mental health disparities in cigarette use increasing? Nicotine Tob Res 22(1):130–134, 2020

Taylor G, McNeill A, Girling A, et al: Change in mental health after smoking cessation: systematic review and meta-analysis. BMJ 348:g1151, 2014

U.S. Department of Health and Human Services: The Health Benefits of Smoking Cessation. Atlanta, GA, Public Health Service, Centers for Disease Control, Center for Chronic Disease Prevention and Health Promotion, Office on Smoking and Health, 1990

U.S. Department of Health and Human Services: The Health Consequences of Smoking—50 Years of Progress: A Report of the Surgeon General. Atlanta, GA, Public Health Service, Centers for Disease Control, Center for Chronic Disease Prevention and Health Promotion, Office on Smoking and Health, 2014

U.S. Public Health Service: Smoking and Health: Report of the Advisory Committee to the Surgeon General of the Public Health Service. Department of Health, Education, and Welfare, Public Health Service, Center for Disease Control (PHS Publ No 1103). Washington, DC, U.S. Government Printing Office, 1964

Whittaker R, McRobbie H, Bullen C, et al: Mobile phone-based interventions for smoking cessation. Cochrane Database Syst Rev 4:CD006611, 2016

Williams GC, McGregor HA, Sharp D, et al: Testing a self-determination theory intervention for motivating tobacco cessation: supporting autonomy and competence in a clinical trial. Health Psychol 25(1):91–101, 2006

Williams JM, Miskimen T, Minsky S, et al: Increasing tobacco dependence treatment through continuing education training for behavioral health professionals. Psychiatr Serv 66(1):21–26, 2014

Wing VC, Wass CE, Soh DW, et al: A review of neurobiological vulnerability factors and treatment implications for comorbid tobacco dependence in schizophrenia. Ann N Y Acad Sci 1248(1):89–106, 2012

World Health Organization: The ICD-10 Classification of Mental and Behavioural Disorders: Clinical Descriptions and Diagnostic Guidelines. Geneva, World Health Organization, 1992

Young-Wolff KC, Henriksen L, Delucchi K, et al: Tobacco retailer proximity and density and nicotine dependence among smokers with serious mental illness. Am J Public Health 104(8):1454–1463, 2014

Zvolensky MJ, Bakhshaie J, Sheffer C, et al: Major depressive disorder and smoking relapse among adults in the United States: a 10-year, prospective investigation. Psychiatry Res 226(1):73–77, 2015

CHAPTER 12

Improving Diet, Activity, and Weight

Katherine D. Hoerster, Ph.D., M.P.H.
Alexander S. Young, M.D., M.S.H.S.

As discussed in Chapter 5, obesity has many detrimental health consequences, making it a major preventable cause of death (Danaei et al. 2009). Adults with serious mental illness (SMI), such as schizophrenia, bipolar disorder, major depression, or persistent posttraumatic stress disorder (PTSD), are at increased risk for obesity and weight-related conditions, including elevated lipids, diabetes, high blood pressure, and cardiovascular disease (De Hert et al. 2011), and for premature mortality (Kilbourne et al. 2009; Olfson et al. 2015). Understanding why individuals with SMI carry this disproportionate disease burden is a key step in addressing this critically important public health issue. Several prior theoretical models outline the many

This work was supported by the U.S. Department of Veterans Affairs (VA) Health Services Research and Development Service (IIR 09-083, CDA 12-263), the National Institute of Mental Health (R34MH090207), the Seattle-Denver VA Center of Innovation for Veteran-Centered and Value-Driven Care, and the VA VISN22 Mental Illness Research, Education and Clinical Center. The contents do not necessarily represent the views of affiliated institutions or the U.S. government.

factors contributing to obesity among people with SMI, helping to identify pathways for effective intervention. However, at present, existing theoretical models tend to be disease specific (e.g., Dedert et al. 2010), do not comprehensively identify all potential intervention targets, and give little attention to relevant factors such as resilience and body image. Thus, in this chapter, we present a novel comprehensive model of obesity among individuals with SMI (Figure 12–1). This can be used to inform targeted, interdisciplinary efforts to reduce obesity and associated disability among individuals with SMI. We include specific recommendations for clinicians and provide a case vignette.

Causes of Overweight and Obesity

Causes of disproportionate obesity and associated chronic disease among people with SMI include psychiatric symptoms, psychological factors, knowledge and beliefs, medications, physiology, and contextual factors. These can directly affect weight or have effects that are mediated by physical activity and healthy diet, which prevent and address cardiovascular disease, diabetes, and obesity (Danaei et al. 2009). Although multiple contributors to weight have strong effects, fortunately, most of them are modifiable and can be important intervention targets. Several key contributors are discussed below.

Psychological Symptoms and Factors, Knowledge, and Beliefs

The symptoms of psychiatric conditions can be substantial barriers to healthy lifestyles. Depressive disorders (Luppino et al. 2010), PTSD (Hall et al. 2015), and psychotic disorders (Vancampfort et al. 2017) are associated with inactivity and poor diet, likely because symptoms of those disorders serve as barriers to healthy lifestyles. For example, PTSD symptoms such as behavioral avoidance, diminished interest in activities, negative beliefs and emotions, social isolation, hyperarousal, and sleep disturbance can be barriers to physical activity and healthy eating behavior (Boutcher and Dunn 2009; Brug 2008; Rutter et al. 2013; St-Onge 2017).

People with mental illness have lower self-efficacy on average, compared with the general population, which can affect health behaviors and well-being. Individuals who are classified as overweight can be subject to stigma related to both mental illness and weight, which can further affect psychological factors (e.g., self-efficacy) and, subsequently, health behaviors and health (Corrigan 2016; Pearl and Puhl 2018). Low self-efficacy can

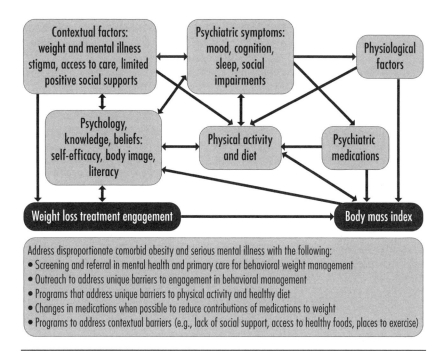

FIGURE 12–1. Model of and strategies for addressing dispropor-tionate weight in those with serious mental illness.

lead to decreased weight intervention participation (Vancampfort et al. 2014). This can be addressed by interventions (Bennett et al. 2018). Additional factors that can act as barriers to weight loss include limited formal education and health literacy, which can be found among people with SMI. Limited knowledge and health literacy can affect understanding and application of information regarding a healthy diet; know-how about preparing healthy foods; and other causes and treatments of health issues, such as diabetes, and their relationships to weight. This poor health literacy is compounded by pervasive misinformation regarding diet in our society, fueled by substantial marketing of foods that are relatively inexpensive but unhealthy. Interventions have been developed that focus on these issues in people with SMI—for example, focusing on improving their ability to shop for, prepare, and choose healthy foods (Faulkner et al. 2007).

Medications

As outlined in Chapter 6, appropriate pharmacological treatment is a necessary component of treatment for most people with SMI. Although significant advances have been made in pharmacological management, the majority of individuals with SMI are prescribed medications that can cause weight gain as a side effect (Young et al. 2010). Some medications are particularly likely to cause weight gain (Table 12–1). The magnitude of the weight gain varies among medications and between individuals. Although medications have associations with weight, there is large variation. Many people can take medications with substantial weight gain liability and experience no weight gain, whereas others gain substantial weight with "low weight gain" medications. Despite this variation, changing to medications with less weight gain potential has been proven to result in lower weight on average (Newcomer et al. 2013). Decisions to change a medication regimen must be made collaboratively by the patient and clinician, considering all relevant trade-offs regarding effectiveness and side effects. For example, clozapine can cause weight gain, but it is also substantially more effective at managing psychiatric symptoms that have not improved with other medications. Engagement with weight management care is critical. Effective treatment can allow individuals to engage in weight management care, successfully improve their diet and activity, and manage or reduce their weight while taking whatever medication is efficacious for them.

Physiology

Various physiological and genetic factors contribute to weight, physical activity, and diet, including satiety, hunger, glucose tolerance, elevated lipids, and energy expenditure. Overactivation of the hypothalamic-pituitary-adrenal stress axis and inflammation are observed among individuals with SMI, which can contribute to obesity and related conditions (Dedert et al. 2010; Marazziti et al. 2014). Sleep disturbance, also common in people with mental illness, has direct physiological effects on weight (St-Onge 2017).

Contextual Factors

The general population has seen substantial gains in health over the past decades, due largely to increased use of preventive services and effective primary care treatments. Unfortunately, similar gains have not occurred in the population with SMI. People with mental illnesses are substantially less likely to receive critical preventive services and high-value, routine primary care treatments (Mitchell et al. 2009). Access to primary care, behavioral services, and services for weight is limited (Liu et al. 2017). Primary care and mental health clinicians have inconsistent knowledge regarding effective medication and psychosocial strategies for management of weight. Weight stigma can affect the experience of and effectiveness of health care, includ-

TABLE 12–1. Common psychiatric medications with substantial weight gain potential

High weight gain potential	
Clozapine	
Olanzapine	
Medium weight gain potential	
Amitriptyline	Paliperidone
Asenapine	Paroxetine
Cariprazine	Quetiapine
Chlorpromazine	Risperidone
Iloperidone	Sertindole
Imipramine	Thioridazine
Lithium	Trifluoperazine
Mirtazapine	Valproate

ing care intended to support obesity management (Pearl and Puhl 2018). Mental health services often lack substantial programs for improving diet, activity, and weight. Few evidence-based programs have been translated to the real-world health care setting (Deenik et al. 2019). Limited financial resources and social, physical, and policy environments also play an important role. For example, in the United States, production of unhealthy foods is subsidized by the federal government, contributing to healthy foods being more expensive than unhealthy choices (Story et al. 2008). Because people with SMI have lower income on average, such policies can make it challenging to purchase and consume healthy foods. People also have competing demands on their time and attention. A focus on subsistence or maintaining income can reduce attention to healthy behaviors and limit positive social supports.

Addressing Weight and Related Conditions in People With Serious Mental Illness

To prevent and treat the myriad causes of obesity among individuals with SMI, health care systems and public health and community programs can apply a stepped approach that includes screening and monitoring, primary prevention, in-person or technology-based behavioral weight management programs, and bariatric surgery. There are additional important considerations when attempts are being made to prevent and reduce obesity among those with SMI. These include barriers to engagement and effectiveness, the risk of compounding weight and mental illness stigma, and capitalizing on resilience. This chapter outlines these stepped-care approaches, highlighting several program examples that have established effectiveness or warrant study.

Screening and Monitoring

To facilitate early intervention, people with SMI should be regularly screened for obesity and common comorbid conditions such as diabetes and cardiovascular disease (De Hert et al. 2011) in primary care, mental health, and community (e.g., senior center, mental health support and advocacy group) settings. Although the schedule for and components of metabolic monitoring depend on an individual's history, preexisting conditions, medications, risk factors, and health status, national treatment guidelines include recommendations for metabolic monitoring (American Psychiatric Association 2019). At intake and after initiation of new treatments, the following should be assessed: weight and height to calculate body mass index, blood pressure, hemoglobin A1c or fasting blood glucose, and lipid levels (not necessarily via a fasting panel). Follow-up assessments should be made within 4 months after starting a new treatment and at least annually thereafter.

When metabolic problems, obesity, or weight gain of at least 5 pounds is identified, clinicians should consider behavioral weight management, primary care management, medication interventions, and/or changes to medications with less weight gain liability (Newcomer et al. 2013). Clinicians can consider adding metformin, which has been shown to reduce body weight and reverse metabolic abnormalities in patients with obesity or other metabolic problems. It is safe in people who do not have hyperglycemia (American Psychiatric Association 2019). Other nonstimulant medications have been successfully used for weight in some patients, including orlistat, topiramate, naltrexone-bupropion, and liraglutide.

Mental health offices should be equipped with tools for assessing blood pressure and weight, and ease of lab access should be prioritized. People with SMI should also monitor their own weight regularly. Including medical-grade scales in waiting areas, coupled with easy-to-read health information, can facilitate self-monitoring of weight and body mass index, given that not all people have home scales or know what to monitor. Likewise, health care organizations should provide home scales whenever possible to individuals with psychiatric conditions who are classified or diagnosed as overweight or with obesity.

To be effective, screening needs to lead to intervention. A successful example of this approach is the Enhancing QUality of Care in Psychosis (EQUIP) project. EQUIP was a controlled trial conducted with 801 patients with schizophrenia at eight U.S. Department of Veterans Affairs (VA) mental health clinics across four states. It deployed patient-facing kiosks in waiting rooms and used patient-reported outcomes (measurement-based care) to track weight and weight intervention participation in patients at these clinics (among other outcomes). Data were used by quality improvement teams to inform delivery of a behavioral weight intervention, patient and staff education, and phone care management. Efforts resulted in a modest decrease in overall health care costs and substantially lower weight among patients at the clinics (Young et al. 2019).

Primary Obesity Prevention

Obesity prevention is a top public health priority and can be achieved through various means, including encouraging healthy diet and physical activity among normal-weight individuals, particularly those who may be at risk for developing obesity. Although interventions are available that increase activity in people with SMI (Muralidharan et al. 2018), implementation of effective lifestyle interventions into mental health treatment settings has been limited (Deenik et al. 2019). Thus, additional research and programs should promote healthy diet and physical activity among normal-weight individuals with SMI to prevent overweight and obesity and related conditions from developing.

Behavioral Weight Management

Individuals with obesity or classified as overweight with a related condition (e.g., cardiovascular disease) can meaningfully reduce cardiovascular disease, diabetes, and mortality risk by losing at least 5% of baseline weight (Jensen et al. 2014). Treatment guidelines recommend that individuals with SMI and who are classified as overweight or with obesity be offered evidence-based weight loss interventions, including behavioral interventions. There are numerous options in the private sector (including in-person and internet-based programs), and some health care organizations have made substantial efforts to provide evidence-based programs. Although the mode and structure of delivery vary, according to obesity management guidelines, key elements of effective behavioral weight loss interventions include encouraging a reduced-calorie diet and increased physical activity through psychoeducation and support; goal setting; and self-monitoring of weight, diet, and activity (Jensen et al. 2014). More intensive, comprehensive interventions have been demonstrated to produce more clinically meaningful outcomes. Importantly, improving physical activity, diet, and weight through behavioral weight management can have mental health benefits, likely due in part to the mood-enhancing and anxiolytic effects of exercise (Hall et al. 2015). Thus, behavioral weight management among people with SMI not only may improve health but may synergistically improve mental health as well.

There are currently available services that clinicians can make use of with their clients with SMI. Recent systematic literature reviews support the acceptability and efficacy of behavioral interventions to promote weight loss among individuals with SMI and who are classified as overweight or with obesity (Naslund et al. 2017). Although some interventions target those with psychiatric conditions using an existing behavioral weight management program, others specifically address unique barriers to weight loss among those with SMI. For example, an 18-month tailored behavioral weight loss intervention in adults with SMI produced significantly better weight loss outcomes compared with control condition participants (Daumit et al. 2013). The Integrated Coaching for Better Mood and Weight intervention synergistically combines evidence-based depression and obesity treatments to treat both conditions simultaneously, with modest improvements observed for both weight and depression (Ma et al. 2019). Similarly, a novel program called MOVE+UP was developed that includes tailored behavioral weight management for overweight veterans with PTSD by coupling traditional weight loss intervention with cognitive-behavioral therapy skills and community-based walking to address unique barriers to weight loss driven by PTSD symptoms (e.g., insomnia, hypervigilance interfering with physical activity) (Hoerster et al. 2020). Also, although these have not been as extensively studied, clinicians have had success referring clients to commercial meal delivery services and programs, nutritionists, personal trainers, and commercially available online weight management programs.

Technology-Based Behavioral Weight Management

There has been proven success with internet-based, audio, computer-assisted, self-administered technologies that meet the needs of individuals with SMI (Young et al. 2017). Researchers have demonstrated that much of the content from evidence-based cognitive-behavioral and psychoeducational intervention practices can be delivered technologically, allowing clients to access a weight management program at convenient locations and/or times. These approaches can result in minimal clinician burden while achieving good clinical outcomes (Young et al. 2017).

One project took an in-person weight intervention tailored for individuals with SMI and adapted it for delivery by kiosk or internet, with inclusion of structured telephonic peer coaching (Young et al. 2017). Patients at a community mental health center and VA mental health clinic were invited to participate. Called WebMOVE, the intervention included internet-based provision of 30 interactive educational modules, tracking of activity and weight, individualized homework, and weekly telephonic peer coaching. Some modules presented summaries or repeated material. Table 12–2 lists the unique module topics. Each module took about 30 minutes to complete, although participants could proceed as slowly as they liked and repeat content as necessary. Individuals were provided with a pedometer and instructed how to use the online system. They were encouraged to complete two online modules per week. The internet-based program was tailored to accommodate cognitive deficits. It included limited text, and all text was read aloud by the computer system. The system utilized a fifth-grade reading level, had explicit navigational aids, and presented information clearly. The program included audio and text-based education, video, pedometer tracking, goal setting, homework, automated diet plans, and quizzes with content repetition if needed for retention. A peer wellness coach was assigned to each participant. Weekly manualized peer coaching was delivered by phone using a strengths-based approach with motivational interviewing. A peer coach manual supported service delivery. Coaches received training in the manual, experiential training in coaching, and weekly supervision from a skilled clinician. Materials supporting the intervention are available online (SMI Adviser: https://smiadviser.org/knowledge_post/how-can-i-implement-a-diet-activity-weight-and-wellness-program-for-patients-or-clients-with-serious-mental-illness).

Researchers compared three modalities for delivering weight services to people with SMI and classified as overweight: WebMOVE, tailored in-person weight services with the same curriculum, and usual care. Participants in the usual-care group took part in wellness or weight programs that were routinely available if they desired. WebMOVE resulted in significantly lower weight than in-person care or usual care, with WebMOVE averaging 6 pounds greater weight loss (Young et al. 2017). No change was seen in weight among those receiving in-person services or usual care. Participants were also more likely to lose at least 5% of body weight in the WebMOVE group than in the in-person group. In terms of treatment retention, 31% completed the WebMOVE program, whereas no one in the in-person group completed the entire program.

TABLE 12–2. WebMOVE weight education module topics

1. Introduction to good nutrition
2. Introduction to physical activity
3. Choosing healthy foods
4. Becoming physically active
5. Portion control and serving sizes
6. Benefits of walking
7. Water and liquid calories
8. Stretching
9. Reading food labels
10. Barriers to exercise
11. Fruits and vegetables
12. Exercising safely
13. Salts and fats
14. Exercising on a budget
15. Thinking about what we eat
16. Making time to exercise
17. Eating good grains
18. Pain, medical conditions, and exercise
19. Fast food
20. Medications and exercise
21. Eating at home and eating out
22. Eating control and hunger management

Combining computerized education with structured coaching is a high-value approach to improving weight. Because traditional interventions require very high levels of staff resources that are often not feasible, this approach is both feasible and effective in the context of usual care.

Mobile phones can now also successfully deliver behavior change interventions, including diet and physical activity promotion information and support (Krishna et al. 2009). Mobile delivery of health services is an appealing strategy because it can reduce clinician burden while being available to the client at the point of decision making. In the United States, most adults (95%) own a cell phone, 95% use their phone for messaging, and the average adult spends about 3 hours on his or her smartphone per day (Pew Research Center 2019). As of 2014, a study found that 60% of 276 patients with SMI had a smartphone (Young et al. 2020), a rate that is comparable to what is found in the general population. Smartphone ownership has increased to 77% of the general population, and almost all new phones are smartphones. Studies have found that it is acceptable and feasible to use mobile phones as part of mental health care in people with SMI (Bell et al. 2017). This presents an opportunity for addressing weight and health behaviors among those with SMI, including delivery of internet-based interventions.

Smartphones can also be used to assess physical activity, making use of continuously generated data from these phones regarding location and movement. Data from mobile phone sensors have been used to accurately assess day-to-day routines, including locations visited, activities, and exercise types, holding promise for applications supporting those with mental health conditions (Mohr et al. 2017). Efforts could be made to use smartphone technology to understand associations between psychiatric symptoms and health, to promote healthy behaviors, and to encourage physical activity and other health behavior self-monitoring among those with SMI.

Bariatric Surgery

Bariatric surgery is an effective practice for severe obesity, being widely disseminated in some health care systems to avert the complications of obesity. It is a viable option for patients with SMI (Shelby et al. 2015). Weight loss outcomes appear to be comparable between those with and without SMI. Bariatric surgery is an important offering for individuals with SMI who have not achieved clinically meaningful weight loss via less expensive and invasive alternative methods such as behavioral weight management. Still, there are important factors when considering bariatric surgery for those with SMI, given that it can be followed by psychiatric symptom exacerbation. Although many people experience improvements in psychological health after bariatric surgery, possibly caused by improved body image and self-esteem, some experience increased psychological distress (Kubik et al. 2013). Thus, mental health assessment and management are important activities prior to and subsequent to bariatric surgery. A video teleconferencing support group program showed promise as a treatment option for addressing mental health among those with depression who underwent bariatric surgery (Wild et al. 2015). Further research is needed to understand how to best support the mental health needs among those with SMI who are preparing to undergo or have undergone bariatric surgery.

Barriers to Behavioral Weight Loss Engagement and Effectiveness

Unfortunately, an insufficient proportion of persons with SMI participate in obesity treatments (Liu et al. 2017). This reduced engagement may be due in part to barriers to care that are common among those with SMI, including cognitive deficits, lower self-efficacy, financial hardship, lack of reliable housing and transportation, and lack of social support (Bennett et al. 2018; Olmos-Ochoa et al. 2019).

Several studies have evaluated the reach and effectiveness of the VA national behavioral weight management program, which is called MOVE!. Although MOVE! is effective for approximately one-third of participants who have sufficient participation (Kahwati et al. 2011), in a study examining national MOVE! data, individuals with SMI were less frequently screened for obesity and were less likely to lose a clinically meaningful amount of weight (Littman et al. 2015). Moreover, among those with intense and sustained participation, individuals with PTSD lost significantly less weight than those without mental health conditions at 6 and 12 months despite comparable participation. Meanwhile, those with other mental conditions lost significantly less weight than those with no mental health diagnoses only at 6 months (Hoerster et al. 2014). Another study found that among people with prediabetes, those with SMI lost less weight in MOVE! than did those without those psychiatric conditions (Janney et al. 2018). Reduced program effectiveness may be due to the various barriers described in the section "Causes of Overweight and Obesity" (e.g., psychiatric symptoms, medications, physiology). Weight loss programs may benefit from being tailored for individuals with SMI in order to better address this public health issue.

Addressing Weight Stigma

Some research has shown that weight stigma has its own independent negative effects on health and well-being (Tomiyama et al. 2018). Thus, health care systems and clinicians should prioritize public health messages and campaigns and health care interactions that are compassionate, patient-centered, and collaborative when discussing recommended lifestyle changes, emphasizing realistic behavioral goals that encompass all aspects of well-being, rather than exclusively focusing on weight. This is particularly important among individuals with SMI, who may experience a double burden of mental illness and weight-related stigma (Corrigan 2016; Pearl and Puhl 2018).

Capitalizing on Resilience

Although SMI is a risk factor for poor diet, inactivity, and increased weight, this is not always the case. Powerful examples are found in the literature on individuals with PTSD. In one cross-sectional study, PTSD symptoms were only associated with poorer health behaviors in the context of comorbid depression symptoms and associated health behaviors; otherwise, PTSD symptoms were associated with *better* physical activity and diet (Hoerster et al. 2019). Likewise, in one rigorously conducted longitudinal analysis, PTSD was associated with prospective weight gain, as expected, but also with a weight *loss* trajectory (Leardmann et al. 2015). Some people with PTSD may use healthy lifestyles as a way of coping. Another important consideration is that effectively treating psychiatric conditions through evidence-based practices (e.g., psychotherapy) may prevent or reduce weight gain when symptoms that interfere with healthy lifestyles decrease; however, this requires further study. Findings suggest some people are resilient with respect to the potential challenges associated with SMI, which could be capitalized upon to promote the health of individuals.

The following fictional vignette presents actions a clinician can take to support a patient presenting with comorbid psychiatric conditions and obesity.

Case Vignette

A psychiatrist meets with Ms. Jones, a single 45-year-old veteran who separated from the military 1 year ago after 20 years of service. During the separation, she was diagnosed with PTSD, secondary to military sexual trauma she had experienced 15 years earlier, and comorbid major depressive disorder. She was prescribed paroxetine, which she has been taking as prescribed since, managed by her primary care clinician. She remains symptomatic and is particularly troubled by her low energy and anhedonia. She also notes that she has gained 20 pounds this year, putting her in the low range of obesity. She reports this affects her self-esteem, and she worries about her health. She presents for assessment and treatment planning, expressing interest in medications and therapy.

Assessment: As with all of his new patients, the psychiatrist performs a thorough assessment of Ms. Jones's psychiatric and health history, including a history of behaviors like physical activity and healthy eating; psychological symptoms and beliefs that may interfere with those behaviors; and contextual factors (e.g., access to healthy foods, access to care, including weight management services). The psychiatrist discovers that although Ms. Jones was never diagnosed with psychiatric conditions prior to last year, she has long experienced PTSD symptoms and had several major depressive episodes. She reports that she previously coped with mental health symptoms using high-intensity exercise, normative and expected in the military context. However, since separation, she has not been able to find the motivation. She says she fears trusting others, which interferes with running in her neighborhood. She also notes that she has recently turned to eating high-calorie foods, especially at night, to cope with painful feelings. She believes eating these foods at night helps her to sleep, which is disrupted many nights. She has adequate access to healthy foods with a nearby grocery store and sufficient income and knowledge to purchase healthy foods. Still, she has little motivation to cook because of her depressive symptoms; trauma-related beliefs such as "I don't deserve good things to happen to me because I let myself be assaulted"; and the fact that she never learned how to cook for herself. Her psychiatrist formulates diagnoses and shares them with Ms. Jones. He confirms that her symptoms meet diagnostic criteria for PTSD and major depressive disorder. He also informs her that her weight and problems with being active and eating a healthy diet are common, understandable responses to what she has been through and might be worsened by her current medication regimen.

Treatment plan: The psychiatrist makes several treatment recommendations to address Ms. Jones's psychiatric, social, and health issues and schedules a future appointment. He orders blood work and takes vitals, including in-office weight and blood pressure, which will be monitored at future visits. He recommends that Ms. Jones participate in a behavioral weight loss program to support her in pursuing a 5% weight loss, noting the health and mental health benefits of doing so. He also encourages her to work toward an attitude of acceptance and compassion about her weight and to focus on all aspects of her health, not just the numbers on the scale. He shares a resource sheet listing various in-person, community, health care system, and technology-based programs, and they discuss how the various options align with her goals, priorities, and barriers to care. In particular, he highlights a community-based program that integrates weight management and depression care. They also explore the potential role of enhanced relationships for improving both her mood and health behaviors. Finally, they identify an alternative antidepressant to try (bupropion) that has less weight gain liability.

Key Points

- Individuals with serious mental illness (SMI) are at risk for obesity, related conditions, and premature mortality due to physiological, behavioral, psychological, and contextual factors.

- Numerous contributors to increased disease burden are modifiable.

- Many feasible and effective interventions are available, with a range of delivery approaches—from screening to comprehensive behavioral intervention.

- Health care organizations should translate evidence into practice and make services available that could substantially improve the health and well-being of individuals with SMI.

References

American Psychiatric Association: Practice guideline for the treatment of patients with schizophrenia. 2019. Available at: www.psychiatry.org/psychiatrists/practice/clinical-practice-guidelines. Accessed October 16, 2020.

Bell IH, Lim MH, Rossell SL, et al: Ecological momentary assessment and intervention in the treatment of psychotic disorders: a systematic review. Psychiatr Serv 68(11):1172–1181, 2017

Bennett LL, Cohen AN, Young AS: Factors associated with weight intervention participation among people with serious mental illness. J Nerv Ment Dis 206(11):896–899, 2018

Boutcher SH, Dunn SL: Factors that may impede the weight loss response to exercise-based interventions. Obes Rev 10(6):671–680, 2009

Brug J: Determinants of healthy eating: motivation, abilities and environmental opportunities. Fam Pract 25 (suppl 1):i50–i55, 2008

Corrigan PW: Lessons learned from unintended consequences about erasing the stigma of mental illness. World Psychiatry 15(1):67–73, 2016

Danaei G, Ding EL, Mozaffarian D, et al: The preventable causes of death in the United States: comparative risk assessment of dietary, lifestyle, and metabolic risk factors. PLoS Med 6(4):e1000058, 2009

Daumit GL, Dickerson FB, Wang NY, et al: A behavioral weight-loss intervention in persons with serious mental illness. N Engl J Med 368(17):1594–1602, 2013

Dedert EA, Calhoun PS, Watkins LL, et al: Posttraumatic stress disorder, cardiovascular, and metabolic disease: a review of the evidence. Ann Behav Med 39(1):61–78, 2010

Deenik J, Czosnek L, Teasdale SB, et al: From impact factors to real impact: translating evidence on lifestyle interventions into routine mental health care. Transl Behav Med June 6, 2019 [Epub ahead of print]

De Hert M, Correll CU, Bobes J, et al: Physical illness in patients with severe mental disorders, I: prevalence, impact of medications and disparities in health care. World Psychiatry 10(1):52–77, 2011

Faulkner G, Cohn T, Remington G: Interventions to reduce weight gain in schizophrenia. Cochrane Database Syst Rev (1):CD005148, 2007

Hall KS, Hoerster KD, Yancy WS Jr: Post-traumatic stress disorder, physical activity, and eating behaviors. Epidemiol Rev 37:103–115, 2015

Hoerster KD, Lai Z, Goodrich DE, et al: Weight loss after participation in a national VA weight management program among veterans with or without PTSD. Psychiatr Serv 65(11):1385–1388, 2014

Hoerster KD, Campbell S, Dolan M, et al: PTSD is associated with poor health behavior and greater body mass index through depression, increasing cardiovascular disease and diabetes risk among US veterans. Prev Med Rep 15:1000930, 2019

Hoerster KD, Tanksley L, Simpson T, et al: Development of a tailored behavioral weight loss program for veterans with PTSD (MOVE!+UP): a mixed methods uncontrolled iterative pilot study. Am J Health Promot 34(6):587–598, 2020

Janney CA, Greenberg JM, Moin T, et al: Does mental health influence weight loss in adults with prediabetes? Findings from the VA Diabetes Prevention Program. Gen Hosp Psychiatry 53:32–37, 2018

Jensen MD, Ryan DH, Apovian CM, et al: 2013 AHA/ACC/TOS guideline for the management of overweight and obesity in adults: a report of the American College of Cardiology/American Heart Association Task Force on Practice Guidelines and the Obesity Society. Circulation 129(25 suppl 2):S102–S138, 2014

Kahwati LC, Lance TX, Jones KR, et al: RE-AIM evaluation of the Veterans Health Administration's MOVE! weight management program. Transl Behav Med 1(4):551–560, 2011

Kilbourne AM, Morden NE, Austin K, et al: Excess heart-disease-related mortality in a national study of patients with mental disorders: identifying modifiable risk factors. Gen Hosp Psychiatry 31(6):555–563, 2009

Krishna S, Boren SA, Balas EA: Healthcare via cell phones: a systematic review. Telemed J E Health 15(3):231–240, 2009

Kubik JF, Gill RS, Laffin M, et al: The impact of bariatric surgery on psychological health. J Obes 2013:837989, 2013

Leardmann CA, Woodall KA, Littman AJ, et al: Post-traumatic stress disorder predicts future weight change in the Millennium Cohort Study. Obesity (Silver Spring) 23(4):886–892, 2015

Littman AJ, Damschroder LJ, Verchinina L, et al: National evaluation of obesity screening and treatment among veterans with and without mental health disorders. Gen Hosp Psychiatry 37(1):7–13, 2015

Liu NH, Daumit GL, Dua T, et al: Excess mortality in persons with severe mental disorders: a multilevel intervention framework and priorities for clinical practice, policy and research agendas. World Psychiatry 16(1):30–40, 2017

Luppino FS, De Wit LM, Bouvy PF, et al: Overweight, obesity, and depression: a systematic review and meta-analysis of longitudinal studies. Arch Gen Psychiatry 67(3):220–229, 2010

Ma J, Rosas LG, Lv N, et al: Effect of integrated behavioral weight loss treatment and problem-solving therapy on body mass index and depressive symptoms among patients with obesity and depression: the RAINBOW randomized clinical trial. JAMA 321(9):869–879, 2019

Marazziti D, Rutigliano G, Baroni S, et al: Metabolic syndrome and major depression. CNS Spectr 19(4):293–304, 2014

Mitchell AJ, Malone D, Doebbeling CC: Quality of medical care for people with and without comorbid mental illness and substance misuse: systematic review of comparative studies. Br J Psychiatry 194(6):491–499, 2009

Mohr DC, Zhang M, Schueller SM: Personal sensing: understanding mental health using ubiquitous sensors and machine learning. Annu Rev Clin Psychol 13:23–47, 2017

Muralidharan A, Niv N, Brown CH, et al: Impact of online weight management with peer coaching on physical activity levels of adults with serious mental illness. Psychiatr Serv 69(10):1062–1068, 2018

Naslund JA, Whiteman KL, McHugo GJ, et al: Lifestyle interventions for weight loss among overweight and obese adults with serious mental illness: a systematic review and meta-analysis. Gen Hosp Psychiatry 47:83–102, 2017

Newcomer JW, Weiden PJ, Buchanan RW: Switching antipsychotic medications to reduce adverse event burden in schizophrenia: establishing evidence-based practice. J Clin Psychiatry 74(11):1108–1120, 2013

Olfson M, Gerhard T, Huang C, et al: Premature mortality among adults with schizophrenia in the United States. JAMA Psychiatry 72(12):1172–1182, 2015

Olmos-Ochoa TT, Niv N, Hellemann G, et al: Barriers to participation in web-based and in-person weight management interventions for serious mental illness. Psychiatr Rehabil J 42(3):220–228, 2019

Pearl RL, Puhl RM: Weight bias internalization and health: a systematic review. Obes Rev 19(8):1141–1163, 2018

Pew Research Center: Mobile fact sheet. June 12, 2019. Available at: www.pewinternet.org/internet/fact-sheet/mobile/. Accessed July 15, 2020.

Rutter LA, Weatheril RP, Krill SC, et al: Posttraumatic stress disorder symptoms, depressive symptoms, exercise, and health in college students. Psychol Trauma 5(1):56–61, 2013

Shelby SR, Labott S, Stout RA: Bariatric surgery: a viable treatment option for patients with severe mental illness. Surg Obes Relat Dis 11(6):1342–1348, 2015

St-Onge MP: Sleep-obesity relation: underlying mechanisms and consequences for treatment. Obes Rev 18 (suppl 1):34–39, 2017

Story M, Kaphingst KM, Robinson-O'Brien R, et al: Creating healthy food and eating environments: policy and environmental approaches. Annu Rev Public Health 29:253–272, 2008

Tomiyama AJ, Carr D, Granberg EM, et al: How and why weight stigma drives the obesity "epidemic" and harms health. BMC Med 16(1):123, 2018

Vancampfort D, Vansteenkiste M, De Hert M, et al: Self-determination and stage of readiness to change physical activity behaviour in schizophrenia. Ment Health Phys Act 7(3):171–176, 2014

Vancampfort D, Firth J, Schuch FB, et al: Sedentary behavior and physical activity levels in people with schizophrenia, bipolar disorder and major depressive disorder: a global systematic review and meta-analysis. World Psychiatry 16(3):308–315, 2017

Wild B, Hunnemeyer K, Sauer H, et al: A 1-year videoconferencing-based psycho-educational group intervention following bariatric surgery: results of a randomized controlled study. Surg Obes Relat Dis 11(6):1349–1360, 2015

Young AS, Niv N, Cohen AN, et al: The appropriateness of routine medication treatment for schizophrenia. Schizophr Bull 36(4):732–739, 2010

Young AS, Cohen AN, Goldberg R, et al: Improving weight in people with serious mental illness: the effectiveness of computerized services with peer coaches. J Gen Intern Med 32 (suppl 1):48–55, 2017

Young AS, Cohen AN, Hamilton AB, et al: Implementing patient-reported outcomes to improve the quality of care for weight of patients with schizophrenia. J Behav Health Serv Res 46(1):129–139, 2019

Young AS, Cohen AN, Niv N, et al: Mobile phone and smartphone use by people with serious mental illness. Psychiatr Serv 71(3):280–283, 2020

CHAPTER 13

The COVID-19 Pandemic

Patrick W. Corrigan, Psy.D.
Sang Qin, M.S.

It is mid-May 2020, and we have been on lockdown in the Chicago area to escape the COVID-19 infection for almost 2 months. Although all chapters for the book are finished, the publisher and I (P.W.C.) agreed that a chapter was needed to make sense of COVID-19, not only because we are in the midst of the crisis but because infections and pandemics will have enduring prominence in the health of everyone in general and people with mental illness more specifically. We offer this chapter, however, with a bit more caution than those preceding it because empirical literature related to COVID-19 and mental illness are obviously lacking. Still, there are lessons that may be learned from research on related pathophysiology. Public health research on addressing past pandemics also has value here. In this light, we seek to address several questions in this chapter. What is known about infectious and respiratory diseases related to mental illness? What effect does living through a pandemic have on mental health, especially for people already vulnerable to psychiatric illness? What might providers consider when addressing the needs of people with serious mental illness (SMI) vis-à-vis pandemics? How does the new normal of infectious disease and pandemics impact health care for this vulnerable population? Although the book has sought an overall international perspective on health and wellness, this discussion on COVID-19 focuses on the United States because the information is ever evolving and distributed mostly through local channels.

Infectious Disease, Pandemics, and Mental Illness

Pandemics are not new; perhaps what is different about COVID-19 is the degree to which it has invaded American consciousness. Pandemics have plagued the world throughout history, with significant examples over the past century. A little more than 100 years ago, humans were bombarded by the 1918 Spanish flu epidemic caused by the H1N1 influenza A virus. It led to more than 500 million confirmed cases, with between 17 and 50 million deaths (Morens and Fauci 2007). Seasonal influenza has the potential to be pandemic every year (Lowen et al. 2007). Epidemics and/or pandemics have emerged in the past 20 years related to, among others, H1N1 (Dawood et al. 2012), severe acute respiratory syndrome (SARS; Likhacheva 2006), and Middle East respiratory syndrome (MERS; Zumla et al. 2015). World health continues to be challenged by HIV (Douek et al. 2009).

People with SMI seem to be at increased risk for infectious disease (Happell et al. 2012). Ample, in-depth research examining risk related to HIV (Blank et al. 2002; Cournos and McKinnon 1997; Rosenberg et al. 2001; Sewell 1996) exists. Reasons for the high rate of HIV in this population may include a lack of knowledge about how people are infected by HIV through sexual transmission and difficulties in maintaining stable relationships (Robson and Gray 2007).

COVID-19 is transmitted through the respiratory system, as are related viruses such as SARS and MERS; thus, the greatest morbidity and mortality are related to symptoms associated with the respiratory system. Of note, people with SMI show a higher risk of lung- and pulmonary-related illness (Copeland et al. 2007; Himelhoch et al. 2004; Hsu et al. 2013; Partti et al. 2015), leading to higher mortality rates, although these illnesses are not all infectious processes. Still, COVID-19 may be especially dangerous for people with SMI because it is both an infectious and a respiratory illness.

Stress, Isolation, and Exacerbation of Mental Health Symptoms

Sheltering in place and social distancing are among widely agreed-on standards for preventing the spread of COVID-19 (Centers for Disease Control and Prevention 2020). Unfortunately, the demands of this kind of lifestyle change are likely to be stressful for people in general (Druss 2020; Santos 2020). In addition, prevention practices necessary to avoid infection (e.g., social distancing) lead to social isolation, heightening one's vulnerability to being overwhelmed. Even worse, SMI is often defined by a stress vulnerability; that is, the mental illness of people with serious psychiatric conditions is likely exacerbated by genetically endowed hypersensitivity to stress (Goh and Agius 2010; Rudnick and Lundberg 2012). Risk is heightened when people with SMI are separated from their support system (Harris 2010). Hence, the stress of COVID-19 social distancing may be increasing psychiatric disorders in people with SMI. Providers need to be alert not only to the risks of COVID-19 for physical health but also to related prevention and treatment needs for mental health and wellness.

Health Care Decisions Related to COVID-19: Three Essential Questions

In light of these patterns, people with SMI face three important issues, which we refer to as the essential questions.

1. How do people with SMI prevent becoming infected? The Centers for Disease Control and Prevention (CDC) updates evidence-based recommendations related to sheltering in place and social distancing regularly. These are currently being qualified as "appropriate" guidelines to describe how proscriptions will be relaxed to return to normal.
2. What should people do if they believe they are infected? Once again, the CDC regularly lists empirically based steps people might take (testing, treatment, and quarantine) if they believe they are positive for the virus. However, people need to consult with local public health authorities about how these steps are realized in their area (e.g., where they should go for testing; whether they must be hospitalized; what can be medically done).
3. What should people do about worsening mental health challenges? The Substance Abuse and Mental Health Services Administration (SAMHSA) and multiple advocacy groups (such as Mental Health America and the National Council for Behavioral Health) are regularly updating guidelines for mental health. These include wellness ideas to prevent stress and social isolation, and interventions when psychiatric symptoms in fact seem to be worsening. Access to care is an especially big hurdle as mental health care providers have socially distanced themselves per public health guidelines.

Trust and Perceived Threat

Information is key to addressing the three essential questions. What are a person's options? Note that we qualified "appropriate" guidelines as evidence based; recommendations and information that are not based on medical science are making the pandemic even more challenging. Trust in public health recommendations is vital to the population's response. Patients who are uncertain about health care recommendations find corresponding care decisions difficult (Goold 2002; Mechanic 1996), a dilemma that is especially exacerbated in the midst of health crises (Gamble 1997; Leavitt 2003; Meredith et al. 2007). Trust in public health messaging has been described in terms of exchanges between provider and health care users (Meredith et al. 2007; Rose et al. 2004):

1. *Fiduciary responsibility* involves the perception that an agent promotes another's well-being first. The concern here is when provider interest is perceived to not comply with person-centered practice.
2. *Honesty* means that health care users have a fundamental need to believe providers and their recommendations.
3. *Competency* is exemplified by the perception that health providers know the research and that practice is based on the evidence.
4. *Consistency* is defined as uniformity in messaging.

Trust is diminished when health communications vary in content and tone. The COVID-19 pandemic is a new, foreign, and demanding experience for most people. Trust in the health care system is key to participation in prevention and clinical services.

The newness of the pandemic is going to impact perceived threat and vulnerability, which will in turn influence health decisions and behaviors (Duncan et al. 2009; Faulkner et al. 2004; Hodson and Costello 2007). People who perceive a health situation as threatening are more likely to engage in protective behaviors (Maddux and Rogers 1983; Rogers and Prentice-Dunn 1997). On the one hand, people who perceived SARS as threatening engaged in avoidance-based precautionary actions (Jiang et al. 2009). Low perceived threat of MERS corresponded with unfavorable attitudes toward quarantine in a South Korean sample (Kim et al. 2016). Interestingly, there seem to be national differences in perceived threat, with one study on SARS reporting Europeans expressing a higher rate of concern than Asians (de Zwart et al. 2009). Threat may include expected susceptibility to disease and fear in the presence of possible infection (Maddux and Rogers 1983).

Perceived Threat and Trust in Health Guidelines

Trust in health guidelines and perceived threat related to a pandemic will impact health behaviors. Perceived threat and trust in health communications seem to independently and positively influence health decisions (Lin and Bautista 2016). In fact, perceived threat and trust interact to influence readiness to act on health advice (Harris et al. 2011). Hence, trust is going to vary with the degree to which the public views a health condition as threatening. Research has applied these constructs specifically to attitudes about vaccines and quarantines. Confusion about vaccine efficacy undermines acceptance of vaccines for self and others (Ballada et al. 1994). More broadly, a systematic review showed mistrust of the health care system inversely related to pro-vaccine views (Yaqub et al. 2014). Generally, people react to calls for quarantine with fear and dismay. One qualitative study showed that the public's first reactions to calls for quarantine yielded concern about overcrowding, infection, and inability to communicate with family members (Blendon et al. 2006).

There are unpublished data on a measure of COVID-19 and perceived threat from three separate groups (N=279, 285, and 413) (Conway et al. 2020). Items reflected threat, worry, stress, and avoidance related to the coronavirus per se, with analyses supporting a single-factor solution. The study also assessed public perceptions of government response to the coronavirus on six dimensions, reflecting, among other things, restrictions (limiting social movement of citizens), punishment (punishing citizens for violating social distancing rules), reactance (anger that government was taking away freedoms), research (desire for funding for research on COVID-19), stimulus (wanting money incentives to support citizens affected by COVID), and informational contamination (trusting government to provide accurate information during the crisis). Perceived threat demonstrates significant positive correlations on all dimensions of government responses except for reactance. Perceived threat and reactance are in fact negatively correlated. Another paper in review has shown the pernicious effects of stigma on COVID-19; namely, those who anticipate stigma related to the coronavirus were less likely to seek testing (Earnshaw et al. 2020).

Ethnic Disparities in Trust of Health Information

Trust in health information often wanes among America's ethnic minority groups, with research repeatedly showing African Americans are mistrustful of the health care system (Gamble 1997); wariness undermines their participation in prevention programs (O'Malley et al. 2004). This is somewhat of a haunting realization given research that shows significantly greater COVID-19 morbidity among African Americans (Hooper et al. 2020). We do not mean to imply that mistrust in health care messaging alone is leading to worse COVID-19 infection and mortality among this population.

Instead, we encourage the reader to keep in mind the recurring messages of social determinants in this book when trying to understand how ethnic and other forms of disparities influence the impact of pandemics on people with SMI.

Status of Health Literacy in the Midst of the Pandemic

People are starving for evidence-based information to deal with the three essential questions discussed in the previous section. Groups like the CDC (with the latest science from the National Institute of Allergy and Infectious Diseases) regularly update guidelines for staying safe and managing infection. In addition, SAMHSA provides guidelines for addressing mental health and wellness (with insights from the National Institute of Mental Health findings). The challenge to the CDC and SAMHSA is that COVID-19 research is limited, and new findings that emerge lead to evolving recommendations. Among other things, scientists are still trying to determine the extent of infection spread, the pattern of immunity for those infected, and effective tests and treatments. The evolving way in which this information is made available is anxiety-arousing for the population because, for example, the time when restrictions can be lifted seems to be extended as new circumstances arise; we are facing longer periods of stress and isolation.

Decisions about staying safe and social distancing are not made in a vacuum. Other social forces impact decisions about society's response to the pandemic. Social distancing has brought about unparalleled harm to the labor force. As of mid-May 2020, more than 30 million Americans have filed for unemployment benefits, signaling the worse unemployment rates since the Great Depression (Marketplace 2020). Social distancing has practically shut down the restaurant and entertainment sectors, putting many people out of work. Prognosticators are grim about America's economic rebound once social restrictions are lifted (Gelles 2020). Many political leaders say we need to limit restrictions so people can get back to work.

In addition, government recommendations related to social distancing have been criticized for limiting constitutionally protected civil rights. Of special concern is the impact on religious freedoms, limiting the congregation of faith-based communities to practice their religion. The issue of civil rights has led to court cases throughout the country (Wolf 2020); for example, Representative Darren Bailey from our home state of Illinois filed an injunction to block Governor J.B. Pritzker's continued directive blocking business in key sectors. Judge Michael McHaney found for the plaintiff (O'Connor 2020).

Leadership is needed in times of great social change with competing voices. Unfortunately, the U.S. administration has failed mightily. Directives coming out of the White House frequently contradict what the government's scientists recommend. For example, on May 19, 2020, President Donald Trump announced that he was taking hydroxychloroquine as a prophylactic against COVID-19 (Carvalho 2020), even though the U.S. Food and Drug Administration explicitly warned misuse of the medication for COVID-19 could lead to lethal cardiovascular side effects. Perhaps even more alarming, President Trump suggested at the end of April that injection of disinfectants—"almost a cleaning"—should be entertained as a COVID-19 treatment. Such mercurial and egregious statements and acts make it difficult for anyone, including people with mental illness, to look to federal guidelines for guidance.

State governments have stepped up to make public health recommendations, which may lead to clearer information but can still yield mixed messages, especially when neighboring states are taken into account. Governor Pritzker in Illinois directed residents to shelter in place through the end of May, whereas similar recommendations by Governor Tony Evers in neighboring Wisconsin were overturned in court, and many businesses opened by ignoring social distancing recommendations. Moreover, counties and municipalities throughout states often differ on guidelines, making it unclear what information the individual should heed.

Implications for Providers

We consider what psychiatrists and other mental health providers might do to help people with SMI cope with COVID-19 in terms of the three essential issues.

1. *Staying safe*: People with SMI need to sift through evolving information to understand guidelines for avoiding infection. The task here is prevention, relying partly on health education, which requires a different set of skills for many clinically focused providers. Hence, provider groups should decide among themselves who will remain up-to-date on guidelines. However, the task involves much more than bestowing information. The person with SMI may need help in sorting out different options and in problem-solving how to put them into effect. For example, how does the person shelter in place and yet not feel overwhelmed by the solitude? Peer service providers may be exceptionally skilled at handling this task.

2. *Managing infection*: As with the other physical health challenges reviewed in this book, mental health providers need to sort out services

that their clinic might provide in an integrated fashion versus those that need to be relegated to the primary or specialist care team. In terms of COVID-19, this begins by accessing tests and acting on positive results. Infectious disease experts can then advise the patient and team on how to respond if the test result is positive, including the need for quarantine at home versus more aggressive interventions in the hospital. As a result, mental health providers need to communicate frequently and freely with all involved in care.

3. *Addressing mental health and wellness*: Psychiatrists and other mental health care providers should consider ways to promote wellness and health as people cope with social distancing. This may include specific strategies related to stress management as well as broader lifestyle changes related to diet, exercise, and other ways to promote well-being. This may also include educating people to be mindful of the impact of social distancing on their mental health. Providers in collaboration with their patients may also need to reevaluate medication or psychotherapy plans.

Virtual Mental Health Care

Providers may need to take advantage of online and other forms of telecommunication to offer services to people in the midst of this and future pandemics. Although virtual mental health treatment has been discussed for more than a decade (Griffiths 2013), in the past few months the COVID-19 pandemic has propelled clinicians into using this tool. A survey of about 2,100 mental health providers identified several concerns, including confidentiality, level of technical skill, and inequity of patient access (Wells et al. 2007). The COVID-19 experience will likely further the establishment of virtual services in the care system. Research and program development need to continue to ensure that best practices are formulated and implemented for this treatment mode.

Online support groups may also be an important approach to deal with the social isolation of sheltering in place. The Depression and Bipolar Support Alliance, for example, has shifted to an online platform to provide virtual support groups (www.dbsalliance.org/support/chapters-and-support-groups/online-support-groups).

Taking Care of Oneself

A recent review highlighted the stress experienced by health care workers working with patients and the coronavirus (Shiozawa and Uchida 2020). Symptoms included new reports of insomnia, anxiety, and feelings of hopelessness, as well as exacerbation of existing disorders. Shiozawa and Uchida identified important factors for addressing mental health challenges arising from clinical practice addressing COVID-19, including multidisciplinary teams, up-to-date communication, and counseling services for the helper. Lessons noted throughout this book about providers taking care of themselves need to be heeded.

The New Normal

Perhaps most remarkable about COVID-19 is neither the pandemic nor sheltering in place per se. Pandemics have been a recurring experience around the world throughout history. We experience an annual influenza outbreak each year, although it very rarely leads to the level of morbidity and mortality that comes from the coronavirus. However, if we use the annual flu bug as a measure of future expectations, we expect COVID-19 will soon burn out, social restrictions will be lifted, and we will return to normal. Unfortunately, as of this writing, a clear end to the pandemic is unknown. Anthony Fauci from the National Institute of Allergy and Infectious Diseases opined that COVID-19 may reemerge later this year in the fall (Behrman 2020). There were two waves of the H1N1 flu (swine flu) outbreak in 2009 and the 1918 Spanish flu pandemic. Hence, a second wave of COVID-19 is conceivable. Moreover, the scientific community has not yet concluded that a COVID-19 infection confers immunity to subsequent infection.

Over the next year, we will be impacted by the new normal. We will all consider social distancing and related cautions as we get back to interacting with others. We will be mindful of the health risks in gathering places and on public transportation. We will experience heightened concern about recurring infections, such as season-related flu. The fear that future shelter-in-place restrictions may lead yet again to crippling social isolation will be present. This kind of background stress will exacerbate mental illness. As a people, we realize that government officials will not someday blast an all-clear signal. This experience will be with us for years to come.

References

Ballada D, Biasio LR, Cascio G, et al: Attitudes and behavior of health care personnel regarding influenza vaccination. Eur J Epidemiol 10(1):63–68, 1994
Behrman S: "Convinced": Fauci says there will be coronavirus in the fall after Trump says "it may not come back." USA Today April 22, 2020. Available at: www.usatoday.com/story/news/politics/2020/04/22/coronavirus-dr-anthony-fauci-says-i-am-convinced-second-wave/3009131001. Accessed November 2, 2020.

Blank MB, Mandell DS, Aiken L, Hadley TR: Co-occurrence of HIV and serious mental illness among Medicaid recipients. Psychiatr Serv 53(7):868–873, 2002

Blendon RJ, DesRoches CM, Cetron MS, et al: Attitudes toward the use of quarantine in a public health emergency in four countries. Health Aff (Millwood) 25(2):w15–w25, 2006

Carvalho TG: Donald Trump is taking hydroxychloroquine to ward off COVID-19. Is that wise? The Conversation, May 21, 2020. Available at: https://theconversation.com/donald-trump-is-taking-hydroxychloroquine-to-ward-off-covid-19-is-that-wise-139031. Accessed June 5, 2020.

Centers for Disease Control and Prevention: Social Distancing. Centers for Disease Control and Prevention, May 6, 2020. Available at: www.cdc.gov/coronavirus/2019-ncov/prevent-getting-sick/social-distancing.html. Accessed June 5, 2020.

Conway LG III, Woodard SR, Zubrod A: Social psychological measurements of COVID-19: Coronavirus Perceived Threat, Government Response, Impacts, and Experiences Questionnaires. Working paper, University of Montana, April 7, 2020. Available at: https://psyarxiv.com/z2x9a. Accessed June 5, 2020.

Copeland LA, Mortensen EM, Zeber JE, et al: Pulmonary disease among inpatient decedents: impact of schizophrenia. Prog Neuropsychopharmacol Biol Psychiatry 31(3):720–726, 2007

Cournos F, McKinnon K: HIV seroprevalence among people with severe mental illness in the United States: a critical review. Clin Psychol Rev 17(3):259–269, 1997

Dawood FS, Iuliano AD, Reed C, et al: Estimated global mortality associated with the first 12 months of 2009 pandemic influenza A H1N1 virus circulation: a modelling study. Lancet Infect Dis 12(9):687–695, 2012

de Zwart O, Veldhuijzen IK, Elam G, et al: Perceived threat, risk perception, and efficacy beliefs related to SARS and other (emerging) infectious diseases: results of an international survey. Int J Behav Med 16(1):30–40, 2009

Douek DC, Roederer M, Koup RA: Emerging concepts in the immunopathogenesis of AIDS. Annu Rev Med 60:471–484, 2009

Druss BG: Addressing the COVID-19 pandemic in populations with serious mental illness. JAMA Psychiatry 77(9):891–892, 2020 32242888

Duncan LA, Schaller M, Park JH: Perceived vulnerability to disease: development and validation of a 15-item self-report instrument. Pers Individ Dif 47:541–546, 2009

Earnshaw VA, Brousseau NM, Hill CE, et al: Anticipated stigma, stereotypes, and COVID-19 testing. Submitted for publication, 2020

Faulkner J, Schaller M, Park JH, Duncan LA: Evolved disease-avoidance mechanisms and contemporary xenophobic attitudes. Group Process Intergroup Relat 7(4):333–353, 2004

Gamble VN: Under the shadow of Tuskegee: African Americans and health care. Am J Public Health 87(11):1773–1778, 1997

Gelles D: Coronavirus shut down the "experience economy." Can it come back? New York Times, May 20, 2020. Available at: www.nytimes.com/2020/05/20/business/public-gathering-events-coronavirus.html. Accessed June 5, 2020.

Goh C, Agius M: The stress-vulnerability model how does stress impact on mental illness at the level of the brain and what are the consequences? Psychiatr Danub 22(2):198–202, 2010

Goold SD: Trust, distrust and trustworthiness. J Gen Intern Med 17(1):79–81, 2002

Griffiths KM: A virtual mental health community: a future scenario. Aust NZ J Psychiatry 47(2):109–110, 2013

Happell B, Scott D, Platania-Phung C: Provision of preventive services for cancer and infectious diseases among individuals with serious mental illness. Arch Psychiatr Nurs 26(3):192–201, 2012

Harris PR, Sillence E, Briggs P: Perceived threat and corroboration: key factors that improve a predictive model of trust in internet-based health information and advice. J Med Internet Res 13(3):e51, 2011

Harris T: A Stress-vulnerability model of mental disorder: implications for practice, in Reflective Practice in Mental Health: Advanced Psychosocial Practice With Children, Adolescents and Adults. Edited by Webber M, Nathan J. London, Jessica Kingsley Publishers, 2010, pp 64–81

Himelhoch S, Lehman A, Kreyenbuhl J, et al: Prevalence of chronic obstructive pulmonary disease among those with serious mental illness. Am J Psychiatry 161(12):2317–2319, 2004

Hodson G, Costello K: Interpersonal disgust, ideological orientations, and dehumanization as predictors of intergroup attitudes. Psychol Sci 18(8):691–698, 2007

Hooper WM, Nápoles AM, Pérez-Stable EJ: COVID-19 and racial/ethnic disparities. JAMA 32391864 2020 [Epub ahead of print]

Hsu J-H, Chien I-C, Lin C-H, et al: Increased risk of chronic obstructive pulmonary disease in patients with schizophrenia: a population-based study. Psychosomatics 54(4):345–351, 2013

Jiang X, Elam G, Yuen C, et al: The perceived threat of SARS and its impact on precautionary actions and adverse consequences: a qualitative study among Chinese communities in the United Kingdom and the Netherlands. Int J Behav Med 16(1:)58–67, 2009

Kim EY, Liao Q, Yu ES, et al: Middle East respiratory syndrome in South Korea during 2015: risk-related perceptions and quarantine attitudes. Am J Infect Control 44(11):1414–1416, 2016

Leavitt JW: Public resistance or cooperation? A tale of smallpox in two cities. Biosecur Bioterror 1(3):185–192, 2003

Likhacheva A: SARS revisited. Virtual Mentor 8(4):219–222, 2006

Lin TTC, Bautista JR: Predicting intention to take protective measures during haze: the roles of efficacy, threat, media trust, and affective attitude. J Health Commun 21(7):790–799, 2016

Lowen AC, Mubareka S, Steel J, Palese P: Influenza virus transmission is dependent on relative humidity and temperature. PLoS Pathog 3(10):1470–1476, 2007

Maddux JE, Rogers RW: Protection motivation and self-efficacy: a revised theory of fear appeals and attitude change. J Exp Soc Psychol 19(5):469–479, 1983

Marketplace: 30 million have sought U.S. unemployment aid since COVID-19 hit. Marketplace, April 30, 2020. Available at: www.marketplace.org/2020/04/30/covid-19-us-unemployment-state-benefits/. Accessed June 5, 2020.

Mechanic D: Changing medical organization and the erosion of trust. Milbank Q 74(2):171–189, 1996

Meredith LS, Eisenman DP, Rhodes H, et al: Trust influences response to public health messages during a bioterrorist event. J Health Commun 12(3):217–232, 2007

Morens DM, Fauci AS: The 1918 influenza pandemic: insights for the 21st century. J Infect Dis 195(7):1018–1028, 2007

O'Connor J: Pritzker: Stay-home lawsuit a 'stunt,' should be overturned. AP News, April 28, 2020. Available at https://apnews.com/be5299a40b728e0cc951d2bd3fc65b21. Accessed June 5, 2020.

O'Malley AS, Sheppard VB, Schwartz M, Mandelblatt J: The role of trust in use of preventive services among low-income African-American women. Prev Med 38(6):777–785, 2004

Partti K, Vasankari T, Kanervisto M, et al: Lung function and respiratory diseases in people with psychosis: population-based study. Br J Psychiatry 207(1):37–45, 2015

Robson D, Gray R: Serious mental illness and physical health problems: a discussion paper. Int J Nurs Stud 44(3):457–466, 2007

Rogers RW, Prentice-Dunn S: Protection motivation theory, in Handbook of Health Behavior Research 1: Personal and Social Determinants. Edited by Gochman DS. New York, Plenum, 1997, pp 113–132

Rose A, Peters N, Shea JA, Armstrong K: Development and testing of the Health Care System Distrust Scale. J Gen Intern Med 19(1):57–63, 2004

Rosenberg SD, Goodman LA, Osher FC, et al: Prevalence of HIV, hepatitis B, and hepatitis C in people with severe mental illness. Am J Public Health 91(1):31–37, 2001

Rudnick A, Lundberg E: The stress-vulnerability model of schizophrenia: a conceptual analysis and selective review. Curr Psychiatry Rev 8(4):337–341, 2012

Santos CF: Reflections about the impact of the SARS-COV-2/COVID-19 pandemic on mental health. Braz J Psychiatry 42(3):329, 2020

Sewell DD: Schizophrenia and HIV. Schizophr Bull 22(3):465–473, 1996

Shiozawa P, Uchida RR: An updated systematic review on the coronavirus pandemic: lessons for psychiatry. Braz J Psychiatry 42(3):330–331, 2020

Wells M, Mitchell KJ, Finkelhor D, Becker-Blease KA: Online mental health treatment: concerns and considerations. Cyberpsychol Behav 10(3):453–459, 2007

Wolf R: Government intrusions on civil liberties during pandemic raise risks, rewards. USA Today, April 9, 2020. Available at: www.usatoday.com/story/news/ politics/2020/04/09/coronavirus-pandemic-restrictions-limit-church-gunsabortion-travel/2968516001. Accessed June 5, 2020.

Yaqub O, Castle-Clarke S, Sevdalis N, Chataway J: Attitudes to vaccination: a critical review. Soc Sci Med 112:1–11, 2014

Zumla A, Hui DS, Perlman S: Middle East respiratory syndrome. Lancet 386(9997):995–1007, 2015

CHAPTER 14

Final Thoughts: Moving Forward

Patrick W. Corrigan, Psy.D.
Sonya L. Ballentine, B.A.

The 13 preceding chapters of this book put forth an important agenda meant to describe problems of physical health and wellness among people living with serious mental illness (SMI) as well as steps to rectify the problems. The content is steeped in the existing empirical literature. In this final chapter, we highlight three especially important lessons that emerged for us—Sonya and Pat, individuals who are living with SMIs and who are psychiatric service providers and work as scientists in this area—in proposing directions to move forward.

Looking Beyond the Mental Illness

We have noticed an important trend in research over the past decade or so: problems occur in the lives of people with mental illness that do not reflect the illness per se. As psychiatric service providers, we are grounded in DSM definitions of symptoms and dysfunctions that describe psychiatric disorders leading to significant harm. These are not trivial matters. But people with SMI also get sick and die at inordinate rates. Authors in this book did not ask "What is it about the DSM diagnosis, or accompanying symptoms, that causes the person to get physically sick?" The issue of morbidity and mortality is a prominent public health issue in its own right deserving of concerted Herculean efforts.

In fact, much of what leads to poor health reviewed in this book is not traced back to a person's symptoms and disabilities. The social determinants of health, such as the following, are as likely, if not more so, to account for the health challenges of people living with SMI:

1. Ethnic, gender, and sexual orientation disparities: services that fail to reflect the priorities of patients of color and those who do not identify as heterosexual
2. Poverty: failure of a payer system to cover all the health needs of people, especially those at the lowest income level
3. Homelessness: an even worse outcome due to income inequity, with the health of people worsening because of living on the streets
4. Criminalization: sending people unnecessarily into jails and prisons, which exacerbate health conditions and ignore wellness
5. Victimization: failing to sensitively address the needs of those traumatized or otherwise harmed by crime or abuse

These barriers lead to grossly unequal distribution of culturally sensitive clinics and services. Some neighborhoods (usually of higher socioeconomic status) are rich in health options, whereas others lack resources or have clinics hindered by long wait lists. In this light, most of the recommendations in this book are couched with a sense of realism; significant social change is needed to fully realize the health and wellness of this group affected by mental illness.

The effects of social determinants on the lives of people living with SMI are not new. More than 80 years ago, sociologists framed the problem as *downward drift*, the empirical finding that people with schizophrenia, for example, are overrepresented with respect to lower socioeconomic status (Faris and Dunham 1939). Scientists have argued since then whether downward drift represents the necessary result of severe symptoms (e.g., people with psychotic symptoms are not able to earn a good income because they cannot keep a job) or the societal impact of factors like the five listed above. An important quote by Draine and colleagues (2002) sums up the issue well.

> In other words, persons with mental illness experience social problems more frequently because they live in a world in which these problems are en-

demic, not just because they are mentally ill. Thus social problems become erroneously simplified as psychiatric problems, resulting in the creation of overly simple interventions and policies to address a complex phenomenon. (p. 565)

Empowerment and Self-Determination

Clinical research resting on symptom description and biological etiology is no longer sufficient in modern medicine. Patient-centered care has emerged as a central value in the development and implementation of effective health and wellness services in the real world (Stanton and McClughen 2017). The Institute of Medicine (2001) called for bridging the chasm between profession-focused values (where the cold rigors of science dictate best practice) and care that reflects the essential perceptions of the person. The Institute of Medicine listed several principles that sustain this bridge, including respect for personal preferences, provision of full information and options, emotional support, and inclusion of family and friends when requested. Subsumed in these ideas are two additional values, empowerment and self-determination, especially important when considering the journey of many people with SMI in the health care system. Patients' perspectives have often been discounted by providers believing "patient health complaints" are inaccurate, caused by cognitive symptoms rather than being genuine priorities. Other providers believe recovery is not a likely outcome for people with SMI, thereby robbing service users of future hope and aspirations.

A somewhat dated literature stressed compliance with or adherence to medication regimens as essential goals (Corrigan et al. 1990, 2012). This was based on provider beliefs that failure to take prescribed medications leads to irrevocable harm and catastrophe. As a result, providers learned how to "incentivize" medication decisions such that people were less likely to reject prescriptions. Self-determination emerged in the past decade as a person-centered approach to health care (Rudnick and Roe 2018). Self-determination is about choice! This is partly ethical manifesto—by the very essence of being human, people have the right to choose where they want to live, what they want to do, with whom they wish to affiliate, and how they wish to address their health and wellness goals. This, however, is also empirical reality; research shows control of one's health decisions leads to better outcomes (Champion and Skinner 2008; Rosenstock 1966, 1974; Tanner-Smith and Brown 2010).

Concern about the egregious effects of ignoring prescriptions may rob the person of dignity, of an individual agency that allows for failure. Attempting to make life "risk free" can undermine future opportunities. People do not land a better job, move to a nicer neighborhood, build more intimate relationships, or enjoy fewer medication side effects if they do not consider and pursue the risks that accompany the option. One of the things that make these pursuits a risk is the absence of prior clear results. For example, it is uncertain whether meeting new people at a synagogue will broaden one's support network or cause more social anxiety. Many of a person's best achievements come the hard way: falling flat, picking oneself up, and moving on. Without these flops, people are unclear about their potential limits and miss out on unforeseen alternatives that may benefit them. This applies to health and wellness. Health choices in one direction that do not bear fruit teach personal lessons about the potential of other directions.

Additional research is needed to test these assumptions. However, just as change in the health care system must reflect empowerment and self-determination, so the research enterprise must strategically embrace inclusion and authority of people with lived experience as partners. In Chapter 2, "Research Considerations and Community-Based Participatory Research," Sheehan and colleagues proposed community-based participatory research (CBPR) as one way to act. As stated in the preface, CBPR is how we—Sonya and Pat—met. It drastically changed worldviews about research and health care for both of us. Readers need to remember the key concept of CBPR: partnership. People with lived experience on the CBPR team are not research subjects; they are investigators working with the "official" scientists on tasks of empirical description and analysis. This can add a strange dynamic for scientists on the team who are also psychiatric service providers and who have had to use their "authority" to make decisions inconsistent with empowerment (e.g., necessary inpatient hospitalization for a person contemplating suicide). They need to check concerns like these at the CBPR door and embrace working together to understand health and wellness goals. They need to be mindful of past clinical responsibilities as they embrace working together with the CBPR team to understand health and wellness goals.

Act in the Person's World

Transformational ideas of recovery, empowerment, and self-determination make a real difference in the lives of people with SMI, but that is not enough. Psychiatric service providers need to partner with people living with SMI and peer advocates to *act*. The last half of our book describes strategies that may yield meaningful action. Dissemination efforts have sprung up across the United States at national (e.g., governmental, such as the Department of Veterans Affairs and Substance Abuse and Mental Health Services Administration's Center for Mental Health Services, as well as professional groups, such as the National Association of State Mental Health Program Directors and the National Council for Behavioral Health), state, and city levels to train peer and professional providers on evidence-based tools like those discussed in the second half of this book. However, implementation remains a hurdle to broad success, just as it often undermines widespread use of most psychosocial interventions.

Funding bodies need the will to implement, among other things, shared decision making, service navigators, and skills training within integrated care settings. This requires funders to demand changes in providers and systems that are reluctant to promote patient-centered care. Political efforts of people with lived experience and like-minded providers are a start in guiding policy makers and administrators toward this end. The Patient Protection and Affordable Care Act, for example, highlighted patient-centered outcomes in modern medicine. Alas, health care providers are not necessarily skilled in political action. They must learn from advocates about how to join the fray and change the status quo.

Conclusion

Our book is a call for providers of psychiatric care to facilitate health and wellness goals of people living with serious mental health challenges. It similarly is meant for people with lived experience, those who will benefit from an improved system as well as from the grassroots efforts that are happening right now. Together, insights related to integrated care, one-stop services, and in-the-field interventions will become standard practice and significantly improve the health and wellness outcomes of this group.

References

Champion VL, Skinner CS: The health belief model, in Health Behavior and Health Education: Theory, Research, and Practice, 4th Edition. Edited by Glanz K, Rimer BK, Viswanath K. San Francisco, CA, Jossey-Bass, 2008, pp 45–62

Corrigan PW, Liberman RP, Engel JD: From noncompliance to collaboration in the treatment of schizophrenia. Psychiatr Serv 41(11):1203–1211, 1990

Corrigan PW, Angell B, Davidson L, et al: From adherence to self-determination: evolution of a treatment paradigm for people with serious mental illnesses. Psychiatr Serv 63(2):169–173, 2012

Draine J, Salzer MS, Culhane DP, et al: Putting social problems among persons with mental illness in perspective: crime, unemployment, and homelessness. Psychiatr Serv 53(5):565–572, 2002

Faris REL, Dunham HW: Mental Disorders in Urban Areas: An Ecological Study of Schizophrenia and Other Psychoses. Chicago, IL, University Chicago Press, 1939

Institute of Medicine, Committee on Quality of Health Care in America: Crossing the Quality Chasm: A New Health System for the 21st Century. Washington, DC, National Academy Press, 2001

Rosenstock IM: Why people use health services. Milbank Q 44(3):94–127, 1966

Rosenstock IM: The health belief model and preventive health behavior. Health Educ Monogr 2(4):354–386, 1974

Rudnick A, Roe D: Serious Mental Illness: Person-Centered Approaches. Boca Raton, FL, CRC Press, 2018

Stanton M, McClughen DC: The CDC guideline and its impact on delivering patient-centered care. Pain Manag Nurs 18(5):270–272, 2017

Tanner-Smith EE, Brown TN: Evaluating the Health Belief Model: a critical review of studies predicting mammographic and pap screening. Soc Theory Health 8:95–125, 2010

Index

Page numbers printed in **boldface** type refer to tables or figures.

AAR (ask, advise, refer) model, 96, 98

AARC Tobacco-Free Lifestyle Roundtable, 96

Accidents
  rates of for homeless, 89
  risk of injury in individuals with SMI, 8–9

Achieving Healthy Lifestyles in Psychiatric Rehabilitation (ACHIEVE), **179**

Adherence, to treatment
  healthy living skills and, 168–169
  shared decision making and, 148

Advocacy, by health care professionals, 92

African Americans. *See also* Race
  access to health care and, 75
  community-based participatory research and, **30, 31, 33,** 38–41
  peer navigator programs and, 230
  prevalence of smoking and, 241
  trust of health information by, 289

Age. *See also* Age at onset; Children and adolescents; Older adults
  prevalence of smoking by, 240
  smoking cessation and, 244

Agency for Healthcare Research and Quality (AHRQ), 67, **134**

Age at onset, of diabetes in individuals with SMI, 113

Agranulocytosis, 123

Alcohol use disorder, 50, 95

Alzheimer's disease, **6,** 11

Ambulatory care–sensitive conditions (ACSCs), 67

Amenorrhea, **7**

American Academy of Family Physicians, 135

American Association of Clinical Endocrinologists, 68

American Diabetes Association, 68

American Indian/Alaska Natives, and prevalence of smoking, 241

American Psychiatric Association (APA), 56, 68, 245–246, 250, 256

Americans with Disabilities Act, 41

Amisulpride, 104

Amitriptyline, **271**

Antidepressants. *See also* Selective serotonin reuptake inhibitors; Tricyclic antidepressants
  diabetes and, 114–115
  hypertension and, 113
  myocardial infarction and, 109
  osteoporosis and, 117
  risk of falls and fractures, 8
  smoking cessation and, 254
  weight gain and, 106, 107–108

Antipsychotics. *See also* Clozapine; Olanzapine
  bone mineral density and, **5, 7**–8
  cancer and, 120
  cardiovascular disease and, 9, 108, 109, 110, 111
  diabetes mellitus and, 113–115

Antipsychotics (*continued*)
  diabetic ketoacidosis and, 116
  dyslipidemia and, 107
  hypertension and, 113
  metabolic syndrome and, 104
  osteoporosis and, 116–117
  pneumonia and, **6,** 12, 118–119
  screening for metabolic syndrome
    and, 68
  sexual dysfunction and, 13
  smoking and smoking cessation,
    243, 254
Anxiety disorders, and heart disease, **5**
Aripiprazole, 104, 105, 110
Asenapine, **271**
Asian Americans, and community-
    based participatory research, **32,**
    35. *See also* Race
Aspiration pneumonia, 118–119
Assessment, and smoking cessation,
    247
Asthma, **6,** 11, 12
Autoimmune disease, **7,** 14–15

Bariatric surgery, 277
Barriers
  to health and health care for people
    with SMI, 16, 66–70, 166, 298
  health navigators and systemic,
    232, 234
  to mental health care in patient-
    centered medical homes, 136
  to physical activity for people with
    SMI, 95
  to smoking cessation, 245
  to weight loss, 269, 278
Behavioral health care manager, and
    collaborative care model, 56
Behavioral interventions
  for smoking cessation, 250–253
  for weight management, 273–277
Beta-blockers, 70
Bipolar disorder
  access to health care and, 66–67
  asthma and, **6,** 12

chronic kidney disease and, **7,** 13
diabetes and, 113
metabolic syndrome and, 104
pneumonia and, 118
smoking and, 240, 241, 243
Blood-borne viruses. *See also* HIV;
    Infectious diseases
  medical screening tests for, 69
  SMI as risk factor for contracting,
    50
Blood pressure, monitoring of, 124.
    See also Hypertension
Bone fracture, and antipsychotics, 116,
    117
Bone mineral density (BMD), **5,** 7–8,
    116, 117
Boston University Center of
    Psychiatric Rehabilitation, 17
Bridge model
  peer-led health navigation for
    psychiatric disability and,
    229–230
  programs for healthy living skills
    and, 190, **198–200,** 210
Buprenorphine, 54
Bupropion, 253, 254, 256

Canadian Task Force on Preventive
    Health Care, 248
Cancer, 68–69, 119–121, 224–225, 243
Cannabis, 49
Carbamazepine, 118
Cardiomyopathy, 112–113
Cardiovascular disease
  poverty and, 87
  psychotropic medications and,
    108–113
  quality of care and, 69
  screening for risk factors in persons
    with SMI, 68
  smoking and, 243
Cardiovascular system, and morbid-
    ities in people with SMI, **5,** 9–10
Care management, and patient-
    centered medical homes, 136–137

Cariprazine, **271**
Case examples
  of access to health care, 75–77
  of antipsychotic-related diabetes,
    115
  of cardiovascular disease and
    psychotropic medications,
    110–111, 112–113
  of co-occurring SMI, substance use
    disorder, and physical illness,
    50–51, 57–58, 59–60
  of health navigators, 221–222
  of healthy living skills, 212–213
  of implementation of community-
    based participatory research,
    38–41
  of kidney disease and psychotropic
    medications, 122–123
  of obesity and weight management,
    279–280
  of patient-centered medical homes,
    138
  of physical illness comorbid with
    SMI, 15
  of shared decision making, 156–157
  of smoking cessation, 257–258
  of weight gain from psychotropic
    medications, 106–107
Celiac disease, 12–13
Centers for Disease Control and
  Prevention (CDC), 16, 287, 290
Children and adolescents, and
  antipsychotics
  bone formation in, 117
  cardiovascular damage in, 108
  diabetes in, 114–115
  risk of weight gain in, 105
Chlorpromazine, **271**
Chronic care model, patient-centered
  medical home as extension of, 134
Chronic Disease Self-Management
  Program (CDSMP), 190, **204**
Chronic kidney disease (CKD), **7**,
  13–14, 121–123

Chronic obstructive pulmonary disease
  (COPD), **6**, 11
Civil rights, and COVID-19 pandemic,
  290
Clinical Practice Research Datalink
  Registry, 13
Clinician's Guide to Treating Tobacco
  Dependence (AARC Tobacco-Free
  Lifestyle Roundtable 2014), 96
Clozapine. *See also* Antipsychotics
  diabetes mellitus and, 114
  diabetic ketoacidosis and, 116
  dyslipidemia and, 107
  metabolic syndrome and, 104
  myocarditis and, 112
  neutropenia and, 123
  pneumonia and, 12, 118
  skin neoplasms and, **5**, 7
  sudden cardiac death and, 111
  weight gain and, 106, 270, **271**
Cognitive-behavioral therapy
  Bridge program and, 229
  healthy living skills and, 170
Cognitive deficits
  health care and, 166
  smoking cessation and, 245, 247
Collaboration
  community-based participatory
    research and, 27
  shared decision making and, 148
Collaborative care model
  for co-occurring SMI, substance
    use, and physical illness, 56
  healthy living skills and, **197**
  patient-centered medical home
    model and, 135
Communication
  health care utilization and, 222,
    223–224
  healthy living skills and, 169
  integrated care models and, 58
Community, concept of in
  community-based participatory
    research, 26

Community-based participatory
  research (CBPR)
  case study of implementation,
    38–41
  critical assessment of, 36–38
  description of, 24–25
  future of, 41–43, 300
  principles of, 25–28
  summary of literature on, 28–36
Community Health Scholars Program,
  24
Community health workers (CHWs),
  225–226, **227**
Community partnered participatory
  research (CPPR), 25
Comorbidity, of mental disorders.
  See also Physical illness
  prevalence of in individuals with
    SMI, 3
  smoking and, 240
Compliance, and shared decision
  making, 147, **148**
Computers. *See* Internet
Context, of community-based
  participatory research, 27
Coordination, and health care
  utilization, 222, **223**, 224
Coping skills, and healthy living skills,
  168
Coronary heart disease, **5**, 9, 108–109
Costs, of co-occurring substance use,
  SMI, and medical disorders,
  53–54. *See also* Funding
Counseling, for smoking cessation, 250
COVID-19
  health care decisions related to,
    287–290
  health literacy and, 290–291
  implications for mental health care
    providers, 291–293
  as new normal, 293
  stress, isolation, and exacerbation of
    mental disorders, 286–287
Criminal justice system
  access to health care and, 74

health challenges of people living
    with SMI and, 298
  life choices of individuals with SMI
    and, **85–87**, 90
Culture
  definition of "significant life goal"
    and, 2
  health navigators and, 225, 234
  shared decision making and, 151

Danish National Patient Registry, and
  Danish Psychiatric Registry, 14
Death, from respiratory disease in
  individuals with SMI, 118. *See also*
  Mortality
Decision making. *See* Shared decision
  making
Decision support tools, for shared
  decision making, 155–157
Deinstitutionalization, and
  homelessness, 89
Deliberation, as stage of shared
  decision making, 150–151
Dental health. *See* Tooth decay
Depression. *See also* Major depressive
  disorder
  asthma and, 12
  domestic violence and, 88
  heart disease and, **5**, 9
  homeless population and, 89
  obesity and, 268
  as risk factor for diabetes, 114
  smoking and, 240, 243
Depression and Bipolar Support
  Alliance, 292
Diabetes Awareness and Rehabilitation
  Training (DART), **185**
Diabetes Management Program, **209**
Diabetes mellitus (DM), 4, **5**, 7,
  113–115, 124
Diabetes Prevention Program Group
  Lifestyle Balance intervention
  plus mobile health (mHealth),
  173
Diabetic ketoacidosis, 115–116

Diagnostic and Statistical Manual of Mental Disorders (DSM-5; American Psychiatric Association 2013), 246

Diathesis-stress model, of co-occurring SMI, substance use disorder, and physical illness, 51–53

Diet
behavioral weight management and, 274
health literacy and, 269
lifestyle choices of individuals with SMI and, **85,** 94, 170

Digestive system, and morbidities in people with SMI, **6,** 12–13

Disability, definition of by Social Security Administration, 2

Domestic violence
community-based participatory research and, 28, **29, 34,** 35
people with SMI as victims of, 88

Downward drift, and socioeconomic status of people with schizophrenia, 298

Dyslipidemia, 107–108

Eating disorders, 94

E-cigarettes, 255

Ecological perspective, and community-based participatory research, 26

Economics. *See* Costs; Funding; Poverty; Socioeconomic status

Edentulousness, **5,** 8

Education
Bridge program and, 229
for health navigators, 227, **232,** 233
healthy living skills and, 167
of patients about psychotropic medications, 92
poverty of individuals with SMI and, 84
prevalence of smoking and level of, 240–241

on shared decision making for health care professionals, 154–155
tobacco treatment training for psychiatry residents, 256

Electrocardiogram (ECG), baseline, 124

Emergency departments (EDs), use of by persons with SMI, 67. *See also* Hospitals

Empowerment
future of care for people with SMI, 299–300
shared decision making and, 147

Endocrine system diseases
comorbidities in people with SMI and, **7,** 14
psychotropic medications and, 113–116

Engagement, and shared decision making, 148

Enhancing QUality of Care in Psychosis (EQUIP) project, 273

Epidemics, history of, 286, 293. *See also* COVID-19

Epidemiology. *See* Prevalence

Epilepsy, **5,** 10

Estrogen, and psychotropic medications, 8, 13, 120–121

Ethnicity. *See* Race

Evaluating Adverse Events in a Global Smoking Cessation Study (EAGLES), 254

Exercise
behavioral weight management and, 274, 277
lifestyle choices of individuals with SMI and, **86,** 94–95, 170

Extrinsic motivation, 168

Falls, risk of fractures and, 8

Family history, of early cardiac death, 124

5 A's and 5 R's models, for smoking cessation and weight management, 96, 98, 248–250

Food and Drug Administration, 291
Fear
avoidance of health care and, 165, 166
extrinsic motivation for healthy
living skills and, 168
Finger prick tests, 124
Focus groups, and community-based
participatory research, 39–40
Funding, of peer health navigation,
231, **232**. *See also* Costs

Gender, and community-based
participatory research, 28, **30**.
See also Women
GLOBOCAN 2018, 119

Haloperidol, 111
Harm reduction, and alternatives to
cigarettes, 255
Health. *See also* Health care; Obesity;
Physical illness
challenges for people living with
SMI, 298
COVID-19 pandemic and literacy
on, 290–291
ethnic disparities in trust of
information on, 289–290
motivation as key factor in
maintaining, 165
Health belief model, and healthy living
skills, 165
Health care. *See also* Barriers;
Community-based participatory
research; COVID-19; Emergency
departments; Health; Health care
professionals; Health navigators;
Hospitals; Integrated care;
Nursing homes; Patient-centered
medical home; Shared decision
making
challenges to utilization of and
wellness, 222, **223–224**
costs of co-occurring substance use,
SMI, and medical disorders,
53–54

factors contributing to disparities
in, 70–77
fear and avoidance of, 165, 166
life choices of individuals with SMI
and, **85–86,** 90–91
medical screening tests for
individuals with SMI, 68–69
prisons and, 90
psychological side effects of, 52
standard of care and quality
treatments, 69–70
systemic issues in, 222, 234
traditional medical care models of,
132
weight stigma and, 270–271
Health care professionals
lifestyle choices and
recommendations for, 96–98
recommendations for treatment of
people with SMI, 91–92
smoking cessation and, 242
training in shared decision making
for, 154–155
Health navigators
case example of, 221–222
challenges for, 231–234
community health workers and,
226, **227**
description of model, 224–225
for psychiatric disability, 226–230
Health and Recovery Peer Program
(HARP), **194, 195**
Healthy living skills. *See also* Lifestyle
choices
creation and maintenance of,
164–167
definition of, 164
future of programs for, 213–214
health in general population
compared to individuals with
SMI, 169–171
research on, 190, **191–209,** 210–213
specific programs for, 171–172,
173–188, 189
targets for intervention, 167–169

Heart disease, 87. *See also*
Cardiovascular disease
Heart rate variability, 10
Helping Older People Experience
Success (HOPES), 190, **192, 206,**
210
Hematological diseases, and
psychotropic medications, 123
Hepatitis C, 50, 69, 95
Heroin use disorder, 49
Hip fracture, and antidepressants, 8
HIV
as epidemic or pandemic, 286
prevalence of in individuals with
SMI, 50, 96
screening tests for, 69
substance use and, 95
Homelessness
access to health care and, 67, 74,
75
community-based participatory
research and, **30, 31,** 38–41
health challenges of people living
with SMI and, 298
life choices of individuals with SMI
and, **85,** 88–89
Homicide, people with SMI as victims
of, **85,** 88
Hospitals, smoking by patients in
psychiatric, 242, 256–257. *See also*
Emergency departments; Health
care
Housing, and co-occurrence of SMI
and substance use disorders, 53.
See also Homelessness
Hyperglycemia, 124
Hyperprolactinemia, 13
Hypertension, and psychotropic
medications, 113. *See also* Blood
pressure
Hypoalgesia, **6,** 11
Hypogonadism, 8
Hypothyroid disorder, **7,** 123
Iloperidone, **271**
Imipramine, **271**

Immigrants and refugees, and
community-based participatory
research, 28, **34,** 35
Immune system
combined impact of mental illness
and substance use on, 52
morbidities in people with SMI and,
7, 14–15
Infectious diseases, and homelessness,
89. *See also* Blood-borne viruses;
COVID-19; Skin infections
Influenza, and epidemics, 286, 293
Information exchange, and shared
decision making, 150, 151
InSHAPE intervention, 172, **174–175,**
188, 189, 190
Institute of Medicine, 299
Insurance, and health care, 66, 256
Integrated care. *See also* Patient-
centered medical home
access to health care and, 71
co-occurrence of SMI with
substance use and physical
illness, 55–58
peer health navigation and, 231,
232
Integrated Coaching for Better Mood
and Weight intervention, 274
Integrated Illness Management and
Recovery (IIMR), **191,** 210
Integumentary system, and morbidities
in people with SMI, 4, **5,** 7
Intensive primary care, and patient-
centered medical homes, 136
Interactive, multimedia approach, to
shared decision making, 154
Interferon-alfa, 52
International Agency for Research on
Cancer, 119
International Classification of Diseases
(ICD-10), 246
International Group for The Study of
Lithium Treated Patients, 123
International Patient Decision Aids
Standards (IPDAS), 156

Internet
  behavioral weight management
    and, 275
  COVID-19 pandemic and support
    groups, 292
  shared decision making and, 154
  smoking cessation and, 253
Interpersonal relationships, and
  healthy living skills, 169. *See also*
  Family history; Social factors
Intrinsic motivation, 167
In vivo supports, health navigators as,
  228–229
Irritable bowel syndrome (IBS), 12–13
Iterative process, community-based
  participatory research as, 27

Kidney disease, and psychotropic
  medications, 121–123. *See also*
  Chronic kidney disease
Kraepelin, Emil, 2

Latinos. *See* Race and ethnicity
  access to health care and, 75
  community-based participatory
    research and, **29, 33**
  peer navigator programs and, 230
Leukocytopenia, 123
LGBT population
  community-based participatory
    research and, 28, **33,** 35
  health challenges of people living
    with SMI, 298
Life expectancy, of individuals with
  SMI, 3–4, 65, 84, 87. *See also*
  Mortality
Life Goals Collaborative Care
  (LGCC), 190, **201, 203**
Lifestyle Balance program, **180**
Lifestyle choices. *See also* Healthy
  living skills
  chronic medical conditions in
    individuals with SMI, 52
  consequences of in individuals with
    SMI, **85–87,** 92–98

multiple poor habits in individuals
    with SMI, 169, 170
  osteoporosis and, 116
  recommendations for health care
    professionals, 96–98
Lithium. *See also* Mood stabilizers
  chronic kidney disease and, 14,
    121–123
  hypothyroidism and, 123
  reduced fracture risk and, 117
  skin conditions and, 7
  weight gain and, **271**
Lived experience leaders, and
  community-based participatory
    research, 42–43
Living Well intervention, 190, **196,
  205,** 210

Major depressive disorder (MDD). *See*
  Depression
  access to health care and, 66–67
  metabolic syndrome and, 104
  smoking cessation and, 244, 248
Manualized curriculum, for peer
    navigator program in community-
    based participatory research, 40
Medicaid, 54, 66, 67, 68, 70, 72, 256
Medical conditions. *See* Physical illness
Medical screening tests, 68–69
Medications. *See also* Antidepressants;
    Antipsychotics; Mood stabilizers
  cancer and, 119–121
  cardiovascular disease and, 108–113
  dyslipidemia and, 107–108
  healthy living skills and, 168–169
  hematological diseases and, 123
  kidney diseases and, 121–123
  metabolic syndrome and, 103–104,
    123–124
  obesity and, 104–107, 269–270, 272
  psychiatrists and education of
    patients about, 92
  respiratory tract diseases and,
    118–119
  risk of falls and fractures, 8

sexual dysfunction and, 13
smoking cessation and, 253–254
weight gain and, 94, **271**
Mental disorders, impact of COVID-9
on symptoms of, 286–287. *See also*
Bipolar disorder; Depression;
Personality disorders;
Posttraumatic stress disorder;
Psychotic disorders;
Schizoaffective disorder;
Schizophrenia; Serious mental
illness
Mental health care. *See* Psychiatrists
Metabolic syndrome
as medical comorbidity in
individuals with SMI, 49–50
psychotropic medications and,
103–104, 123–124
screening tests for, 68
substance use disorder as risk factor
for, 50
Metformin, 272
Middle East respiratory syndrome
(MERS), 286, 288
Migraines, **6**, 10–11
Mirtazapine, **271**
MISSION (Maintaining
Independence and Sobriety
through Systems Integration,
Outreach, and Networking), 57
Monitoring, of weight gain in people
with SMI, 272–273
Monoamine oxidase inhibitors
(MAOIs), 109
Mood stabilizers. *See also* Lithium
osteoporosis and, 117
pneumonia and, 118
weight gain and, 106, 108
Morbidity. *See also* Health; Physical
illness
multimorbidity and, 48
poverty and, 87
smoking and, 243
types of in individuals with SMI,
4–15

Mortality. *See also* Death; Life
expectancy
co-occurring mental health disorders and substance abuse, 47–48
homelessness and rates of, 89
people released from prisons and
rates of, 90
rates of for individuals with SMI,
3–4
smoking and, 243
Motivation
healthy living skills and, 167–168
as key factor in maintaining health,
165–166
for smoking cessation, 244
Motivational interviewing, and
smoking cessation, 250–251
MOVE intervention, 172, **182**, 278
MOVE+UP program, 274
Myocardial infarction (MI), 108,
109–110
Myocarditis, 112–113

National Association of State Mental
Health Program Directors, 301
National Cancer Institute, 248
National Committee for Quality
Assurance (NCQA), 133, **135**
National Council for Behavioral
Health, 301
National Health Interview Survey, 67
National Institute of Allergy and
Infectious Diseases, 290, 293
National Institutes of Health, 16
National Survey on Drug Use and
Health, 48, 240, 241
Nervous system, and morbidities in
people with SMI, **5–6**, 10–11
Neurodegenerative diseases, 11
Neutropenia, clozapine-associated,
123
Nicotine dependence, and nicotine
withdrawal syndrome, 241
Nicotine replacement therapy (NRT),
245, 253–254, 256

North American Association for the Study of Obesity, 68
Nurse care managers, and patient-centered medical homes, 138
Nursing homes
early institutionalization of persons with SMI in, 3
quality of and admission of persons with SMI to, 70

Obesity. *See also* Weight gain
cardiovascular disease and, 108
causes of, 268–271
eating patterns of people with SMI and, 94
prevention and treatment of in people with SMI, 271–280
psychotropic medications and, 104–107
risk of in individuals with SMI, 267–268
as risk factor for sleep apnea, 10
Obstructive sleep apnea, **5,** 10
Olanzapine
diabetes mellitus and, 114
diabetic ketoacidosis and, 116
dyslipidemia and, 107
metabolic syndrome and, 104
sudden cardiac death and, 111
weight gain and, 105, 106, **271**
Older patients. *See also* Age
antidepressants and risk of falls and fractures, 8
dosages of tricyclic antidepressants for, 111
pneumonia in individuals with SMI, 118
Opioid epidemic, and opioid use disorder, 48–49
Osteoporosis, 7–8, 116–117
Ottawa Hospital Research Institute, 156

Pain, schizophrenia and altered perception of, **6,** 11
Paliperidone, **271**

Parkinson's disease, **6,** 11
Paroxetine, **271**
Participatory action research (PAR), 25, 28
Patient activation, and shared decision making, 153–154
Patient-centered medical home (PCMH)
augmentation of, 136–138
challenges to implementation of, 131–132, 135–136
description of, 133–135
MISSION services and, 57
Patient-Centered Outcomes Research Institute, 24
Patient navigators, 224–225
Patient Protection and Affordable Care Act (ACA), 59, 66, 67, 71, 225, 301
Pay-for-performance (P4P), 231
Peer coaching, and behavioral weight management, 275
Peer navigator programs. *See also* Health navigators
community-based participatory research and, 40
models of for psychiatric disability, 229–230
Peers for Progress model, 225
Peer support specialists, and patient-centered medical homes, 136
Personality disorders, and impact of stigma on access to health care, 73
Person-centered care, and shared decision making, 149
Physical illness. *See also* Health; Health care; Morbidity
case example of in individual with SMI, 15
case examples of substance use co-morbid with SMI and physical illness, 50–51, 57–58, 59–60
etiology of substance use comorbid with SMI and physical illness, 51–53

impact of on wellness, 16–17
life choices of individuals with SMI
and, **85–87**
mental health care for substance use
comorbid with SMI and
physical illness, 55–60
mortality, costs, and treatment of
substance use comorbid with
SMI and physical illness,
53–55
mortality rates in individuals with
SMI and, 3–4
prevalence of substance use
comorbid with SMI and
physical illness, 47–50
psychiatric providers and, 15–16
types of in individuals with SMI,
4–15
Physiology, and obesity, 270
Picker Institute, 146–147
Planned behavior, and maintenance of
health, 165
Pneumonia, **6**, 12, 118–119
Polypharmacy, and risk of chronic
kidney disease, 122
Posttraumatic stress disorder (PTSD)
obesity and weight management,
268, 274, 278, 279
smoking and, 240
Poverty
access to health care and, 74, 75
co-occurrence of SMI and
substance use disorders, 53
health consequences of for
individuals with SMI, 84, 87,
93, 298
smoking and, 240
PREMIER study, **178**
President's Commission for the Study
of Ethical Problems in Medicine
and Biomedical and Behavioral
Research (1982), 146
Prevalence
of comorbidity in individuals with
SMI, 3

of co-occurring SMI, substance use
disorder, and physical illness,
48–51
of SMI in general population, 1–2,
47
of smoking in individuals with SMI,
49, 239–243
Prevention Quality Indicators (PQIs), 67
Primary Care Access, Referral, and
Evaluation (PCARE), 137, **193,**
210
Prisons, chronic medical conditions
and health care in, 90. *See also*
Criminal justice system
Provider-patient relationship, and
shared decision making, 148–149
Psychiatrists
access to health care for patients
with SMI, 70
education of patients about
medications, 92
implications of COVID-19 for,
291–293
integrated care for co-occurrence of
SMI with substance use and
physical illness, 55–60
physical illness in patients with SMI
and, 15–16
smoking cessation and, 242,
245–246, 249
stigmatizing attitudes toward
individuals with SMI and
substance use, 55
Psychosocial interventions, for
smoking cessation, 250–253
Psychotic disorders. *See also*
Schizoaffective disorder;
Schizophrenia
access to health care and, 66–67
homeless population and, 89
obesity and, 268
sedentary behavior and, 170
smoking and smoking cessation,
243, 248
PubMed, 171

QTc prolongation, 110–111, 125
Quality of Life for Persons With Bipolar Disorder, **181**
Quality treatments, and health care, 69–70
Quetiapine, 104, 111, **271**
Quitlines, and smoking cessation, 252

Race, and ethnicity. *See also* African Americans; Asian Americans; Latinos
  disparities in trust of health information, 289–290
  as focus of CBPR studies, 28, 35
  health navigators and, 225
  prevalence of smoking and, 241
  social determinants of health and, 74–75, 298
Recovering Energy Through Nutrition and Exercise for Weight Loss (RENEW), **177**
Relapse, and smoking cessation, 248
Reproductive system, and morbidities in people with SMI, **6–7**, 11–12, 13
Research. *See also* Community-based participatory research
  on community health workers, 226
  future of, 300
  on health navigators for psychiatric disability, 227–228, 229–230
  on healthy living skills, 171–172, **173–188**, 189, 190, **191–209**, 210–213
  on homeless population, 89
  influence of tobacco industry on, 242
  on peer navigator programs, 230
Resilience, and weight management, 279
Resistance, and shared decision making, 147, **148**
Respiratory diseases, **6**, 118–119, 243. *See also* Pneumonia
Risperidone, 105, 107, 111, **271**

Schizoaffective disorder, 113, 244
Schizophrenia
  altered pain perception and, **6**, 11
  antipsychotics and risk of bone fracture, 116
  autoimmune disease and, 14–15
  cancer and, 119, 120
  cannabis use and, 49
  celiac disease and, 12–13
  chronic obstructive pulmonary disease and, **6**
  diabetes and, 113
  epilepsy and, **5**, 10
  metabolic syndrome and, 104
  pneumonia and, 118
  response to pain and, 166
  sexual dysfunction and, **6**, 13
  smoking and smoking cessation, 94, 240, 241, 242, 243, 244
  socioeconomic status of people with, 298–299
  stigma as factor in access to health care, 73
  sudden cardiac death and, **5**, 9, 111
Screening, for obesity in people with SMI, 272–273
Sedentary behavior. *See* Exercise
Selective serotonin reuptake inhibitors (SSRIs), 110, 117, 121
Self-determination
  future of care for people with SMI, 299–300
  motivation for improving health behaviors and, 165
  shared decision making and, 147, 150
Self-efficacy
  healthy living skills and, 168
  obesity and, 268–269
Self-management
  health care utilization and wellness, 222, **223**, 224
  healthy living skills and, 168
  shared decision making and programs for, 153–154
Self-Management Addressing Health Risk Trial (SMAHRT), **202**

Self-medication
  smoking cessation and, 245
  substance use in individuals with
    SMI as, 52
Self-monitoring, and healthy living
  skills, 167
Serious mental illness (SMI). *See also*
  Health care; Healthy living skills;
  Medications; Mental disorders;
  Morbidity; Mortality; Obesity;
  Physical illness; Research; Shared
  decision making; Substance use
  concept of acting in person's world,
    300–301
  consequences of lifestyle choices,
    85–87, 92–98
  definition of, 2
  dimensions of wellness specific to,
    16–17
  empowerment and self-
    determination as principles in
    care of, 299–300
  homelessness and, 88–89
  involvement with criminal justice
    system, 90
  mortality rates and, 3–4
  persistence and chronicity of, 2
  poverty and, 84, 87, 93
  prevalence of, 1–2, 47
  rate of HIV in, 286
  substandard medical care and,
    90–91
  violent victimization and domestic
    violence, 87–88
Serotonin-norepinephrine reuptake
  inhibitors (SNRIs), 109, 113
Sertindole, **271**
Severe acute respiratory syndrome
  (SARS), 286, 288
Sexual behaviors, and life choices of
  individuals with SMI, **87,** 95–96
Sexual dysfunction, **6,** 13
Sexually transmitted diseases, 96
Shared decision making (SDM)
  foundation and ethics of, 146–150

health navigators and, 228
history of concept, 145–146
impact of, 152–153
model of, 150–152
tools and interventions to support,
  153–157
Simplified Intervention to Modify
  Physical Activity, Lifestyle and
  Eating (SIMPLE), **187**
Skeletal system, diseases of, 4, **5,** 7–9,
  116–117
Skin infections, 4, **5**
Sleep disturbance, and weight gain,
  270. *See also* Obstructive sleep
  apnea
Smartphone apps. *See* Telephone
Smoking
  cessation of, 243–258
  effects of on morbidity and
    mortality, 243
  exercise and, 95
  life choices of individuals with SMI
    and, **86,** 93–94, 96
  prevalence of in individuals with
    SMI, 49, 239–243
Social determinants of health. *See also*
  Housing; Poverty
  access to health care and, 74–77
  co-occurrence of SMI and physical
    illness, 52–53
  effects of on people living with SMI,
    298–299
Social distancing, and COVID-19, 290
Social factors, and smoking cessation,
  245. *See also* Interpersonal
  relationships
Social media, and smoking cessation, 253
Social Security Administration, 2, 84
Social workers, and patient-centered
  medical homes, 136
Socioeconomic status, and poverty in
  individuals with SMI, 84, 87
Spanish flu epidemic (1918), 286, 293
Specialty medical homes, and patient-
  centered medical homes, 137–138

Special populations, healthy living skills programs for, 210–211. *See also* Children and adolescents; Older adults

Stages of change model, of smoking cessation, 247–248

Stigma

barriers to health care for individuals with SMI and, 166

lifestyle choices of people with SMI and, 98–99

peer health navigation and, **232,** 233

provider-level factors in access to health care and, 72–73

treatment of co-occurring SMI and substance use disorders, 55

weight management and, 270–271, 278

STRIDE intervention, 172, **183, 184**

Structural interventions, for smoking cessation, 255–258

Study of Lithium Treated Patients, 121

Substance Abuse and Mental Health Services Administration (SAMHSA), 255–256, 287, 290, 301

Substance use, and substance use disorders (SUDs). *See also* Smoking

case examples of co-occurrence with SMI and physical illness, 50–51, 57–58, 59–60

etiology of co-occurrence with SMI and physical illness, 51–53

life choices of individuals with SMI and, **87,** 95

mortality, costs, and treatment implications of co-occurrence with SMI and physical illness, 53–55

prevalence of co-occurrence with SMI and physical illness, 47–50

psychiatric practice and co-occurrence of with SMI, 55–60

Sudden cardiac death (SCD), **5,** 9, 111, 124, 125

Suicide, and homelessness, 89

Supervision, and peer health navigation, **232,** 233

Support groups, COVID-19 pandemic and online, 292

System-level factors, in access to health care, 71–72

Targeted Training for Illness Management, 190, **207–208**

Technology, and behavioral weight management, 274–277. *See also* Internet; Telephones

Telephones

behavioral weight management and, 276–277

smoking cessation and, 252–253

Thioridazine 110, 111, **271**

Tobacco use, promotion of by industry, 241–241. *See also* Smoking

Tooth decay, **5, 8**

Torsades de pointes (TdP), 110

Training. *See* Education

Transportation, and access to health care, 224

"Treating Tobacco Use and Dependence" (U.S. Public Health Service 2008), 248, 250, 251

Treatment. *See* Adherence; Behavioral interventions; Cognitive-behavioral therapy; Medications; Psychiatrists

Tricyclic antidepressants (TCAs)

coronary heart disease and, 109

hypertension and, 113

sudden cardiac death and dosages of for older adults, 111

Trifluoperazine, **271**

2 A's+R (Ask, Advise, and Refer), 249–250

U.S. Department of Health and Human Services, 246

U.S. Preventive Services Task Force, 149
U.S. Public Health Service, 248, 250, 251
U.S. Surgeon General, 93–94
University of California, Los Angeles, 171
University of Southern California, 171
Urinary system, diseases of, **7,** 13–14

Valproate, 108, **271**
Valproic acid, 118
Varenicline, 253, 254, 256
Veterans Health Administration, 132, 137, 273, 301
Virtual mental health care, and COVID-19 pandemic, 292

Waist circumference, and metabolic syndrome, 124

Walk, Address Sensations, Learn About Exercise, Cue Exercise Behavior for SSDs (WALC-S), **176**
WebMOVE, **186,** 275, **276**
Weight gain and psychotropic medications, 94, 105, 270. *See also* Obesity
Wellness. *See also* Health
challenges to health care utilization and, 222, **223–224**
impact of physical illness on, 16–17
W. K. Kellogg Foundation, 24
Women. *See also* Gender
community-based participatory research and, **30, 34**
depressive disorders and domestic violence, 88
medical screening tests for, 69
World Health Organization, 16, 52